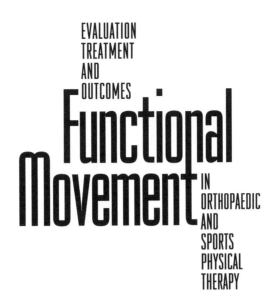

EVALUATION
TREATMENT
AND
OUTCOMES

Functional

Movement

IN
ORTHOPAEDIC
AND
SPORTS
PHYSICAL
THERAPY

EVALUATION TREATMENT AND OUTCOMES

Functional Movement

IN ORTHOPAEDIC AND SPORTS PHYSICAL THERAPY

Edited by

BRUCE BROWNSTEIN, MBA, PT
Administrator
HealthSouth Sports Medicine and Rehabilitation Center
Co-Director
Sports Orthopaedic and Athletic Rehabilitation Research
New York, New York

SHAW BRONNER, PT, MHS,OCS
Academic Adjunct Professor
Physical Therapy Program
Long Island University
Brooklyn, NY
Clinical Coordinator
HealthSouth Manhattan II
Co-Director
Sports Orthopaedic and Athletic Rehabilitation Research
New York, New York

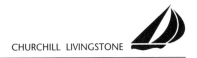

CHURCHILL LIVINGSTONE

New York, Edinburgh, London, Madrid, Melbourne, San Francisco, Tokyo

Library of Congress Cataloging-in-Publication Data

Functional movement in orthopaedic and sports physical therapy :
   evaluation, treatment, and outcomes / edited by Bruce Brownstein,
   Shaw Bronner.
          p.   cm.
      Includes bibliographical references and index.
      ISBN 0-443-07530-1 (alk. paper)
      1. Physical therapy. 2. Sports physical therapy. 3. Human
   mechanics. I. Brownstein, Bruce. II. Bronner, Shaw.
      [DNLM: 1. Movement—physiology. 2. Musculoskeletal System—
   physiopathology. 3. Rehabilitation. 4. Sports Medicine.   WE 103
   F979 1997]
   RD798.F86   1997
   615.8′2—dc21
   DNLM/DLC
   for Library of Congress   96–36811
                                                                 CIP

Distributed in the United Kingdom by Churchill Livingstone, Robert Stevenson House, 1–3 Baxter's Place, Leith Walk, Edinburgh EH1 3AF, and by associated companies, branches, and representatives throughout the world.

Medical knowledge is constantly changing. As new information becomes available, changes in treatment, procedures, equipment and the use of drugs become necessary. The editors/authors/contributors and the publishers have, as far as it is possible, taken care to ensure that the information given in this text is accurate and up to date. However, readers are strongly advised to confirm that the information, especially with regard to drug usage, complies with the latest legislation and standards of practice.

The Publishers have made every effort to trace the copyright holders for borrowed material. If they have inadvertently overlooked any, they will be pleased to make the necessary arrangements at the first opportunity.

Acquisitions Editor: *Carol Bader*
Production Editor: *Colleen Quinn*
Production Supervisor: *Kathleen R. Smith*
Cover Design: *Jeannette Jacobs*

Printed in the United States of America

First published in 1997   7   6   5   4   3   2   1

To Bob Lamb and Bob Mangine, who taught me to ask questions and made me answer them; and Bob Engle, who did both in his own way. My greatest thanks to Shaw, the partner who has seen it all happen—there is more to come.
—BB

To the loving support, patience, and friendship of Stuart and Bruce. Thanks for believing in me. To Alfredo Corvino, who instilled in me his love of movement and dance. May we all dance with grace throughout our lives.
—SB

Contributors

Shaw Bronner, PT, MHS, OCS
Academic Adjunct Professor, Physical Therapy Program, Long Island University, Brooklyn, New York; Clinical Coordinator, HealthSouth Manhattan II, Co-Director, Sports Orthopaedic and Athletic Rehabilitation Research, New York, New York

Bruce Brownstein, MBA, PT
Administrator, HealthSouth Sports Medicine and Rehabilitation Center, Co-Director, Sports Orthopaedic and Athletic Rehabilitation Research, New York, New York

Tony Brosky, Jr., MS, PT, SCS
Assistant Professor of Physical Therapy, Physical Therapy Department, Carroll College, Waukesha, Wisconsin

David Caborn, MD
Professor of Surgery, Department of Surgery, Division of Orthopaedic Surgery, University of Kentucky College of Medicine, Lexington, Kentucky

Andrew R. Einhorn, MS, PT
Los Alamitos Orthopaedic and Sports Physical Therapy, Los Alamitos, California

Walter Jenkins, MS, PT, ATC
Clinical Associate Professor, Department of Physical Therapy, East Carolina University; Coordinator of Physical Therapy Services, Student Health Service, Greenville, North Carolina

Marijeanne Liederbach, MS, ATC
Instructor, Department of Kinesiology, Teachers College, Columbia University; Program Coordinator, Harkness Institute for Dance Injuries, Hospital for Joint Diseases, New York, New York

David Macha, PT
Licensed Assistant Physical Therapist and Knee Specialist, Department of Sports Medicine, HealthSouth Sports Medicine and Rehabilitation Center, Houston, Texas

Michael Mandas, PT
Los Alamitos Orthopaedic and Sports Physical Therapy, Los Alamitos, California

Robert Mangine, MEd, PT, ATC
Clinical Instructor, Jesuit University, Wheeling, West Virginia; Director, Kentucky Rehabilitation Services, Fort Mitchell, Kentucky

Arthur J. Nitz, PhD, PT
Associate Professor of Physical Therapy, Physical Therapy Division, University of Kentucky School of Medicine, Lexington, Kentucky

John Nyland, EdD, PT, ATC
Assistant Professor of Physical Therapy, Physical Therapy Division, University of Kentucky School of Medicine, Lexington, Kentucky

Russell Paine, PT
Associate Professor, School of Physical Therapy, Texas Woman's University; Clinical Director, HealthSouth Sports Medicine Center; Rehabilitation Consultant for the Houston Rockets, Houston, Texas

Ray Plona, PT
President, Plona & Associates Physical Therapy, Inc., Westlake, Ohio

Michael Sawyer
Los Alamitos Orthopaedic and Sports Physical Therapy, Los Alamitos, California

Preface

Q Can grace be taught?

A Yes, absolutely, I would call it coordination. It's not just a physical thing; it's a mental thing—to know what one part is doing while the other part is happening, to have that happen seamlessly and efficiently. I think efficiency has to do with grace, in employing the most direct action to accomplish a task. Like picking up a pen, or folding a piece of paper, or talking on the phone, or tying your shoe, or putting groceries in a sack: functional things.

—Excerpt from an interview with Mark Morris, choreographer, New York Times Magazine, *July 9, 1995 page 10*

Movement underlies every action that we participate in on a day to day basis. As physical therapists, we have learned to focus on the components of movement that are limited by injury—range of motion, strength, and somatosensory functions. Movement scientists have begun to create a new vocabulary for physical therapists. Terms such as strategy and synergy are being redefined and incorporated into the lexicon of orthopaedic and sports physical therapy. Adaptations in gait and sports activities caused by onset and recovery from injury are considered to be movement strategies that develop to accommodate the new environment caused by external and internal changes following an insult to the neuromuscular and somatosensory systems.

A review of physical therapy literature documents this gradual shift toward movement as its own entity. Physical measurements of joint motion and force production remain important, but new efforts focus on other components—balance, somatosensory awareness, movement error detection, sensory effects of somatic injury, etc.—that allow us to *perform* our daily and recreational activities at the levels we wish. This serves as the basis for determining function.

Corresponding changes in the way that we measure success in physical therapy are occurring. Achieving full range of motion or strength is no longer the final goal of treatment. Function, that elusive term, is the new standard. Can the patient return to the same level of movement, perform the same activities, and function at the same level, with the same skill, ease, and enjoyment as before the injury? If this question could be answered at the yes or no level, proving effectiveness of treatment would be simple. Unfortunately, measuring the results of injury and rehabilitation does not occur at that level. Thus, a new aspect of physical therapy has arisen, the measurement of function and outcomes.

We believe that movement is the underlying key to function. The ability to generate movements that can fulfill our intents and purposes of daily work and recreation, as well as the performance of more occasional sports and fitness activities or hobbies, is essential to a satisfactory quality of life. Movement may be the goal (demonstration of skill as in gymnastics or expression of an unspoken emotion as in dance) or the means to achieving a goal (picking up a glass of water or shooting a basketball). Either way, no individual wants to feel limited in his ability to move.

The performance aspect to movement is not limited to athletes and artists. As described by Mark Morris (see previous page), coordination and efficiency are essential to graceful movement. The variables that the central nervous system and the musculoskeletal system use to determine efficiency and coordination are not yet understood, although significant work is now being done in this area.[1,2] Regardless, physical therapists are in a unique position to enhance the ability of our patients to perform movement in a graceful manner and enable them to achieve their desired levels of function.

Functional Movement in Orthopaedic and Sports Physical Therapy deals with the role of physical therapy in addressing movement and function. Three sections discuss the underlying principles of movement and measuring function, treatment and evaluation of movement and function losses, and the special aspects of movement in unique populations: athletes, older individuals, and dancers. It is these groups that present with characteristic qualities of movement that are more consistently observed than in the general population. A special appendix is included that presents outcome data in orthopaedic physical therapy.

We hope that the ideas and information presented here will become part of the growing body of knowledge dedicated to that most basic of human functions—movement.

Bruce Brownstein MBA, PT
Shaw Bronner PT, MHS, OCS

1. Hogan N, Flash T. Moving gracefully: quantitative theories of motor coordination. TINS 10:170–174, 1987
2. Kelso JAS. The informational character of self-organized coordination dynamics. Human Movement Science 13:393–413, 1994

Contents

1

Movement Biomechanics and Control

BRUCE BROWNSTEIN

Movement has been studied by researchers in a variety of disciplines using techniques that range as widely as the different types of movement that exist. Movement itself is the expression of several powerful influences in the human—anatomy, consciousness, biomechanics, physiology, and disease. Movement is both a tool we utilize to manipulate our environment as well a form that exists for artistic expression.

Injury, trauma, and disease affect the body according to the nature of the insult. In all cases, we lose the ability to perform tasks that are part of our daily existence, ranging from throwing a ball to walking comfortably, to lifting a child or a bag of groceries. The loss of purposeful, controlled, effective movement reflects the functional loss as a result of damage to one of our body systems. As physical therapists, we employ a variety of strategies to enable the recovery of strength, motion, and coordination. Our ultimate goal is to facilitate the restoration of movement in order to enable the limbs and body to accomplish desired tasks.

Movement is subject to a number of constraints imposed by internal and external factors. The final presentation of a particular movement is influenced by our intention and purpose of the act, mechanical and physical limits of our joints and muscles, ability to sense and monitor our environment and body, and the capacity to control and correct the resulting movement. Movement is our capacity to change the state of our musculoskeletal system (posture, gait, etc.) in response to internal and external demands.[1-3]

Functional movement depends upon the interaction of multiple sensory systems—visual, vestibular, somatosensory—with the musculoskeletal components. This interaction is guided, mediated, and controlled by central nervous system (CNS) elements ranging from the motor cortex to the spinal cord. Our sensory systems provide information regarding the environment, orientation of our limbs, and the activity of our muscles and joints. The musculoskeletal system supplies force, provides for motion and positioning of the extremities and trunk, and maintains mechanical stability. The CNS is the locus of decision and goal direction, supplies movement strategies and patterns, and translates the information provided by the sensory system into pragmatic responses by the muscles and joints[4] (Fig. 1-1). Movement science is the area where biomechanics, anatomy, and neural sciences overlap.

The element primarily affected in orthopaedic and sports injuries is the musculoskeletal system. The loss of the ability to generate the force to move our joints and perform activities is defined as weakness (as opposed to strength, which is the ability to generate adequate force to meet the muscular task at hand). The interaction between musculoskeletal and neural/sensory components cannot be ignored. Some of the sequelae of injury—effusion, pain, soft tissue dam-

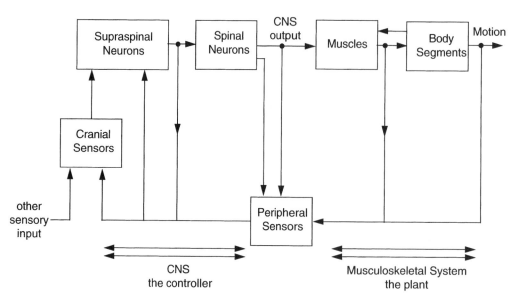

FIGURE 1-1 *Conceptual diagram of the neuromuscular control system, consisting of the linkage between the CNS, or controller, and the musculoskeletal system, or plant. Neural information flows in only one direction. Mechanical interaction between the muscles and body segments can be in both directions due to coupling (From Zajac FE and Winters JM,[4] with permission.)*

age—directly interfere with the functioning of the peripheral nervous system. In this manner, the information provided to the CNS is corrupted. The musculoskeletal system is no longer able to carry out the intentions of the CNS or competently correct for errors in movement, if they are detected. The extent to which movement patterns or highly skilled motions are altered is not known.

This chapter reviews some of the variables in our ability to move in our environment. The focus is on the biomechanical aspects of movement science, but necessarily includes ingredients from other domains. The interplay between systems is now a locus in orthopaedic and sports physical therapy research.

Movement Biomechanics

Shifting the focus to movement and function from strength and range of motion (ROM) means retaining an understanding of the bio-

mechanics of forces and torques, while adding concepts that pertain to movement parameters. For a given movement, the following factors must be taken into consideration: gravitational and inertial properties, forces applied by segments that support the one being moved, forces applied to segments by the one being moved, muscle and soft tissue considerations in the moving and supporting segments, and forces applied by other tissues not directly attached to the moving limb (i.e., leg forces applied to the arm during throwing).[5]

KINEMATICS AND KINETICS

Biomechanics encompasses the study of forces exerted on and by the body under a variety of conditions, both static and dynamic. Statics is the study of bodies at rest or at equilibrium as a result of the forces exerted on them. Dynamics is the study of the motion that occurs as a result of forces that act on an object. Further, kinematics is the study of body motion (translations and rotations), while ignoring the forces that cause the motion.[6] Kinetics is the study of the forces involved in creating motion.

From a mechanical perspective, a rigid body moving in space has six degrees of freedom—three rotations and three translations.[7] Each of these motions can be defined kinematically by describing the displacement, velocity, and acceleration, both linear and angular. Kinetic analysis is either direct or indirect.[8] Direct analysis measures forces applied and then solves for the resulting motion. Indirect analysis measures the motion and then solves for the necessary forces.

From a rehabilitation perspective, we must also consider other aspects of the analysis of forces applied to the body. Is there enough force available to move a joint or limb safely and effectively? Is the musculoskeletal system able to manage the control of the forces necessary for movement? Can mechanical parameters of movement be matched to the sensory data adequately? In a certain sense, we are equipped with an internal motion analysis system via the somatosensory, visual, and equilibrium components of the body. This internal biomechanics laboratory is involved in all our movements during all activities. Understanding the nature of the interactions of the several systems involved in movement and the effects of injury, training, and recovery is the basis for rehabilitation protocols centered around functional movement.

OPEN AND CLOSED MOVEMENT CHAIN

Several articles have recently been written regarding the pros and cons of closed versus open chain rehabilitation,[9–13] based upon interpretations of the work of Steindler.[14] The advantages of reduced knee joint shear, greater potential for joint contraction, greater (perhaps) neuromuscular integration, and multijoint influences cannot be denied. It is important to note, however, that significant movements occur in the open chain, and are more appropriately labeled movable boundary exercise.[13]

The newer classification of kinetic chains according to distal segment boundary limitations (fixed versus moveable) and load (external versus none, axial versus rotary) proposed by Dillman et al.[13] and modified by Lephart et al.[15] may eventually clarify the differences between open and closed kinetic chain exercises based upon the biomechanical environment, rather than the strict mechanical definition. Movement skills demand accurate placement of the distal segment in walking, running, kicking, striking, throwing, and catching. These skills go against the notion, as stated by Rivera,[12] that ". . . rehabilitation exercises, in order to be functional, . . . must be of a closed kinetic chain nature. . . ."

Movement demands a mixture of closed and open chain functions. Supporting structures are placed in the closed chain, promoting stability and ground reaction forces that can be utilized by the musculoskeletal system. Sensory data regarding the *position* of the supporting joints are promoted in the closed chain. Movement of one joint will cause movement of other joints in the chain; isolated joint motion is impossible except at the most proximal joint in the chain. For example, trunk motion may occur without necessarily inducing hip, knee, or ankle movements.

It is important to note that the compressive forces that occur as a result of axial loading throughout the lower extremity are not necessarily mimicked in the upper extremity. The glenohumeral joint is not identical to the articulation of the femur in the acetabulum. Axial loads applied to the arm do not cause only compression of the humerus against the glenoid once the humerus is moved out of 90 degrees of abduction in the pure frontal plane. Some shear force occurs that may be problematic for the capsular tissue of the joint, particularly on the posterior structures. It is relevant to consider that the shoulder is not stabilized by compressive forces like the knee, but by muscle activity. Exercise progressions should consider ways to increase the muscular stability of the joint as an early intervention in treatment, rather than depend upon a mechanical situation that does not readily occur in daily activities.

In the open chain, isolated movements are possible at any link in the chain, allowing for a greater flexibility in movement patterns. Cocontraction occurs to distribute forces throughout the limb, if required.[16] The nature of cocontraction in the open chain is related to force coupling and distribution of force and power throughout the limb, not necessarily to stabilize a joint. This may be the case in the closed chain as well, but cocontraction in the lower limb during weight-bearing is generally examined from a joint stability standpoint in the rehabilitation literature.[9-12] Sensory data regarding the *orientation* of the limb are used by the CNS to effect accurate movements. Joint reaction forces are caused by muscle contraction alone without the compression from the ground; therefore, shear is more likely to occur at any given joint.[9]

The usual comparison between open and closed chain exercise, the squat versus isolated knee extension, represents unique exercise situations, both of which occur in real life. It is more typical, however, that mixtures of open and closed chain functions occur, compelling the need for understanding the movement, sensorimotor, and musculoskeletal differences between these two environments. The natural assumption that closed chain is superior applies only in certain situations. The upper extremity is highly dependant upon open chain, muscularly stabilized placing activities; closed chain training does not mimic these functional demands. Lower extremity movements are comprised of two groups—those requiring closed chain and those requiring open chain. When considered from a movement standpoint, rather than a mechanical one, lower limb open chain placement and orientation exercises may be just as important to functional training as closed chain stabilizing exercises.

MUSCLE MECHANICS

The physiology and mechanical properties of skeletal muscle have been well studied with respect to structure and function. The behavior of muscle under varying conditions and contraction types is well known. Skeletal muscle exhibits consistent length-tension and force-velocity rela-

tion.[17-21] In-depth reviews of muscle mechanics and physiology are available.[19-20]

According to Fitts et al.[22] peak force and power output of a muscle fiber depends upon anatomic/physiologic considerations of (1) muscle and fiber size and length, (2) architecture, (3) fiber type, (4) number of cross bridges in parallel, (5) force per cross bridge, (6) rate of tension development, (7) force-velocity relation, (8) maximal shortening velocity, (9) available free calcium, and (10) force-frequency relation. Afferent input, muscle fiber recruitment, and other neural factors affect the output of muscle tissue.[22]

The most important aspects of muscular architecture are the fiber length and physiologic cross-sectional area.[20,23,24] Pennation of the muscle affects the velocity of fiber contraction and force production.[20,21] Short pennated muscles have high tension generated capacity while longer, more parallel oriented muscles have greater shortening capability. According to Zajac,[23] pennation must be greater than 20 degrees to affect the musculotendinous properties of skeletal muscle. A secondary effect of pennation is the amount of intermuscular pressure generated within the muscle itself,[19] which can contribute to force output. Fusiform muscles generate higher intramuscular pressures as a result of pennation.[25] Unipennate and bipennate muscles have less absolute fiber shortening with less resultant intramuscular pressure. Interference in the function of an active fiber from nearby passive fibers lessens under this type of architecture.

Alexander and Ker[26] propose three types of musculotendinous units, using a teleologic perspective. The three types are:

1. Muscles with long fascicles and relatively short tendons. These muscles are located proximally and tend to be large in size. They can produce large amounts of work and accelerate the limb over a significant range of motion. They can also absorb energy when it is necessary to decelerate the limb.

2. Muscles with long, relatively thick, inelastic tendons. The long tendon allows the muscle

mass to be located proximally and reduce limb inertia. The thick tendons have relatively high stiffness, an important characteristic for position control of the distal segment. The muscle portion of the unit undergoes a relatively large amount of shortening for a given change in muscle force. These musculotendinous units have a relatively large change in the length of the muscle component for a given change in force. This presents the CNS with a challenge in executing the position control required of these muscles.

3. Muscles with short fascicles and long, slender tendons predominate among the antigravity muscles. These tendons are relatively elastic (up to 5 percent extensibility) and can store large amounts of energy. These muscles are metabolically efficient due to the small muscle mass and spring-like elastic tendon. These muscles undergo a relatively small change in length for a given force output, resulting in function in a more efficient band of the length-tension and force-velocity curves. Hof[27] and Chapman and Sanderson[28] have confirmed the metabolic efficiency of these musculotendinous units in walking and running at various speeds, although their explanations as to how this efficiency is maintained differs.

Muscle mechanics and architecture represent one of the morphologic constraints to movement.[2] In conjunction with neural factors, the production of force is determined by the anatomy, physiology, and structure of the musculotendinous unit.[29] In the vast majority of movement situations, we rarely exert the maximal force that muscle is capable of. Generally speaking, in the absence of injury or disease, muscle provides the requisite force to engender functional movement.

STIFFNESS AND SENSORIMOTOR SET

Muscle stiffness is the ratio of force change to length change. Stiffness is controlled by the muscle spindles with influences from Golgi tendon organs and other mechanoreceptors in the joint. Muscle stiffness is a function of the muscle's sensitivity to stretch.[30] Force output can also be mediated by this mechanism. Lorentzon et al.[31] believes that nonoptimal quadriceps function following anterior cruciate ligament (ACL) tear is caused by altered feedback from damaged mechanoreceptors.

Muscle stiffness has two components—intrinsic stiffness and reflex-mediated stiffness. Intrinsic stiffness is dependant on the degree of muscle contraction at a specific point in time.[32] Reflex mediated stiffness can be powerfully influenced by low threshold mechanoreceptors.[33] Nichols[34] states that muscle stiffness under dynamic conditions is a function of reflex mediated stiffness. Control of this variable is important for continuous regulation of muscle and limb stiffness and, therefore, postural adjustments and coordination of limb synergies.[32,35,36]

Lieber and Fridén[37] refer to muscular, neural, and combined factors in stiffness regulation. Muscular factors include muscle activation frequency, muscle fiber recruitment, sarcomere length-tension and force velocity relations, and muscle architecture. Higher stiffness is associated with higher frequency activation, greater fiber recruitment, optimal sarcomere length, isometric or eccentric contraction, and architecture associated with low velocity, high force contractions (quadriceps, gastrocnemius).

Neural factors of stiffness regulation include the stretch reflex and heterogenic reflexes. Muscle spindle sensitivity determines the response of the stretch reflex that, in turn, regulates the stiffness of the muscle. Agonist and antagonist muscles can influence the stretch reflex of another muscle (heterogenic reflex) under certain conditions.[38]

Combined factors refer to the interactions between muscles, tendons, and joints. Muscle fiber length is dependant in part on joint rotation. This can affect the force generation of the muscle and its contribution to joint and limb stiffness. Tendon compliance can accommodate some length changes, depending upon the architecture of the muscle and tendon (see above).[39] Tendon compliance can serve as a mechanism by which sarcomere length is kept within a smaller range around the optimal.

Stiffness properties of the joint and limb can contribute to the patient's ability to move. In sports and orthopaedics, the greater concern is inadequate stiffness as a result of ligament damage, direct muscle or tendon injury, and neuromuscular inhibition due to pain, immobilization, effusion, and overuse. If inadequate stiffness is present in the lower limb, gait deviations, problems with changing direction, and supporting the body weight during walking, running, or landing may occur. In the upper extremity, stiffness is more difficult to evaluate. It is likely that inadequate muscle stiffness as a result of injury will lead to joint overload, and potential problems in shoulder or wrist stability during functional tasks may result. Inadequate stiffness in the trunk as a result of decreased muscle factors can lead to tissue overload of the disk and facet joints as well as other soft tissues.

Prochazka[40] proposed that control of sensorimotor gain is a basic strategy of motor control. He states that the fusimotor set allows for adjustment of feedback under varying conditions. The role of the proprioceptive system (and cutaneous feedback) is to bias and adjust the sensitivity and gain of the γ-spindle system, using muscle and limb stiffness as the control parameter. This theory and the work now being done on the global effects of joint injuries have powerful implications for the style and substance of rehabilitation programs in orthopaedic and sports therapy. Attention to movement patterns and awareness of the influence of the system's responsiveness to exercise interventions are now key factors in our approach to restoration of function. Movement affects the feedback into the sensorimotor, cognitive, and association areas, and other control areas. Abnormal movement perpetuates abnormal sensory and muscle patterns. The use of manual and exercise therapy to normalize motion helps maintain preinjury movement patterns and neuromuscular sensitivity (Fig. 1-2).

MONO AND BIARTICULAR MUSCLES

There are two distinct classes of muscle forms in the body—those muscles that cross only one joint (brachialis, vasti portion of the quadriceps,

short heads of the biceps femoris and triceps brachii, etc.) and those that cross two or more (rectus femoris, gastrocnemius, biceps brachii, etc.). Both of these muscle classes contribute to the generation of force, movement of joints, and control of limbs.[4,24,41,42]

To understand the role of monoarticular muscles, the muscle element first must be adequately described. For all intents and purposes, the muscle is an actuator that produces a linear force.[21,22,43] Yet, we visualize movement as rotational motion of the joints, not linear force production of the muscles.[9,16] The mechanics of the joint (reaction force, friction, geometry, ligamentous restraints) and the anatomy of the musculotendinous attachment produce rotatory motions. The result is a double transformation; linear muscle tension is converted to joint rotations, which are used to translate the body or limb in space.[44–46]

Complex motions generally require the activation of many lower extremity muscles. The mover must generate forces and resultant torques to produce the power necessary to displace the body or limb in space. These tasks have two components—the above mentioned force generation and coordinating/distributing torques throughout the moving limb.

The role of mono- and biarticular muscles has been studied in jumping,[47–49] cycling,[41,50,51] sit-to-stand,[52] and in a theoretical sense, postural and limb synergies.[53] Whatever the multijoint movement being discussed, monoarticular muscles are assigned the role of power generators, both in cats[42,54] and humans.[24,55–57] Monoarticular muscles may also absorb energy at the joint they cross.

Certain monoarticular muscles may also play a major sensory role. Bastide[58] proposed that the smaller, deep muscles are really "active ligaments," which function primarily in a proprioceptive/kinesthetic fashion. Nitz (see Ch. 2) uses the term "kinesthetic monitors" to define the role of smaller uniarticular muscles that act in conjunction with larger, force-producing muscles. The "monitor" muscles have higher densities of muscle spindles. Scott and Loeb[59] modeled the distribution of muscle spindles in

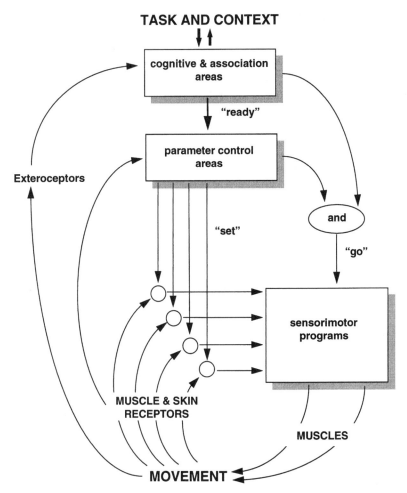

FIGURE 1-2 *Model of movement using central and peripheral information to adjust sensorimotor gain. This determines the responsiveness of muscles and resulting movement to internal and external stimuli. (From Prochazka A,[40] with permission.)*

an idealized two-joint system with both single and biarticular muscles. They used two separate models of mono- and biarticular muscles and varying types of reference frames to predict position and orientation errors. Their model assumed that the muscle spindles provide the bulk of the normal afferent position sense; the CNS makes optimal use of the information available to it; and the fusimotor system is used to adjust the gain of the sensors to match the expected behavioral kinematics. The first model placed the mono- and biarticular muscles on the same side of the joint system. The second model used a biarticular muscle that crossed on opposite sides of the joint (Fig. 1-3). It should be noted that the second model represents a special case. In the human, only the sartorius muscle crosses two joints in such fashion. In most cases, the least error occurred when the majority of spindles were placed in the monoarticular muscles. Based upon the assumptions of the model, Scott and Loeb concluded that spindle distribution is

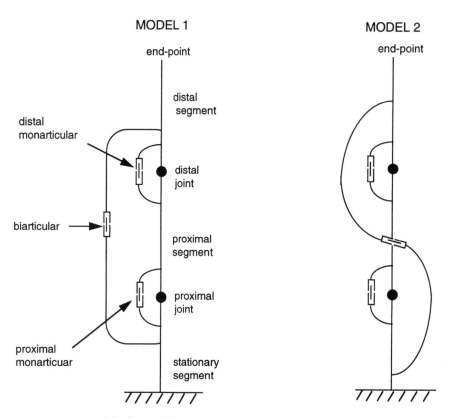

FIGURE 1-3 *Model of possible orientation of mono- and biarticular muscles with respect to the joints crossed. Model 1 represents the common arrangement of mono- and biarticular muscles with all muscles on the same side of the joint. Spindle information is affected by the orientation of the muscle to its respective joint. (From Scott SH and Loeb GE,*[59] *with permission.)*

better suited for information purposes than control purposes, and that no particular frame of reference is favored by the distribution of sensory elements within the muscles.[59]

Another aspect of monoarticular muscles is that they can cause accelerations or decelerations at joints other than the one they cross, depending upon the mechanical state of the entire limb. An external or internal force applied to a limb can produce angular motion at all joints coplanar to the applied force.[60] Zajac and Gordon[24] showed that the joint torque produced by a uniarticular muscle induces angular acceleration of unspanned joints as well. This acceleration either results in movement of the unspanned joint or induces the CNS to produce a stabilizing

muscle contraction if no movement is desired. The model that Zajac and Gordon developed showed that the soleus can cause knee accelerations at almost twice the value of ankle accelerations, assuming an upright posture. The short head of the biceps femoris may cause ankle acceleration as well, assuming that the foot is on the ground. This concept of induced acceleration holds true in activities such as cycling, in which the soleus muscle may be shown to induce acceleration at both the hip and knee.[24,41]

A multisegmented limb comprised solely of monoarticular muscles would prove to be both inefficient[4,26,47,55,61] and limited in its movement capability.[53] Often, a complex movement requires positive work to be performed at one joint while negative work is being performed at another. Gielen et al.[61] and others[42,44] have shown that using monoarticular muscles only results in a large amount of negative work to be performed, causing energy dissipation and resultant inefficiency.

This problem is neatly solved by the use of bi- or multiarticular muscles. The role of these muscles is threefold. They (1) distribute mechanical energy throughout the limb and increase efficiency, (2) couple joint movements, and (3) transform rotation of limb segments into translation of the distal end points or center of mass of the body.

Gregoire et al.[56] showed that the rectus femoris and gastrocnemius muscles were responsible for distributing the force generated by the gluteus maximus during the push-off phase of jumping throughout the leg. Van Soest et al.,[48] using a mathematical model, showed that jumping height was decreased if the gastrocnemius was converted into a monoarticular muscle. The moment arm of the gastrocnemius at the knee was important in contributing to and redistributing forces generated by the leg muscles during the takeoff phase of jumping. Similarly, the hamstrings distribute forces throughout the limb during pedaling motions.[47,50,55] The same phenomenon occurs during speed-skating and other explosive activities.[44] The biarticular muscles transfer power generated by the positively working monoarticular muscles throughout the limb. Energy transfer may occur either distally or proximally.[49]

Multiarticular muscles couple joint motions in both the upper and lower extremities. The gastrocnemius couples knee extension and plantar flexion[4,55] in the leg. In certain movements of the arm, the biceps brachii and or the triceps brachii may couple shoulder and elbow motions, producing elbow motion that may be a result of action at the glenohumeral joint.[47] Happee[62] noted that the biarticular muscles of the arm remained active throughout a goal-directed movement, while the uniarticular muscles did not.

The third function of the multiarticular muscles is to transform rotation into translation. Monoarticular muscles generate the majority of the power required for explosive limb movements. Contractions of this type cause rotation of the joints associated with the contracting muscle. Biarticular muscle contraction is coordinated so that its action serves to counteract the rotation while distributing and preserving the power generated by the monoarticular motor.[61,63] This theory of motor control is unproven, but some evidence exists to support it.[44,45]

Control of mono- and biarticular muscles is indicative of their varied functions. Since monoarticular muscles are used for the same purpose regardless of the task at hand, their activation patterns during activities show remarkable consistency. Van Ingen Schneau et al.[47] demonstrated that the monoarticular muscles of the leg are used to produce work, particularly positive work, with no consideration of the direction of limb motion or force application. The multiarticular muscles (gastrocnemius, hamstrings, rectus femoris) are activated differently depending on the directional aspect of the task (i.e., forward and backward cycling). In a second report, van Ingen Schneau et al.[42] reviewed the work done in cats during forward and backward walking. The monoarticular muscles showed little or no variation in activation patterns, while the multiarticular muscles did. This is reflective of the need to distribute joint moments throughout the limb in a different fashion. Similar activation patterns were noted in the upper extremity, with monoarticular muscles more likely to be operating under when they are in a position to shorten.[61] The multiarticular muscles are capable of more complex contractile behaviors (Fig. 1-4).[16] It also suggests that control mechanisms of multiarticular muscles may receive additional sensory input from cutaneous receptors in the foot or hand. This additional information may provide the basis for instructing the multiarticular muscles as to in which direction to channel the flow of power.[47,64,65] Another factor is the balance between movement and stability required at each joint. Biarticular muscles can be used to transfer power between joints to achieve the necessary balance during changes in posture, such as sit to stand movements.[52]

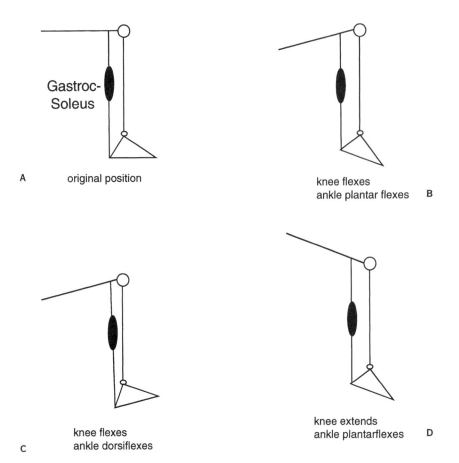

Gastroc-Soleus

A   original position

knee flexes
ankle plantar flexes   B

knee flexes
ankle dorsiflexes
C

knee extends
ankle plantarflexes   D

FIGURE 1-4 *Possible combinations of actions of a biarticular muscle using the gastrocnemius as an example. Knee extension with dorsiflexion would require eccentric action at both ends and does not occur. (From Zajac FE,[16] with permission.)*

DEGREES OF FREEDOM

One of the basic problems in control of multijoint or multisegmental movement is that of redundancy. The issue was formally stated by Bernstein.[1] The combined motions available at the joints of a limb plus the number of muscles that can be selected offer the CNS a choice of movement combinations to achieve the task at hand. Bernstein termed this "redundancy"—more than one combination of muscle activation and joint motion can perform a given task. Bernstein[1] also defined motor coordination as "the process of mastering redundant degrees of freedom of the moving organ, in other words its

conversion to a controllable system." The redundant nature of the neuromusculoskeletal system introduces a great deal of variability in our movements. Bernstein suggested that the solution to the problem of redundancy was motor learning. Learned responses limit the number of independent degrees of freedom by placing constraints on movement choices.[66–69] The available solutions to any motor task are always greater than the number of learned patterns.[67] When the available solutions to a problem are essentially infinite, the problem is indeterminate.[70]

Of course, the CNS is not only faced with the task of limiting degrees of freedom, but also with knowing when to recruit them. One of the tasks of the CNS is to maintain optimal function of the various joints involved in movement. When one link approaches its limit of function, then the CNS may recruit another joint to provide additional degrees of freedom of motion.[3] If the task is to serve a tennis ball, but the ball is tossed too far posteriorly for the customary glenohumeral joint extension, additional motion may recruited by increasing spinal extension.

The degrees of freedom problem is one that is often faced in orthopaedic physical therapy. Observation of the manner and style in which people move is often helpful in identifying when component joints of a multijoint segment are contributory or not. A large part of the evaluation of pelvic and lumbar motions is devoted to identifying when joints are "stuck" or hypomobile. If, for example, the hip or pelvis is relatively immobile in gait, then the loss of a degree of freedom must affect the motion that is available to the limb. Foot placement during heel-strike is a combination of movements from the lumbar spine to the toes[71] (see Gait Review, ch. 5). Reduced or eliminated degrees of freedom will create a problem with one of two solutions. Either the stride must be shortened, or increased motion must be recruited from one or more joints. Since one of the results of a redundant system is that the links can function in a fashion that avoids overstressing any one joint, the accommodation that results will place some tissue at risk. Inadequate hip flexion may result in stress at the knee during gait.

The situation of increased mobility is more familiar in physical therapy. Excessive motion at the subtalar joint has been implicated in pain and problems at every joint proximal to it.[72] Alternatively, excessive lumbar lordosis or hypermobility may be the causative factor in repetitive microtrauma injuries in all joints distal in the kinetic chain.

Frames of Reference

Unfortunately, there is no identifiable "position board" in the CNS that tells the brain where in space the limbs are with respect to themselves and the rest of the body parts. Visual, kinesthetic, vestibular, and proprioceptive inputs relay information about the orientation of body parts and body with respect to some internal and/or external frame of reference. The method by which this is accomplished involves at least one transformation of sensory data into coded, usable information on the state of the joints and muscles. Georgopoulos[73] showed that neuronal pools orient their activity in the direction that mimics the movement vector. Typically, the proprioceptive map of moving limbs within the environment is matched to the visuomotor representation of the environment, so that limb position and position of a targeted object may correspond.[74]

The classic frame of reference problem involves the description of a moving object by an observer (Fig. 1-5). The observed path of the object is dependent upon whether the observer is stationary with respect to the object. Observation in the CNS occurs with respect to some fixed point. Frame of reference can be fixed to the eye, head, trunk, gravity, or any joint that is best suited to aligning the task at hand to the movement that must occur. Jeannerod[74,75] suggested a hierarchical system in which certain pieces of information are considered before others in locating targets and organizing movements. The progression begins with target location on the retina then progresses to eye position in the head, head position on the trunk, and relative positions of the limbs. The end result is knowledge of the position of the end segment (hand or foot) in space and with reference to the target or obstacle. Each progression through the chain uses a different reference frame that is interpreted by the CNS, either through computation[76] (inverse dynamics) or mechanics[77] (equilibrium point hypothesis).

Regardless of how the CNS initiates or controls movement, some frame of reference must be identified in order to create the spatial representations necessary to determine movements. The complexity of the movement involved may determine the reference frames necessary for the CNS to maintain control of the body. Control of hand function based upon elbow joint position[78,79] presents a different problem than con-

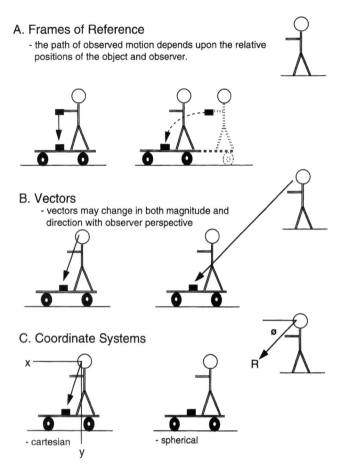

FIGURE 1-5 *Illustration of the differences in motion description depending upon frame of reference, vectors, and coordinate systems. (From Soechting JF and Flanders M,[66] with permission.)*

trol of the arms and limbs required of a dancer, gymnast, diver, or person who has slipped on a banana peel and is in the process of falling. During multijoint, single-limb tasks, the frame of reference can be based around the locus of rotation of the limb.[80-82] During tasks that require coordination of limbs, such as locomotion or jumping, either several reference frames must also be coordinated[83] or the CNS must use some sort of composite reference frame.

Given multiple reference frames, the CNS must have some mechanism by which a frame of reference is selected. Vision plays a major role in this process. Vision identifies objects in the environment[84,85] (including targets and obstacles), locates them with respect to the eye, provides feedback regarding the execution of a movement, and gives additional information regarding the position and orientation of our limbs to augment other sensory data.[84-89] After an object has been identified by the eye (retinocentric frame of reference), its position is coded by the CNS and a movement response can triggered.[85] Considerable processing occurs in the optic system to identify true motion. Supplementary information from head and neck receptors determines head and eye position with respect to the world and body. This enables the CNS to define

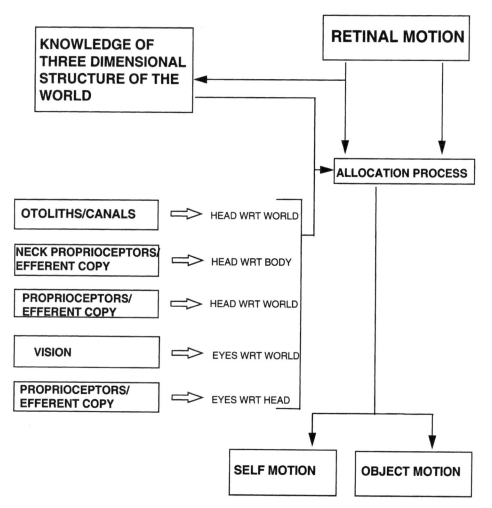

FIGURE 1-6 *Systems involved with determining motion of objects with respect to the eyes and head. (From Harris LR,[213] with permission.)*

external motion versus motion of the eyes and head (Fig. 1-6). The presence or absence of visual input significantly affects movement error in both arm-based tasks,[80,81,90] complex tasks (such as gymnastics),[83] and locomotion.[91]

Conflicting demands upon the visual system often result in collisions or errors in reaching or catching activities. Consider the problem of an athlete who has to run to catch a ball. The eye must provide information about the ball position and location, which is constantly changing. At the same time, the visual system has to update

the environment, which may contain obstacles such as an outfield wall, playing surface contours, or opposing football players defending against a catch. The latter information can prepare the player for what will happen after he catches the ball. If too much attention is focused on the ball, one runs the risk of collision without adequate preparation. Alternatively, if the environment is scanned too often or at the wrong time, one runs the risk of failing to catch the ball.

A similar problem is faced in gait. Enough attention must be paid to the environment to identify obstacles and ensure that proper foot contact is made on the ground (the equivalent task of placing a hand to catch a ball). Failure to adequately perform these tasks may not allow the musculoskeletal system enough time to respond to an unexpected foot placement, resulting in a stumble, ankle sprain, or fall.

Visual data are required for many activities. Vision is generally used only intermittently with respect to a given task.[85,91] During time dependant activities, the visual system updates information at regular intervals, usually at a rate that the CNS judges to be sufficient to enable corrective actions to be taken, if necessary.[92,93] Once a movement has been initiated, the CNS uses a second frame of reference to base the movement on, other than the eye. Generally speaking, the most stable segment is used as the body reference.[90] Usually, the head is the most stable. A series of studies by Pozzo et al.,[83] demonstrated that the angular displacement of the head is less than that of the trunk during balancing activities under nonconstrained visual control. The head position is even more stable when gaze is fixed. Additional information from studies on neck proprioceptors[94,95] suggests that feedback from the neck is important in maintaining an internal representation of posture and the head in space, and correctly utilizing visual data.

The role of vision in locomotion has been studied with respect to a person's ability to avoid obstacles. Thomson[91] found that subjects were able to walk through an obstacle course in the absence of vision without difficulty after being shown the layout of the course. This ability was limited by time, indicating that visual memory of a stable, unchanging environment can persist for some time. Their results contribute to the concept of internal mapping of the external environment as well as an internal representation of the body with respect to the environment. In situations where the environment is not known to be stable, visual guidance must be updated more frequently, to avoid obstacles.[93] Cognitive spatial mapping is one of the key variables in Patla's[96] scheme of factors that influence skilled locomotion (see Fig. 1-7). Mapping sets the stage for control of several variables that are considered by the CNS during ambulatory activities.

Selection of a frame of reference for movement may also be influenced by the mechanical parameters of motion. Soechting and Flanders[80] suggest that distance and direction are important in determining a reference frame for movement. During pointing activities, the shoulder appears to be the reference frame for distance control, while vision is dominant for direction. These experiments were made on stationary subjects. In the absence of vision, a less effective frame of reference must be selected, resulting in greater movement error.[81]

COORDINATE SYSTEMS

As noted earlier, myriad reference frames exist. They can be egocentric (located in some part of the body), allocentric (located in space), or geocentric (referenced to gravity or direction).[83] While the frame of reference identifies motion relative to some fixed axis, the coordinate system identifies the position and orientation of an object or joint with respect to the center of the frame of reference. Position coordinates are the most familiar, generally defined in a Cartesian system based on the x, y, z axes. Cartesian coordinates are generally used to define planar motion, although three-dimensional movement is easily defined with the triaxial system. The International Society for Biomechanics has standardized four Cartesian coordinate systems:[97] (1) the *absolute* or *global reference system* is fixed to the ground, (2) the *local reference system* is fixed to and moves with the body, (3) the *segmental* or *anatomic reference system* is fixed to the body and uses anatomic definitions, and (4) the *joint reference system* is defined for each joint individually. These systems define movement in terms of an outside observer.

Orientation angles include radius (R), elevation (the angle between the radius and the horizontal plane, ϕ), and azimuth (the angle between the radius and the sagittal plane). Orientation angles are generally used in a spherical coordinate systems[66] (Fig. 1-5). Spherical coordinates

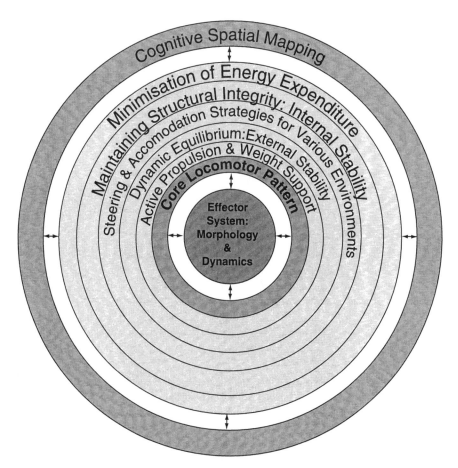

FIGURE 1-7 *Illustration of the variables that influence skilled locomotor activities. Inner circle factors must take into account the outer circle variables. (From Patla AE,[214] with permission.)*

are used commonly in aiming and navigational tasks. Spherical coordinate systems generally define movement in terms of an internal observer, or an observational viewpoint that is the same as the moving subject. The shoulder is often involved in tracking and aiming tasks in three dimensions. It may be helpful to begin thinking of shoulder motion in terms of spherical coordinates rather than traditional planar definitions (Fig. 1-8).[98] This shift in approach to shoulder motion may spur new thinking in how somatosensory information is interpreted by the CNS in the upper extremity.[98,99]

The question of coordinate systems and frame of reference is basic to the problem of determining how the CNS codes information from joint and muscle receptors. Several studies have been performed on peripheral joints to determine the threshold of detecting movement at a single joint.[100-103] Altered function has been noted in some pathologic conditions, such as chronic laxity and postsurgery. Loss of joint proprioception has been implicated in the cycle of functional instability (ch. 2).

The ability of the sensory system to detect joint angle and motion may be a secondary one. Soechting[104] suggests that position sense at the elbow is better suited to match the orientation

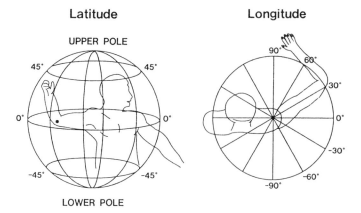

FIGURE 1-8 *Spherical coordinate system used for measuring position of the hand in space. In this model, latitude and longitude are used to describe movement, using the glenohumeral joint as the center of the sphere. In this type of motion system, the focus is on position of the hand in space as well as on the kinematics of the glenohumeral joint. (From Yoshikawa GI,[98] with permission.)*

of the forearm rather than reproducing the joint angle. Similar results have been found at the shoulder.[88,105] Perhaps future work on joint proprioception can add a functional focus regarding joint proprioception (hand and foot placement, knowledge of the body in space, ability to react to changes in the environment) to the traditional studies of joint angle detection.

MOVEMENT CONSTRAINTS

Constraints refer to the type and manner in which an identifiable element affects the manner in which we choose, plan, control, and organize movement. Higgins defines three type of constraints to human movement: environmental, biomechanical, and morphologic.[2] Environmental constraint refers to the ability to coordinate spatial and temporal aspects of movement to the expected environment. The discussion on the use of vision is an example. The rate at which one scans his surroundings and the subsequent influence on movement is dependent upon the expectation of a stable environment. Movements become more reactive and less predictable as the environment becomes less stable. The loss of vis-

ual input, either through the aging process or concentrating on one aspect of the environment, is significant to the execution of movement.

Biomechanical constraint refers to our ability to maintain a mechanical basis for movement. Certain factors must be present in order for movement to be successful. Higgins lists some of the mechanical factors that contribute to successful movement. Time may also be considered a biomechanical constraint. If a movement must occur in a certain length of time, the muscular system must generate adequate force to create the acceleration necessary to complete the task. Rapid movements require different movement strategies to accommodate higher generated forces and velocities.[106–111] Time constrained movements may also be less accurate.[112] Treslian[113] considers time to contact to be a perceived variable and an important constraint during targeted movements of the upper limb. He suggests that perceptual information is an important factor in generating control signals to the musculoskeletal system.[84,113] Accuracy may also be a constraint. Some movements must be very precise and skilled.

Morphologic constraint refers to the structure and design of the musculoskeletal system and how these variables limit or contribute to our movement capabilities. The role of muscle morphology has been discussed earlier. Joint morphology also causes limitation on movement. Joint geometry determines, in part, some of the motion that is possible at a joint.[114] The presence or absence of ligaments and other soft tissue components of a joint contributes to the absolute motion available at a joint as well as the forces that a joint can withstand during movement.[115,116] The ability of the CNS to determine when to recruit extra degrees of freedom during movement is related to one's ability to detect the limit of motion at a given joint. That is one of the major roles of isolated joint position sense. Limited or impaired knowledge of when a joint is at its normal limit can result in mechanical overload and inefficient use of other joints in a limb.

Nashner and McCollum[117] present constraints in a different format in their model of the organization of human postural movements. Neural and mechanical constraints impose different limitations on the selection of movement strategies in response to balance disturbance without stepping. Neural constraints consist of the following:

1. The number of muscles used to execute a movement is minimized. This is one of the mechanisms by which the CNS addresses the degrees of freedom and redundancy issues. The number of muscles selected may depend upon the restrictions imposed by the environment.[118] Kuo and Zajac[118] found that the ankle strategy may require more muscle activation than the hip strategy for a given acceleration.

2. The calculations imposed upon the CNS are minimized. Nashner and McCollum[117] interpret this constraint as meaning that the CNS will choose the movement strategy that requires the least amount of calculations of vectors, positions, and orientation of the limbs by keeping the axes of motion limited.

The mechanical constraints are:

1. Muscle torques and friction forces can limit the effectiveness of a strategy. Support surface conditions and potential ankle torque are factors that influence the CNS to select a hip or ankle strategy or a combination, if necessary. Limited ankle torque potential will result in a hip strategy, while slippery support surfaces will favor an ankle strategy.

2. Selected strategies may be hybrids of the two dominant strategies, but not all possible neural combinations are functionally sufficient. Nashner and McCollum[117] believe that the set of possible combination strategies is limited. Functional limitations are imposed by the dynamics of synergistic muscle actions. Not all combinations can restore balance following a perturbation. The CNS limits the possible combinations by dividing space into regions and knowing what combinations are effective when the center of gravity (COG) is pushed into a given region.

Kuo and Zajac[118] present another view of the biomechanical restraints to movement during posture control. They modeled the human body as a series of links with specific types of muscle motors. Each possible combination of muscle activations resulted in some movement of the linkage with an acceleration. Their method calculates the acceleration set that will produce an adequate postural correction. Constraints exist when joints are limited in motion, which reduces the possible combinations of muscle forces.

COMPUTATION VERSUS MECHANICS IN MOVEMENT CONTROL

As mentioned earlier, two major schools of thought exist regarding the method by which movement is controlled by the CNS. The inverse dynamics model assumes that the CNS contains a detailed model of the kinematic and inertial properties of the musculoskeletal system.[119,120] In this model, the required forces and moments to be generated by the muscular system are computed from the desired trajectories, angular velocities, and angular accelerations. The complexity of this problem given multiple joints and three-dimensional space is enormous. Hogan and Winters[120] note that one author used two pages of text to describe the dynamic equations for a five degree of freedom model of the upper arm. In reality, the arm has almost three times the number of degrees of freedom, so one can begin to appreciate the true computational challenge to the CNS. The complexity and precision expected of the inverse dynamics approach makes it doubtful that the CNS reproduces this mode of control exactly.

Another aspect of the inverse dynamics model is that the CNS must carry out inverse dynamics calculations to generate torques necessary to produce *desired* kinematics.[121] This is different from the biomechanical tool of inverse dynamics analysis, which determines torques based upon *observed* kinematics. Hasan[121] states that the inverse dynamics model requires that kinematic details be preplanned. Hasan also argues that if the CNS uses an internal inverse dynamics computer to produce movement, then the loss of proprioceptive input should not have a major effect, which is clearly not the case. Yet some evidence does exist that the CNS does produce motor neuron activity that mimics the trajectory of the end point of a moving limb. Georgopoulos et al.[73] found that cortical neuron populations have a vector-oriented response that relates to mechanical properties of a segment.

An opposing model of movement is the equilibrium point (EP) hypothesis. Bizzi et al.[122] state that the CNS responds to a sensory stimulus (e.g., a ball to be caught) by first generating a neural code that represents the location of the object with respect to the head and body. Next, the direction, velocity, and amplitude of the required hand movement to catch the ball is planned. This requires some transformation or series of transformations[1,60,123] to represent the

motor behavior in terms of extrinsic space. The EP hypothesis as expressed by Feldman,[77] describes the generation of single and multijoint movements, following the identification of a target and the desired response. The EP model states that the CNS changes the relative activation of agonist-antagonist pairs to generate joint torques. The resulting joint motion will depend upon the torques and external loads.

The equilibrium point model assumes that muscles exhibit spring-like behavior, with force generation determined by the length of the muscle and the neural activation. The equilibrium point is defined by Bizzi et al.[122] as the position at which the limb would rest if, given the last set of CNS instructions, the limb were free to move in the absence of external loads or additional CNS commands. The actual position of the limb is the balance, or static equilibrium, between the CNS activation of the muscles and the external loads. Movement generated follows the shifting equilibrium point as muscle activation and external loads change. Shifting equilibrium points form a path that Bizzi calls a "virtual trajectory."

Although the EP hypothesis presents a much simpler (in terms of computational requirements) means of controlling movement, it fails to account for the sensorimotor transformations that occur in the first two steps mentioned by Bizzi et al.,[122] noted above. The computations necessary to identify the positions of the joints, compute a virtual trajectory, and monitor the activity are not simple. Further, the model addresses the static components of equilibrium but tends to ignore dynamic influences.[70] Experimental evidence exists that both supports[87,124] and opposes[89,125] predictions made by the EP model, depending upon conditions.

Sensory information plays a major role in the control of limb movements. Gandevia and Burke[126] outlined the data provided by the peripheral sensory system. They code and detect changes in joint position, signal the extremes of angular motion, and sense the relative amounts of force being applied. Proprioceptive triggering is discussed in Chapter 2. The EP hypothesis does not account for the role of this sensory information.[127] Cordo and Bevan believe that because of this lack, the EP hypothesis must be limited to the initial planning of normal movement, after which it becomes insufficient.

Clearly, neither model is sufficient to account for or explain the control of all types of movement available to the human body. Part of the problem is that the sensory apparatus is expected to play a dual role—provide information as well as control dynamics.[128] The sensors involved are, by the nature of their multiple roles, "noisy." That is to say that the sensory systems that subserve movement are not maintained at the level of precision necessary to satisfy the rigorous examination of mathematics.

Luckily, that level of precision is not required for movement. Many movements last for 400–500 msec.[127] This allows time for the initiation of movement and for correction based upon visual and kinesthetic information acquired during the time of movement.[85] The implication is that the movement is initiated along a course that is approximately optimal and corrections are made along the way. In the model proposed by Soechting and Flanders,[66,70,123] successive sensorimotor transformations are made during target directed movements. The position of the target is compared to the position and orientation of arm (Fig. 1-9). Appropriate movement kinematics are selected to accomplish the goal of meeting the target with the hand or its tool.[105,123,127]

Both models have given rise to a number of proposed optimized variables, such as maximal smoothness,[119] minimal jerk,[122] minimal neural control,[118] minimal total muscular effort,[129] or any dynamic performance criterion,[4] or a combination of factors.[69] The CNS is capable of selecting a single variable or multiple variables to optimize. In the former case, most optimization criteria predict approximately the same results.[57] In the latter instance, no clear cut solution will be identified by optimization theories,[130] or solutions will be limited by the model assumptions. It appears that task-dependant conditions determine the key performance parameters that affect movement control.[4,46,47,131]

The CNS appears to favor neither the inverse dynamics model nor the equilibrium point hypothesis, since neither can explain the full range of behavior of which the human is capable. The CNS appears to maintain an internal representation of the moving body or limb.[86] The parameters that the CNS uses as control factors are not yet known. The CNS is able to utilize information from several sensory systems (visual, kinesthetic, cutaneous) to select, initiate, monitor, and control multijoint and multisegmental movements. A combination of explanations based upon a series of approximations compared to the internal representation of the CNS may successfully describe movement, once the appropriate control factors are identified.

Other theories have evolved to explain the control of movement. Kelso[128] has developed a dynamic systems theory that he bases on "coordination dynamics." He states that "relevant collective variables or order parameters express the coherent relations between the interacting components of a system and how these evolve under changing ... conditions."[128] His underlying principles are based on the pattern formation and self-organizational behavior of nonequilibrium systems. Dynamic system theory[132] has been used to explain the development of coordinated movements in infants. Dynamic systems are self-organized and capable of changing their attributes.[128,133,134] Neural network theory[135–137] has been used by Droulez and Berthoz[138] to develop their concepts on dynamic memory and sensorimotor control. The attraction of neural network theories is the resemblance between the proposed information processing structure and the biologic organization of the CNS.[120] Neural networks have been shown to be capable of learning[135,137] and are not limited to linear systems (as opposed to a dynamic system), two capabilities of the neuromusculoskeletal system. All of these theories on the organization and control of human movement provide insight into the range of movement expressions available in the human.

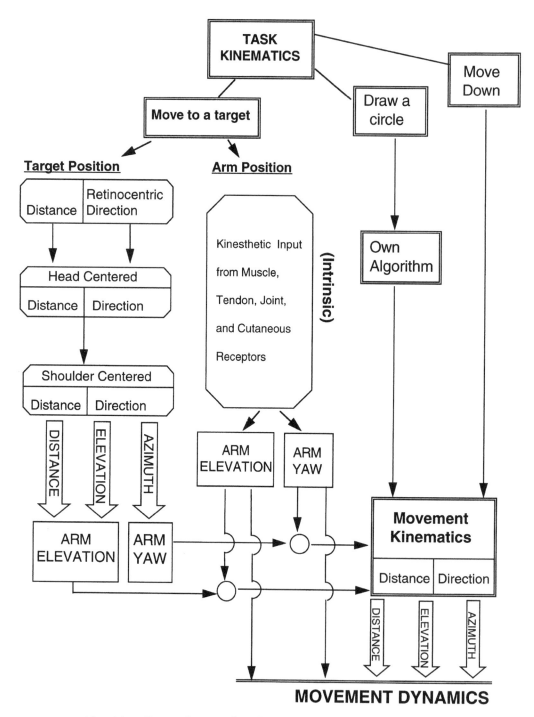

FIGURE 1-9 *Algorithm for tracking tasks of the upper extremity. Each change in frame of reference requires a transformation requiring time and introducing potential error. (From Soechting JF, Flanders M,*[70] *with permission.)*

Single Joint Movement

A great deal of work has been performed in analyzing the function of single joints. The single joint system is used to identify biomechanical and neuromuscular factors that can shed understanding on the control of the neuromuscular system. A single joint system consists of five elements. They are the rigid link, synovial joint, muscle, neuron, and sensory receptors that are associated with these structures.[139]

ORGANIZATION OF MOVEMENT

Several levels of control exist in the single joint model. Muscle mechanics (architecture, contractile properties, etc.) and neural factors (as expressed by muscle mechanics nature of motor unit recruitment[16]) each play a role in the behavior of the single joint system. The elbow and shoulder joints are often selected to study the performance of the single joint model.[106–110, 127,141–144] It is important to note that even though motion may be limited to a single joint, muscle activity is elicited at joints located far from the moving segment.[145–147] In the case of the upper extremity, cervical, trunk, and lower extremity muscles are activated during motor tasks to limit the effect of monoarticular muscles on proximal and distal segments.[24,142,148,149] Massion[160] suggests that even flexion of the arm in standing triggers an expected or real shift in the COG of the body that the CNS acts to counteract. For the purposes of this section we will assume that single joint movement is a special example of how the CNS can control and limit its degrees of freedom of movement. The strategies employed by the CNS to produce movement at only one joint will be discussed.

ORGANIZATION OF SINGLE JOINT MOVEMENTS

Gottlieb et al.[106,108,110] and Corcos et al.[107,109] conducted a series of experiments to determine how single joint movements are organized by the CNS. Their goal was to define principles and rules by which the body regulates movement via the excitation of muscle, recruitment of motor units as expressed by electromyography (EMG), and the kinematics of the motion. The research group used a set of four organizing principles to create their hypothesis. The principles are:[106,111]

1. Elements of a movement task lead to a strategy governing its control.

2. Strategies consist of sets of rules that determine patterns of muscle activation.

3. Rules for muscle activation lead to patterns of muscle torques and EMG. Measures of torque and EMG will be highly and consistently correlated irrespective of task because of their shared causal, neural activation.

4. Muscle torques interact with limb loads to generate kinematics (angle and its derivatives of speed and acceleration, and movement intervals). Because of the role of load in determining kinematics, no general correlations between EMG and purely kinematic measures are possible.

These principles are possible due to the predictability of single joint movements. Limb masses are consistent, muscle mechanics are closer to the classical models of length-tension and force-velocity, and there is no input from other moving joints to either facilitate or inhibit performance at the target joint.

The movement task selected for study was that of moving the elbow (single joint only) to a selected target under varying task conditions.

SINGLE JOINT MOVEMENT STRATEGY

Input into the α-motor neuron pool can be described as a function waveform with duration and intensity.[111] The CNS can vary either or both of these parameters to activate agonist-antagonist pairs to create motion. The key variable to determining how the CNS ordered the movement was whether speed of motion was important. Their dual-strategy hypothesis separated single joint movements into two types. Movement that could be accomplished successfully regardless of speed were termed *speed insensitive*.

This class of movement could include waving goodbye or lifting a piece of paper, either of which can be performed at any speed. *Speed-sensitive* movements were those in which the movement had to be completed within a given time frame (i.e., catching a ball).[108]

In the speed-insensitive strategy,[106] the excitation of the motor neuron pool is controlled by the duration of the input, while the intensity remains constant. The rate of EMG recruitment and torque generation does not vary. In the speed-sensitive strategy,[107] the motor neuron pool is modulated by the intensity of the excitation pulse, while duration is kept constant. In this strategy, the rate of EMG and torque generation is dependant upon the intensity of the effort. Gottlieb et al.[108] go on to state their belief that the speed-insensitive strategy is the default strategy. In other words, when given a choice of speeds to move at, subjects self-select the strength of the movement (intensity) and vary the duration to achieve the desired speed of movement.

Most movements require interaction between agonist-antagonist pairs in order to regulate the extent of the motion. Schmidt et al.[143] and Sherwood et al.[144] found that the CNS uses a variety of control variables during movements, which include a single joint and a reversal of the motion. These researchers found that when a subject is asked to move the elbow joint in one direction, then reverse the motion, movement time, movement amplitude, and inertial load of the limb were all variables that could be controlled by the CNS, producing predictable changes in EMG and kinematic patterns of the functioning muscles.

Proprioceptive Triggering

While Gottlieb et al.[106,108,110] and Corcos et al.[107,109,111] investigated the motor control strategies of single joint motions, Cordo et al.[78,79,141] and Bevan et al.[150] studied the proprioceptive monitoring of single joint movement. Most movements incorporate different phases of motion, particularly when changes in direction, or reversals of joint motion are required. Single joint movements may be coupled to other functions (e.g., hand opening when a particular elbow angle is reached) to trigger activity at another joint, necessitating the need for accurate knowledge of position and orientation of all the segments of a limb. Although these activities involve control of more than one joint, the proprioceptive trigger is based upon single joint movement.

Cordo et al.[141] studied the role of velocity and position information in using passive single joint motion to trigger hand opening. The CNS is able to make use of both velocity and position data to accomplish the triggering task. In fact, if high precision is required, then both inputs are also required. Velocity information is used to compensate for neuromuscular delays by either biasing the internal representation of elbow position or predicting how much rotation will occur during the neuromuscular delay. Knowledge of elbow position can be used to trigger activity in either the ipsi- or contralateral hand, with fair accuracy.[141]

Joint position may be represented in several ways—either as an absolute joint angle or as an angular distance moved from some starting position.[150] It appears that the CNS encodes both parameters from the kinematic data provided by the sensory system.[126] Soechting[104] also proposed that position sense was a measure of limb orientation, not joint angle. Angular distance is probably more precisely discriminated than joint position when triggering or targeting tasks are involved. It also appears that during these types of tasks, the CNS maintains an internal representation of the task at hand and anticipates the movement of the joints.[78,79,85,104,138,145,146,151–153]

The key to trigger type tasks is the ability to discriminate joint positions under dynamic conditions. Several studies have investigated the accuracy of detecting joint movement and position. Static resolution of joint position measured by matching the placement of the contralateral limb ranges from 3 degrees to 14 degrees, depending on the joint. The perception of movement is between 3.5 degrees and 10 degrees, also depending upon the investigated joint. The ability to detect movement is dependant upon the movement velocity, with a wide variation of velocities for optimal detection of position.[154,155] Unfortunately, most of the work done in this area involves purely detection. Except for the studies by Cordo et al., dynamic control as a result of sensory detection of movement has been largely ignored.

The concept of proprioceptive triggering may be applied to more complex multijoint movements such as throwing, locomotion, and grasping. Cordo et al.[141] define a "discrete movement sequence" as multijoint movements with a single functional goal in which the rotations of different joints overlap partially in time. Their belief, as described above, was that kinesthetic information from one joint may be used to cause or alter the activity of another joint during discrete movements. Accurate execution and timing of the task was a result of sequencing of joint rotations with each joint rotation coordinated, in part, upon the spatial and temporal information provided by the joint rotations that preceded it. In an activity such as throwing, ball release may be triggered by the CNS knowledge of the position of the elbow and glenohumeral joints.[85]

Multijoint Movements

The vast majority of movements that we create and use for day to day activities and sports are multijoint. Muscles, joints, and limb segments must be coordinated in space and time in order to have purposeful movements. The control task of moving multiple joints is very different than the single joint situation. The degrees of single joint motions are limited to the three or less that are available to an individual joint. (Note: Grood[7] demonstrated that all joints have six degrees of freedom in the mechanical domain. The degrees of freedom used in this chapter refer to the available *movements* of flexion-extension, medial-lateral rotation, and ab-adduction. Distraction-compression, medial-lateral glide, and anterior-posterior translations are accessory motions and are not considered to be controll-able movements. Thus, the shoulder has three degrees of freedom, the elbow has two, etc.) In single joint movement experiments, movement is generally isolated to the joint and plane of motion being studied. Constraining the experiment to one joint also allows predictable responses of muscle as determined by length-tension and force-velocity relations. Multijoint movements are not planned or controlled by the same mechanisms that operate in the single joint case.[156]

The environment in which we function is a three-dimensional one. The CNS is confronted with the task of coordinating the muscles and joints of the extremities to perform the movements that we need or desire. In order to organize multijoint movements, certain biomechanical factors must be resolved. These include frame of reference, degrees of freedom, coordination of movement elements, interpretation of sensory information from several systems, and regulation of movement.

Most of the voluntary multijoint movements investigated in the laboratory involve the upper extremity. The lower extremity multijoint movements are more stereotypical, with the primary function of the lower limbs being locomotion and stance support. The planning, execution, and monitoring of upper limb functions such as reaching, grasping, holding, throwing, and striking require a level of skill and performance that is generally not required of the lower extremity. This is not to say that the leg is not provided with challenges. Stepping, obstacle avoidance, foot placement, kicking, and stabilization of the trunk, head, and arms place similar demands on the CNS. All multijoint movements require the coordinated effort of the sensory and neuromuscular capabilities at hand.

Multijoint muscle control and mechanics cannot be directly inferred from the study of single joint muscles.[156,157] There are a greater number of degrees of freedom. The movement potential available in a single joint system is limited to an arc in the plane of the joint, while multijoint movements are quite variable. Coupled motions at different joints imposed by limb mechanics and multiarticular muscle function complicate the control problem. In a single joint system, displacement and force are colinear[60] and angular acceleration is proportional to joint torque.[66] This is not the case in multiple joint movements.

POSTURE AND CONTROL

One of the constraints to movement is that a base of support that enables movement must be maintained. Therefore, some postural control must be maintained and coordinated with the movement demands of a given task. Control of body posture involves multisensory pathways, including visual, vestibular, and somatosensory[158,159] data, regulation, and feedback (Fig. 1-10).[160] This sensory information is used to create an internal representation of the body geometry, orientation, and support.[84,118,143,160,161]

Posture has an antigravity function that enables us to maintain an upright position and orientation.[161,162] To accomplish this task, the CNS must regulate either the center of mass[162–164] or center of gravity[160,165,166] of the supported body. Failure to control the effects of gravity under static or dynamic conditions results in a fall or dropping an object. Equilibrium is related to the antigravity function by contributing to knowledge of the head with respect to vertical position

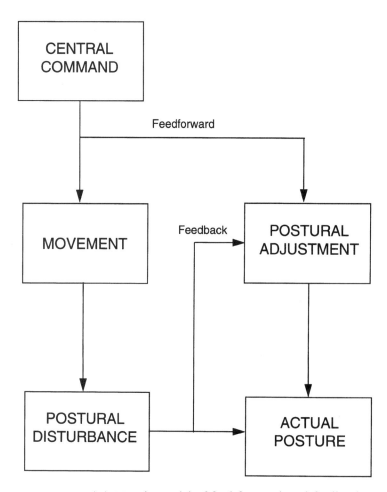

FIGURE 1-10 *(A) Simple model of feed-forward and feedback control of postural adjustments and reactions. A detailed description of postural adjustment is in Figure 10B. Figure 10C offers a more comprehensive view of the two types of control. (From Gahery Y and Massion J,[147] with permission.)*

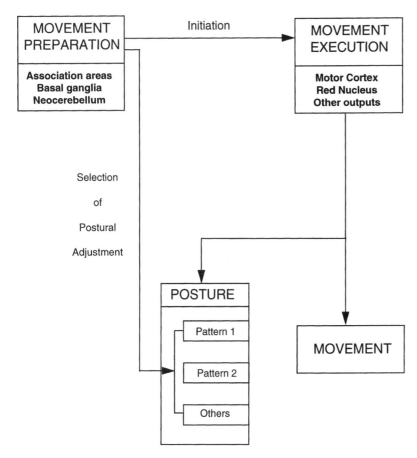

FIGURE 1-10 *(Continued). (B) Central control of postural adjustments. Gahery and Massion suggest that postural adjustments are probably initiated at a relatively "low hierarchical level," with selection of the postural pattern taking place during initiation and selection. (From Gahery Y and Massion J,[147] with permission.)*

and gravity. The vestibular system helps to maintain a gravity-related frame of reference.[83,164]

A second model involves the regulation of body geometry. Lacquinti and Maoli[167] determined that the geometric relations of the limbs in cats is the regulated variable with regard to postural control. Fung and Macpherson[168] also concluded that limb geometry is responsible for maintaining trunk orientation in cats. Preferred limb geometry may also correspond to the posture of least energy consumption.

Certain geometric relations are maintained in the human as well. Head and trunk orientation are stabilized with respect to the vertical position.[83,165,169] The orientation of these segments may enable the human to calculate the position of the arm[70] or leg[170] in space. Representation of segmental geometry is based on muscle spindle input.[94,95] A continuous kinematic chain of spindle input exists from the feet to the eyes. This input helps to create an internal body postural scheme modulated by kinesthetic input.[171,172]

Posture also serves as its own reference frame for perception[84] and movement with respect to the environment. The position of the eyes, head, and trunk can be used to orient

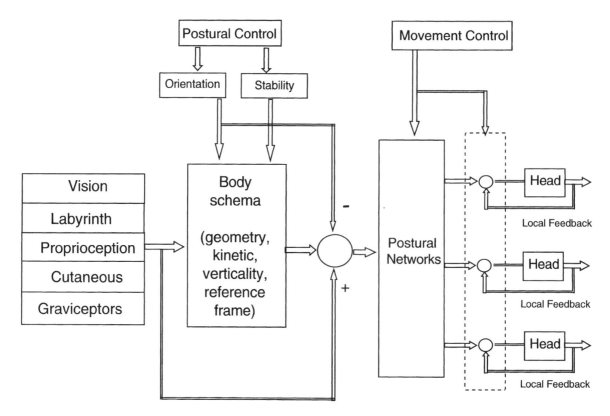

FIGURE 1-10 *(Continued).(C) Comprehensive model of feed-forward and feedback control of posture and movement. See text for description. (From Massion J,[160] with permission.)*

movement of the arms[66,123] and legs.[165,170] Postural orientation is determined by a combination of visual, vestibular, and proprioceptive input.[95,117,160]

One of the goals of the CNS is to maintain an upright position of the head and trunk under most conditions. To achieve this, the CNS maintains its internal reference of where it should be and makes adjustments to varying task conditions. The control of upright stance when the base of support is disturbed has been an area of intense research.[82,117,163,164,166,173–176] Mechanisms by which the CNS activates the musculoskeletal system in order to maintain an upright posture have been termed strategies. The stereotypic muscle pattern that a strategy uses is a synergy.[117] Study of postural disturbances via support surface perturbations has become a powerful paradigm within which motor control can be investigated.

The three "pure" strategies that are available to maintain an upright posture are the hip, ankle, and stepping strategy. These automatic postural responses are used when the base of support is disturbed. The strategy selected for use is dependant upon the nature and intensity of the disturbance and the constraints imposed by the support surface and environmental conditions.[163] The hip strategy is preferred when the support surface is rotated, while the ankle strategy is preferred when the surface is translated.[177] Rogers[178] maintains that the stepping strategy is probably the preferred method of maintaining balance, but this response may not be possible in some situations (e.g., standing on a crowded bus, standing on a balance beam, any situation where stepping is prohibited).

Strategies are not fixed.[179] Humans often select strategies that are mixed with aspects of both muscle synergies.[163] Training can influence the method by which a person responds to perturbed balance. The role of a strategy is to have a learned reaction available to respond to a given situation. The availability of postural synergies/strategies simplifies the task of motor control.[1] The problem of redundancy makes it difficult for the CNS to prepare an instruction set for individual muscles to react to changes in posture. An illustration of this issue was presented by de Bono,[180] in an unrelated area. Consider the problem of dressing when given 11 items to put on. There are 39,916,800 different combinations of clothing possible, although not all are feasible. Our choice of clothing is constrained by perception, previously used combinations that were satisfactory, and the requirements of the activities we are dressing for. The CNS performs all of these interpretive functions for us in terms of movement patterns, defined by the number of possible combinations of muscles that can be activated at any given time.

A more applicable example of redundancy was presented by Collins[69] in his investigation of optimizing models of locomotion. He attacked the problem of indeterminate solutions by limiting the number of unknown forces in the equations of mechanics. In his model, nine unknown forces generated a possible 498 solutions. Using optimization to identify solutions that were feasible, he determined that 18 possible solutions existed, making the problem of selecting muscle activation patterns more manageable for the CNS. It must be noted that his model is a sagittal plane, two-dimensional model. Adding a third dimension increases the difficulty in modeling forces and generates a higher number of unknowns and possible solutions. Collins' work does show that the CNS must have a means of identifying possible solutions to movement pattern selection in order to make the selection process possible in a short time span. Motor learning occurs with exploration of the environment

which, combined with a plastic neuromuscular system, allows us to "know" which muscles to select first for most tasks.

Centrally preprogrammed strategies with their associated synergistic motor patterns relieve the CNS of the burden of having to control all joints and muscles simultaneously. These patterns are not rigidly organized. Instead, the CNS has the freedom to modulate a selected movement pattern based upon existing conditions, constraints, and movement goals.[161,181,182] Additionally, athletes and highly trained individuals may utilize movement strategies that are more efficient than untrained people.[161]

Postural responses are in part triggered and modified by somatosensory inputs.[176,182] Allum et al.[182] found that leg afferents contributed to the selection of muscle synergies. Inglis et al.[176] found that sensory neuropathy affected the ability of individuals to respond to balance perturbations and to vary their response based on the velocity and amplitude of the perturbation. Di Fabio et al.[183] found that subjects with anterior cruciate ligament (ACL) deficiency were able to alter their postural response to decrease quadriceps activity and increase hamstring activity. Age-related changes in postural responses have been noted,[161] but the problem of balance control in the elderly involves performance deterioration in almost every aspect of balance control—visual, vestibular, and somatosensory deficits, strength loss, and attention demands (ch. 9).

Orthopaedic injuries also cause reduced performance. Johansson[32] discusses the changes in muscle α-gamma regulation as a result of damage to the anterior cruciate ligament (Fig. 1-11). Loss of afferent input may lead to delayed, altered, or less effective movement strategies.[184] Changes in proximal muscle activation following ankle injuries were noted by Bullock-Saxton.[185] Zätterström et al.[186] found that control of balance in ACL deficient subjects was altered in both the normal and affected limbs. This effect persisted for up to 12 months. Postural responses in ACL deficient limbs can be restructured to account for the altered mechanics of the

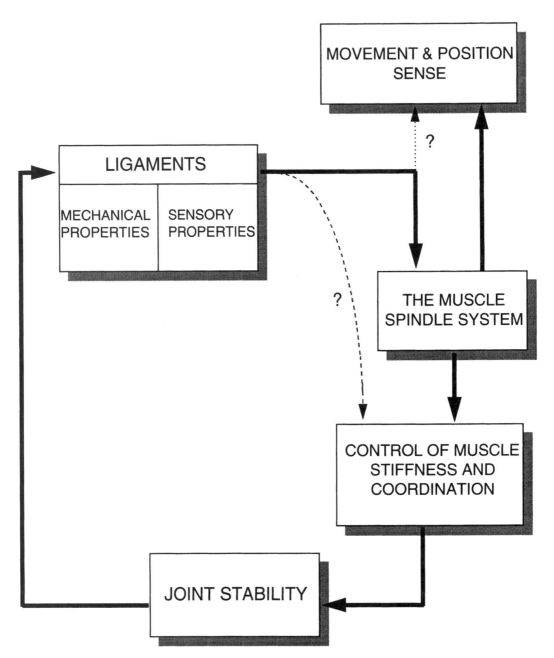

FIGURE 1-11 *Mechanism by which the cruciate ligaments contribute to regulation of joint stability and proprioception. (From Johansson H,[32] with permission.)*

joint.[183] This may account for lack of functional instability in some ACL deficient knees.

Clearly, loss of somatosensory input from a link in the lower extremity via joint or muscle damage from orthopaedic injuries effects sensorimotor control of the entire limb. Damage only to joint receptors is probably not enough to alter most movement skills.[100] Barrack found no change in gait pattern in subjects with normal knees, but anesthetized joints. Individuals with ACL deficient knees, however, demonstrate altered muscle patterns during gait and pivoting activities.[187,188] It appears that more significant involvement of sensorimotor control, such as concurrent nerve injury,[189] or affected fusimotor modulation[40,184] combined with complex tasks can force alterations in movement strategy or synergy. Impaired postural and synergistic responses may place an individual at greater risk of injury if these changes are not taken into consideration and treated appropriately. Until a new synergy can be learned that is as effective as the one being replaced, complex movements or effective responses to mechanical disturbances can be impaired.

COORDINATION OF POSTURE AND MOVEMENT

All movements begin and end with a postural adjustment.[158] According to Massion,[161] "Anticipatory postural adjustments mean that the onset of the postural changes occurs prior to the onset of the postural disturbance due to movement and that a feedforward postural control is associated with the movement control which prevents the posture and equilibrium disturbances associated with movement performance from taking place." Movement requires a postural response for two reasons. First, changes in limb geometry are accompanied by shifts in the center of gravity. Raising the arm[147] or leg[165] alters the projection of the COG on the ground, which must be compensated. Second, internally generated forces from initiation of movement exert reaction forces in the opposite direction on the proximal supporting segments and trunk. Slow movements do not require high acceleration and may not entail postural adjustments,[190] but faster, more dynamic movements do.[142] Postural adjustments associated with rapid movements are dependent upon the velocity of the voluntary motion.[191]

Postural adjustments occur in the 100 or so milliseconds before occurrence of movement.[146,192] Bouisset and Zattera[145] found that anticipatory muscle activity and acceleration of the legs preceded active flexion of the arms in a standing posture by 50 msec. Frank and Earl[146] noted that activation of the biceps during a lever pulling task was preceded by gastrocnemius and trunk muscle activity by 120 ± 16 and 44 ± 12 msec, respectively. Rapid trunk flexion movements are preceded by activation of the anterior tibialis and vastus medialis by approximately 100 msec, while backward trunk movement is preceded by hamstrings and gastrocnemius contraction by about 60 msec.[173]

Frank and Earl[146] (after Gahery[140]) make the distinction between postural preparations, postural accompaniments, and postural reactions (Fig. 1-12), based upon the perceived trade-off between safety and efficiency. Postural accompaniments are the same as the anticipatory postural adjustments just discussed. They occur via a mechanism of "feedforward control"[160,161] (Fig. 1-10). Postural preparations include movements in which the posture is altered before making a voluntary movement. Examples of this are the setting of stance that a soccer goalie may make before attempting to block a shot, or an elderly person who widens their base of support in order to walk. Postural reactions occur after a disturbance, generally within 100–150 msec later. They are controlled by multisensory feedback (vision, proprioception, etc: see Fig. 1-10C and 1-13) and include the postural strategies for correction—ankle, hip, and stepping.

FEEDFORWARD AND FEEDBACK CONTROL

Feedforward is the mechanism by which the CNS anticipates a change in state and activates muscles to adapt to and enable effective voluntary movement. The purpose of feedforward control in posture is to maintain the reference frames necessary for posture and awareness of body and limb orientation.[161] In the hierarchy of reference frames, gravity is primary. The CNS

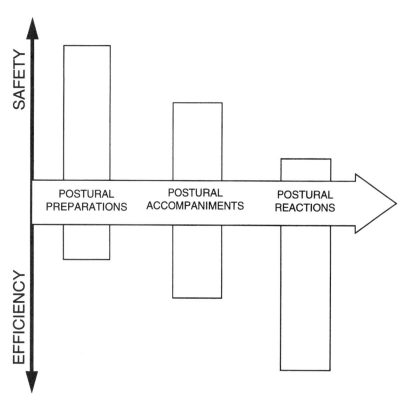

FIGURE 1-12 *Hypothetical relationship between different postural mechanisms used to maintain control of the center of gravity and balance. For definitions, refer to text. (From Frank JS and Earl M,[146] with permission.)*

prepares against a disturbance in the COG by shifting it. Second is the maintenance of the position of the head and trunk in an egocentric reference frame. The head and trunk are stabilized in almost all locomotor and complex movements.[83] Finally, the CNS maintains a link between egocentric and exocentric (external environment) frames via sensorimotor transformations in terms of the retina and then the head and trunk (via proprioceptors).[94,95,160] Feedforward stabilization of the head has been noted in both arm[80,81] and leg[165,170] movements.

Feedforward mechanisms may also function in the peripheral joints. Voight and Weider[193] found that the reflex response times in the vastus medialis oblique (VMO) were faster than the vastus lateralis (VL) in normal subjects, yet slower in patients with extensor mechanism dysfunc-

tion. The temporal advantage of the normal VMO was considered to be a form of feedforward control. Grabiner et al.,[194] however, failed to find statistical evidence of feedforward control, but noted that the VMO was activated earlier than the VL in all normal isometric conditions.[194,195] Patterns of altered muscle activation are evident at the shoulder and knee, with changes in timing due to pain or pathology.[187,196] The role of the CNS in this phenomenon has yet to be defined, beyond inhibition due to inflammation, if any.

Feedback from somatosensory monitors is used to trigger and scale postural responses to perturbation. A feedback loop means that response will occur after the disturbance and after sensors have signaled that an event is happening that requires an action. Feedback can be initiated from proprioceptors located in the lower

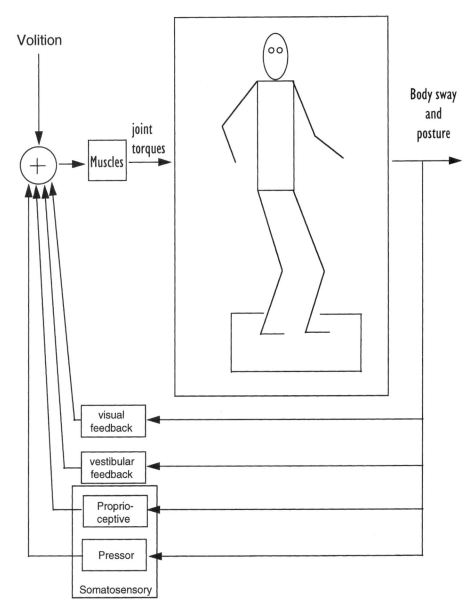

FIGURE 1-13 *Model of sensory mechanisms in feedback control of posture. (From Johansson H, Magnusson M,[215] with permission.)*

limb[117,163,170] and/or neck,[197,198] and/or receptors in the foot.[94] Visual and vestibular information can influence the postural reactions, but do not appear to be primary in this type of response.[158] Visual and vestibular information appear to be more important in feedforward control and when afferent input from other sources is impaired.

Inputs from multisensory pathways are then compared to the body's internal representation of its position/posture/schema[118,160] and groups of muscles or postural networks are activated to restore equilibrium or control body displacement (Fig. 1-10). In cases where the sensory feedback is impaired, then new strategies must be created or existing ones altered. The work of Di Fabio,[183] Zätterström et al.,[186] and Bullock-Saxton,[185] noted earlier, indicates that injuries that disrupt the proprioceptive system in one joint can have systemic effects.

Johansson[32] proposed the mechanism by which ligamentous injuries can affect the control joints and, perhaps, limbs. (Fig. 1-11) He suggests that low threshold joint afferents influence the γ-spindle system rather than the α-motoneurons. The effect of this influence is to alter control of muscle stiffness and coordination, two factors important in functional joint stability.

Training and Adaptation

Perhaps the most obvious adaptations of movement capabilities are age-related. The development of purposeful movement is related to the maturation of several systems, in conjunction with the ability of the child to explore her environment.[132] The development of sensory systems mimics the hierarchical order of reference frames—vision, vestibular, head stabilization, and somatosensory. Increasingly complex movements are possible as the musculoskeletal and somatosensory systems develop. Aging has different effects on movement capabilities.[199,200] For a review, please see Chapter 9, Geriatrics.

Sensory Receptors

Proprioceptors, muscle spindles, and Golgi tendon organs all show short-term adaptation to muscle contraction. Spindles and proprioceptors appear to be more sensitive to stretch following a conditioning contraction,[153,201] while Golgi organs experience a brief desensitization after a contraction.[202] The implication is that muscles may react faster and with greater output following a "setting" contraction. This may be one of the reasons why athletes use postural preparations in certain instances, as noted in the section on Coordination of Posture and Movement. A secondary result of this "preset" is that force reg-ulation may not be as precise, resulting in potential movement errors.[201]

Exercise does not cause hypertrophy of muscle spindles similar to that of extrafusal muscle fibers. There were no reports found on the effect of training on tendon organ function. Some evidence exists that stretch reflex gain can be trained, but this has been accomplished under limited conditions.[203] Gandevia and Burke[204] found that spindle afferents could not be selectively activated. This remains a questionable area.

In a review article on the topic of fatigue, Hutton et al.[205] proposed that muscle sensory receptors may be able to compensate for neuromuscular fatigue by providing increased excitation. This proposal should be reviewed with respect to comments by Enoka[131] on task dependency, motivation, and central mechanisms during fatigue.

Motor neuron pool sensitivity (as measured by the H-reflex) can be modulated according to the task at hand. Dyhre-Poulsen et al.[36] found that the soleus H-reflex is low during touch-down from a downward jump and high during touch-down while hopping. The value of the H-reflex correlated to muscle stiffness in the limb, indicating the ability of the CNS to adapt the mechanical properties of the musculoskeletal system depending on the activity.

Training may also affect the sensitivity of the motor neuron pool. Koceja et al.[206] found that trained dancers exhibited different properties in unilateral and conditioned Achilles tendon tap responses than untrained individuals. They hypothesized that differences in muscle stiffness, tissue compliance, or neural organization may account for their results. Trained athletes generally have smaller H-reflexes than untrained subjects. This has also been noted in volleyball players[207] and sprinters.[208] This may be a result of motor unit specificity; however, other explanations, based upon synapse transmission or motor neuron pool excitability, may exist.[209]

Postural Strategies

Perhaps the greatest adaptations in postural control occur as a result of aging. Development of the musculoskeletal and sensorimotor systems, awareness of environment, and psychological changes in behavior and motivation create the ability to modify and control our posture.[160] At the opposite end of the spectrum are the losses that occur as a result of aging. Decreased attention span,[199] limited musculoskeletal capabilities,[210] reduced competence of the visual and equilibrium systems, and degradation of the postural responses associated with movement[200] lead to poorer balance control.

Long-term training can lead to changes in both muscle synergies and postural strategies. Pedotti et al.[129] found that the temporal pattern of muscle activation changed in gymnasts from proximal-distal to distal-proximal during backward upper trunk reaction time tasks. This resulted in better velocity and equilibrium control. They hypothesized that the gymnasts' training in backward movements gave them a better awareness of the space behind the body, enabling a more efficient pattern. Mouchnino et al.[165] found that dancers used a postural strategy that was not available to untrained subjects during the task of raising one leg in an upright posture. The dancers were able to use a feedforward rather than a feedback mechanism to maintain posture and compensate for the change in their base of support. The researchers suggested that the new strategy was more effective in reducing the number of degrees of freedom that needed to be coordinated in order to maintain control of equilibrium. They suggest that the trained dancer's awareness of head-trunk orientation is better than untrained subjects, allowing for new strategies to develop.

Massion[161] suggests long-term training allows short-term adaptations to occur. Training can influence the central set of the neuromuscular system,[40] which in turn affects the biomechanical response to movement.[212] The greater the degree of control of muscle activation, the greater the ability to select and create movement patterns.

Rehabilitation Implications

The shift to a movement paradigm has several implications for the way that we approach rehabilitation of function. We must move our think-

ing away from joints and focus on limbs. Greater understanding of the integration of sensory and musculoskeletal functions is required as we begin to explore the concepts of limb orientation instead of joint position, frames of reference, multijoint muscle function, the use of visual and sensory feedback, muscle synergies, and movement strategies to prevent injury. The traditional teaching of ROM-strength-function is becoming a progression of ROM-movement control-movement strategy-function as we begin to integrate movement science into our knowledge of anatomy, biomechanics, and physiology. Gambetta[211] correctly stated the basic principles of conditioning of the shoulder by emphasizing performance (intensity and quality of an exercise), muscular balance, movements over muscles, core strength before extremity strength, synergists before prime movers, joint integrity before joint mobility, and fundamental movement skill before sports skill. These principles can be applied to rehabilitation of any injury. The emphasis on movement and the components of movement necessitate a focus on multiple systems and adequate training of the muscles that *generate* the force used in movement as well as the muscles used to *direct* the force. These muscle groups may not be the same. Rehabilitation of movement implies that we are reconditioning several joints simultaneously, not only the injured one.

References

1. Bernstein N: The Coordination and Regulation of Movement. Pergamon Press, Oxford, 1967
2. Higgins JR: Human Movement: An Integrated Approach. CV Mosby, St Louis, 1977
3. Kelso JAS: Biological coordination dynamics of complex systems. Presented at Multisegmental Motor Control: Interfaces of Biomechanical, Neural, and Behavioral Approaches. New Hampshire, 1995
4. Zajac FE, Winters JM: Modeling musculoskeletal movement systems: joint and body segmental dynamics, musculoskeletal actuation, and neuromuscular control. p. 121. In Winters JM, Woo

SL-Y (eds): Multiple Muscle Systems: Biomechanics and Movement Organization. Springer-Verlag, New York, 1990

5. Butler PB, Major RE: The learning of motor control: biomechanical considerations. Physiother 78:6–11, 1992

6. Torzilli PA: Basic biomechanical principles: forces, moments, and equilibrium. p. 122. In DeLee JC, Drez D (eds): Orthopedic Sports Medicine, Volume 1. WB Saunders, Philadelphia, 1994

7. Grood ES, Suntay WJ: A joint coordinate system for the clinical description of three-dimensional motions: applications to the knee. J Biomechanical Engineering 105:136–144, 1983

8. Seliktar R, Bo L: The theory of kinetic analysis in human gait. p. 223. In Craik RL, Oatis CA (eds): Gait Analysis: Theory and Application. Mosby, St Louis, 1995

9. Palmatier RA, An K-N, Scott SG et al.: Kinetic chain exercise in knee rehabilitation. Sports Med 11:402–413, 1991

10. DeCarlo M, Porter DA, Gehlsen G et al.: Electromyographic and cinematographic analysis of the lower extremity during closed and open chain exercise. Isokinetics Exer Sci 2:24–29, 1992

11. Lutz GE, Pamitier RA, An K-N et al.: Comparison of tibiofemoral joint forces during open kinetic chain and closed kinetic chain exercises. J Bone Joint Surg 75A:732–738, 1993

12. Rivera JE: Open versus closed kinetic chain rehabilitation of the lower extremity: a functional and biomechanical analysis. J Sport Rehab 3: 154–167, 1994

13. Dillman CJ, Murray TA, Hintermeister RA: Biomechanical differences of open and closed chain exercises with respect to the shoulder. J Sport Rehab 3:228–238, 1994

14. Steindler A: Kinesiology of the Human Body. Charles Thomas, Springfield, 1955

15. Lephart SM, Henry TJ: The physiologic basis for open and closed chain rehabilitation for the upper extremity. J Sport Rehab 5:71–87, 1995

16. Zajac FE: Muscle coordination of movement: a perspective. J Biomechanics 26(supp 1):109–24, 1993

17. Hof AL, van Der Berg JW: EMG to force processing I–IV. J Biomechanics 747–788, 1981

18. Edgerton VR, Roy RR: Regulation of skeletal muscle fiber size, shape, and function. J Biomechanics, Suppl. 24:123–133, 1991

19. Baratta RV, Solomonow M: The dynamic performance model of skeletal muscle. CRC Crit Rev Biomed Engineer 19:419–454, 1992

20. Zajac FE: Muscle and tendon: properties, models, scaling, and applications to biomechanics and motor control. CRC Crit Rev Biomed Engineer 17:359–411, 1989

21. Lieber RL, Bodine-Fowler SC: Skeletal muscle mechanics: implications for rehabilitation. Phys Ther 73:844–856, 1993

22. Fitts RH, McDonald KS, Schluter JM: The determinants of skeletal muscle force and power: their adaptability with changes in activity pattern. J Biomechanics, Suppl. 24:111–122, 1991

23. Zajac FE: How musculotendon architecture and joint geometry affect the capacity of muscles to move and exert force on objects: a review with application to arm and forearm transfer design. J Hand Surg 17A:799–804, 1992

24. Zajac FE, Gordon ME: Determining muscle's force and action in multi-articular movement. Exerc Sport Sci Rev 17:187–230, 1989

25. Korner L, Parker P, Almstrom C et al.: Relation of intramuscular pressure to the force and output EMG of skeletal muscle. J Orthop Res 2: 289–296, 1984

26. Alexander R, Ker RF: The architecture of leg muscles. p. 568. In Winters JM, Woo SL-Y (eds): Multiple Muscle Systems: Biomechanics and Movement Organization. Springer Verlag, New York, 1990

27. Hof AL: Effect of muscle elasticity in walking and running. p. 591. In Winters JM, Woo SL-Y (eds): Multiple Muscle Systems: Biomechanics and Movement Organization. Springer Verlag, New York, 1990

28. Chapman AE, Sanderson DJ: Muscular coordination in sporting skills. p. 608. In Winters JM, Woo SL-Y (eds): Multiple Muscle Systems: Biomechanics and Movement Organization. Springer Verlag, New York, 1990

29. Wickiewicz TL, Roy RR, Powell PL, et al.: Muscle architecture of the human lower limb. Clin Orthop Rel Res 179:275–283, 1983

30. Sinkjær T, Hayashi R: Regulation of wrist stiffness by stretch reflex. J Biomechanics 22: 1133–1140, 1989

31. Lorentzon R, Elmqvist L-G, Sjöström M et al.: Thigh musculature in relation to chronic anterior cruciate ligament tear: muscle size, morphology, and mechanical output before reconstruction. Am J Sports Med 17:423–429, 1989

32. Johansson H: Role of ligaments in propriocep-

tion and regulation of muscle stiffness. J Electromyog Kinesiol 1:158–179, 1991

33. Sojka P, Johansson H, Sjolander P et al.: Fusimotor neurons can be reflexly influenced by activity in receptor afferents from the posterior cruciate ligament. Brain Res 483:177–183, 1989

34. Nichols TR: The regulation of muscle stiffness. Implications for the control of limb stiffness. Med Sports Sci 26:36–47, 1987

35. Vincken MH, Denier van der Gon JJ: Stiffness as a control variable in motor performance. Hum Movement Sci 4:307–319, 1985

36. Dyhre-Poulsen P, Simonsen EB, Voight M: Dynamic control of muscle stiffness during hopping and jumping in man. J Physiol 437: 237–304, 1991

37. Lieber RL, Fridén J: Neuromuscular stabilization of the shoulder girdle. p. 91. In Matsen FA, Fu FH, Hawkins RJ (eds): The Shoulder: A Balance of Mobility and Stability. American Academy of Orthopaedic Surgeons, Rosemont, IL, 1992

38. Nichols TR, Houk JC: Improvement in linearity and regulation of stiffness that results from actions of stretch reflex. J Neurophysiol 39: 119–142, 1976

39. Rack PM, Ross HF, Thilmann AF et al.: Reflex responses at the human ankle: the importance of tendon compliance. J Physiol 344:503–524, 1983

40. Prochazka A: Sensorimotor gain control: a basic strategy of motor systems? Progr Neurobiol 33: 281–307, 1989

41. Zajac FE: How computer simulations of motor tasks help us understand muscle coordination. Presented at Multisegmental Motor Control: Interfaces of Biomechanical, Neural, and Behavioral Approaches. New Hampshire, 1995

42. Van Ingen Schneau GJ, Pratt CA, Macpherson JM: Differential use and control of mono- and biarticular muscles. Hum Movement Sci 13: 495–517, 1994

43. Hannaford B, Winters J: Actuator properties and movement control: biological and technologic models. p. 101. In Winters JM, Woo SL-Y (eds): Multiple Muscle Systems: Biomechanics and Movement Organization. Springer Verlag, New York, 1990

44. Van Ingen Schnau GJ: From rotation to translation: constraints on multi-joint movements and the unique action of bi-articular muscles. Hum Movement Sci 8:301–337, 1989

45. Van Ingen Schnau GJ: From rotation to translation: implications for theories of motor control. Hum Movement Sci 8:423–442, 1989

46. Gielen CCAM: If mono- and bi-articular muscles do have a different functional role, is their activation different and task dependent? Hum Movement Sci 8:375–380, 1989

47. Van Ingen Schneau GJ, Boots PJM, de Groot G et al.: The constrained control of force and position in multi-joint movements. Neurosci 46: 197–207, 1992

48. Van Soest AJ, Schwab AL, Bobbert MF, van Ingen Schnau GJ: The influence of the biarticularity of the gastrocnemius muscle on vertical-jumping achievement. J Biomechanics 26:1–8, 1993

49. Pandy MG, Zajac FE: Muscular coordination of jumping. J Biomechanics 24:1–10, 1991

50. Van Ingen Schneau GJ, Bobbert MF, van Soest AJ: The unique action of bi-articular muscles in leg extensions. p. 639. In Winters JM, Woo SL-Y (eds): Multiple Muscle Systems: Biomechanics and Movement Organization. Springer Verlag, New York, 1990

51. Redfield R, Hull ML: On the relation between joint moments and pedalling rates at constant power cycling. J Biomechanics 19:317–329, 1986

52. Doorenbosch CAM, Harlaar J, Roebroeck ME, et al.: Two strategies of transferring from sit-to-stand; the activation of monoarticular and biarticular muscles. J Biomechanics 27:1299–1307, 1994

53. McCollum G: Reciprocal inhibition, synergies, and movements. J Theor Biol 165:291–311, 1993

54. Perret C, Cabelguen JM: Main characteristics of the hindlimb locomotor cycle in the decorticate cat with special reference to bifunctional muscles. Brain Res 187:333–352, 1980

55. Van Ingen Schneau GJ, Bobbert MF, Rozendal RH: The unique action of bi-articular muscles in complex movements. J Anat 155:1–5, 1987

56. Gregoire L, Veeger HE, Huijing PA, et al.: Role of mono- and biarticular muscles in explosive movements. Int J Sports Med 5:301–305, 1984

57. Gielen S: Muscle activation patterns and joint-angle coordination in multijoint movements. p. 293. In Berthoz A (ed): Multisensory Control of Movement. Oxford University Press, Oxford, 1993

58. Bastide G, Zadeh J, Lefèbvre D: Are the "little muscles" what we think they are? editorial. Surg Radiol Anat 11:256, 1989

59. Scott SH, Loeb GE. The computation of position

sense from spindles in mono- and multiarticular muscles. J Neurosci 14:7529–7540, 1994

60. Lacquinti F, Carrozzo M, Borghese N: Planning and control of limb impedance. p. 314. In Berthoz A (ed): Multisensory Control of Movement. Oxford University Press, Oxford, 1993

61. Gielen CCAM, van Ingen Schneau GJ, Tax AAM, et al.: The activation of mono- and bi-articular muscles in multi-joint movements. p. 302. In: Winters JM, Woo SL-Y (eds): Multiple Muscle Systems: Biomechanics and Movement Organization. Springer Verlag, New York, 1990

62. Happee R: Goal-directed arm movements: I. Analysis of EMG records in shoulder and elbow muscles. J Electromyogr Kinesiol 2:165–178, 1992

63. Bobbert M, van Ingen Schnau GJ: Coordination in vertical jumping. J Biomechanics 21:249–262, 1988

64. Aniss AM, Gandevia SC, Burke D: Reflex changes in muscle spindle discharge during a voluntary contraction. J Neurophysiol 59:908–920, 1988

65. Pierror-Desilligny E, Bergego C, Katz R, et al.: Cutaneous depression of Ib reflex pathways to motoneurons in man. Exp Brain Res 42: 351–361, 1981

66. Soechting JF, Flanders M: Moving in three dimensional space: frames of reference, vectors, and coordinate systems. Ann Rev Neurosci 15: 167–191, 1992

67. Sporn O, Edelman GM: Solving Bernstein's problem: a proposal for the development of coordinated movement by selection. Child Development 64:960–981, 1993

68. Young RP, Marteniuk RG: Changes in inter-joint relationships of muscle movements and powers accompanying the acquisition of a multi-articular kicking task. J Biomechanics 28:701–713, 1995

69. Collins JJ: The redundant nature of locomotor optimization laws. J Biomechanics 28:251–267, 1995

70. Soechting JF, Flanders M: Arm movements in three-dimensional space: computation, theory, and observation. Exerc Sport Sci Rev 19: 389–418, 1991

71. Winter DA: Foot trajectory in human gait: a precise and multifactorial motor control task. Phys Ther 72:55–66, 1992

72. Tiberio D: The effect of excessive subtalar joint pronation on patellofemoral mechanics: a theo-retical model. J Ortho Sports Med 9:160–165, 1987

73. Georgopoulos AP, Kettner RE, Schwartz AB: Primate motor cortex and free arm movements to visual targets in three dimensional space. II. Coding of the directions of movements by a neuronal population. J Neurosci 8:2928–2937, 1988

74. Jeannerod M: A neurophysiological model for the directional coding of reaching movements. p. 49. In Paillard J (ed): Brain and Space. Oxford University Press, Oxford, 1991

75. Jeannerod M: The interaction of visual and proprioceptive cues in controlling reaching movements. p. 277. In Humphrey DR, Freund H-J (eds): Motor Control: Concepts and Issues. John Wiley & Sons, New York, 1991

76. Hollerbach JM: Computers, brains and the control of movement. Trends Neurosci 6:189–192, 1982

77. Feldman AG: Once more for the equilibrium point hypothesis (l-model). J Motor Behavior 18: 17–54, 1986

78. Cordo PJ: Kinesthetic coordination of a movement sequence in humans. Neurosci Lett 92: 40–45, 1988

79. Cordo PJ: Kinesthetic control of a multijoint movement sequence. J Neurophysiol 63: 161–172, 1990

80. Soechting JF, Flanders M: Sensorimotor representations for pointing to targets in three-dimensional space. J Neurophysiol 62:582–594, 1989

81. Soechting JF, Flanders M: Errors in pointing are due to approximations in sensorimotor transformations. J Neurophysiol 62:595–608, 1989

82. Gollhofer A, Horstmann GA, Berger W, et al.: Compensation of translational and rotational perturbations in human posture: stabilization of the centre of gravity. Neurosci Lett 105:73–78, 1989

83. Berthoz A, Pozzo T: Head and body coordination during locomotion and complex movements. p. 147. In Swinnen SP, Massion J, Heuer H, Casaer P (eds): Interlimb Coordination: Neural, Dynamical, and Cognitive Constraints. Academic Press, San Diego, 1995

84. Viviani P, Stucchi N, Laissard G: Issues in perceptuo-motor coordination. p. 394. In Berthoz A (ed): Multisensory Control of Movement. Oxford University Press, Oxford, 1993

85. Cordo PJ, Flanders M: Sensory control of target acquisition. TINS 12:110–116, 1989

86. Helms Tillery SI, Flanders M, Soechting JF: A

coordinate system for the synthesis of visual and kinesthetic information. J Neurosci 11:770–778, 1991

87. Soechting JF, Lacquinti F: Invariant characteristics of a pointing movement in man. J Neurosci 1:710–720, 1981

88. Soechting JF, Ross B: Psychophysical determination of coordinate representation of human arm orientation. Neurosci 13:595–604, 1984

89. Lacquinti F, Soechting JF, Terzuolo C: Path constraints on point-to-point arm movements in three dimensional space. Neurosci 17:313–324, 1986

90. Vanden Abeele S, Crommelinck M, Roucoux A: Frames of reference used in goal directed movement. p. 363. In Berthoz A (ed): Multisensory Control of Movement. Oxford University Press, Oxford, 1993

91. Thomson JA: How do we use visual information to control locomotion? TINS 3:247–250, 1980

92. Gentile AM: Skill acquisition. p. 93. In Carr JH, Sheperd RB (eds): Movement Science. Foundations for Physical Therapy in Rehabilitation. Aspen Publishers, Rockville, 1987

93. Patla AE: Understanding the roles of sensory input, particularly vision, in controlling and adapting locomotion for various environments. Presented at Multisegmental Motor Control: Interfaces of Biomechanical, Neural, and Behavioral Approaches. New Hampshire, 1995

94. Roll JP, Vedel JP, Roll R: Eye, head, and skeletal muscle spindle feedback in the elaboration of body references. Prog Brain Res 80:113–123, 1989

95. Roll R, Velay JL, Roll JP: Eye and neck proprioceptive messages contribute to the spatial coding of retinal input in visually oriented activities. Exp Brain Res 85:423–431, 1991

96. Patla A: A framework for understanding mobility problems in the elderly. p. 436. In Craik RL, Oatis CA (eds): Gait Analysis: Theory and Application. Mosby, St Louis, 1995

97. International Society of Biomechanics Newsletter: No. 45, 1992. From Wu G: Kinematics theory. p. 159. In Craik RL, Oatis CA (eds): Gait Analysis: Theory and Application. Mosby, St Louis, 1995

98. Yoshikawa GI: A spherical model analyzing shoulder motion in overhand and sidearm pitching. J Shoulder Elbow Surg 2:198–208, 1993

99. Pearl ML, Jackins S, Lippitt SB et al.: Humeroscapular positions in a shoulder range-of-motion examination. J Shoulder Elbow Surg 1:296–305, 1992

100. Barrack RL, Skinner HB, Brunet ME, et al.: Functional performance of the knee after intra-articular anesthesia. Am J Sports Med 11:258–261, 1983

101. Barrack RL, Skinner HB, Brunet ME, et al.: Proprioception in the anterior cruciate deficient knee. Am J Sports Med 17:1–6, 1991

102. Borsa PA, Lephart SM, Kocher MS, et al.: Functional assessment and rehabilitation of shoulder proprioception for glenohumeral instability. J Sport Rehab 3:84–104, 1994

103. Clark FJ, Horch KW, Bach SM, et al.: Contributions of cutaneous and joint receptors to static knee joint position sense in man. J Neurophysiol 42:877–888, 1979

104. Soechting JF: Does position sense at the elbow represent a sense of elbow joint angle or one of limb orientation? Brain Res 248:392–395, 1982

105. Hore J, Watts S, Tweed D: Arm constraints when throwing in three dimensions. J Neurophysiol 72:1171–1180, 1994

106. Gottlieb GL, Corcos DM, Agarwal GC: Organizing principles for single joint movements: I. A speed-insensitive strategy. J Neurophysiol 62:342–357, 1989

107. Corcos DM, Gottlieb GL, Agarwal GC: Organizing principles for single joint movements: II. A speed-sensitive strategy. J Neurophysiol 62:358–368, 1989

108. Gottlieb GL, Corcos DM, Agarwal GC, et al.: Organizing principles for single joint movements: III. Speed sensitive strategy as a default. J Neurophysiol 63:625–636, 1990

109. Corcos DM, Agarwal GC, Flaherty BP, et al.: Organizing principles for single joint movements: IV. Implications for isometric contractions. J Neurophysiol 64:1033–1042, 1990

110. Gottlieb GL, Latash ML, Corcos DM et al.: Organizing principles for single joint movements: V. Agonist-antagonist interactions. J Neurophysiol 67:1417–1427, 1992

111. Corcos DM: Strategies underlying the control of disordered movement. Phys Ther 71:25–38, 1991

112. Brown JMM, Bronks R: Electromyographic basis of inaccurate movement; its dependence upon the mode of muscle contraction. Eur J Appl Physiol 62:162–170, 1991

113. Treslian JR: Perceptual and motor processes in interceptive timing. Hum Move Sci 13:335–373, 1994

114. Warwick R, Williams PL: Gray's Anatomy. 35th British edition. WB Saunders, Philadelphia, 1973

115. Woo SL-Y, McMahon PJ, Debski RE et al.: Factors limiting and defining shoulder motion: what keeps it from going farther? p. 141. In Matsen FA, Fu FH, Hawkins RJ (eds): The Shoulder: A Balance of Mobility and Stability. AAOS, Rosemont, 1993

116. Lew WD, Lewis JL, Craig EV: Stabilization by capsule, ligaments, and labrum: stability at the extremes of motion. p. 69. In Matsen FA, Fu FH, Hawkins RJ (eds): The Shoulder: A Balance of Mobility and Stability. AAOS, Rosemont, 1993

117. Nashner LM, McCollum G: The organization of human postural movements: a formal basis and experimental hypothesis. Behav Brain Sci 8: 135–172, 1985

118. Kuo AD, Zajac FE: Human standing posture: Multi-joint movement strategies based on biomechanical constraints. Prog Brain Res 97: 349–358, 1993

119. Hogan N: Planning and execution of multijoint movements. Can J Physiol Pharmacol 66: 508–517, 1988

120. Hogan N, Winters JM: Principles underlying movement organization: upper limb p. 182. In Winters JM, Woo SL-Y (eds): Multiple Muscle Systems: Biomechanics and Movement Organization. Springer Verlag, New York, 1990

121. Hasan Z: Role of proprioceptors in neural control. Curr Op Neurobiology 2:824–829, 1992

122. Bizzi E, Nogan N, Mussa-Ivaldi FA, et al.: Does the nervous system use equilibrium-point control to guide single and multiple joint movements? p. 1. In Cordo P, Harnad S (eds): Movement Control. Cambridge University Press, Cambridge, 1994 (Reproduced from Brain Behav Sci 15:603–613, 1992)

123. Soechting JF, Flanders M: Deducing algorithms of arm movement control from kinematics. p. 293. In Humphrey DR, Freund H-J (eds): Motor Control: Concepts and Issues. John Wiley & Sons, New York, 1991

124. Morasso P: Spatial control of arm movements. Exp Brain Res 42:223–237, 1981

125. Atkeson CG, Hollerbach JM: Kinematic features of unrestrained vertical arm movements. J Neurosci 5:2318–2330, 1985

126. Gandevia SC, Burke D: Does the nervous system depend on kinesthetic information to control natural movements? Brain Behav Sci 15: 614–632, 1992

127. Cordo PJ, Bevan L: Successive approximation in targeted movement: an alternative hypothesis, (commentary). p. 127. In Cordo PJ, Harnad S (eds): Movement Control. Cambridge University Press, Cambridge, 1994 (Reproduced from Brain Behav Sci 15:739–740, 1992)

128. Kelso JAS: The informational character of self-organized coordination dynamics. Hum Movem Sci 13:393–413, 1994

129. Pedotti A, Crenna P, Deat A et al.: Postural synergies in axial movements: short and long term adaptations. Exp Brain Res 74:3–10, 1989

130. Stein RB, Oguztoreli MN, Capaday C: What is optimized in muscular movements? p. 131. In Jones NL, McCartney N, McComas AJ (eds): Human Muscle Power. Human Kinetics, Champaign, IL, 1986

131. Enoka RM: Mechanisms of muscle fatigue: central factors and task dependancy. J Electromyogr Kinesiol 5:141–150, 1995

132. Thelen E: A dynamical systems view of the development of multisegmental motor tasks. Presented at Multisegmental Motor Control: Interfaces of Biomechanical, Neural, and Behavioral Approaches. New Hampshire, 1995

133. Clark JE: Dynamical systems perspective on gait. p. 79. In Craik RL, Oatis CA (eds): Gait Analysis: Theory and Application. Mosby, St Louis, 1995

134. Higgins JR, Higgins S: The acquisition of locomotor skill. p. 65. In Craik RL, Oatis CA (eds): Gait Analysis: Theory and Application. Mosby, St. Louis, 1995

135. Holreitzer SH, Köhle ME: Assessment of gait patterns using neural networks. J Biomechanics 26:645–651, 1993

136. Robinson DA: Implications of neural networks for how we think about brain function. Behav Brain Sci 15:644–655, 1992

137. Sepulveda F, Wells DM, Vaughan CL: A neural network representation of electromyography and joint dynamics in human gait. J Biomechanics 26:101–109, 1993

138. Droulez J, Berthoz A: The concept of dynamic memory in sensorimotor control. p. 137. In Humphrey DR, Freund H-J (eds): Motor Control: Concepts and Issues. John Wiley, New York, 1991

139. Enoka RM: Neuromechanical Basis of Kinesiology. 2nd Ed. p. 22. Human Kinetics, Champaign, IL, 1994

140. Gahéry Y. Associated movements, postural adjustments and synergies: some comments about the history and significance of three motor concepts. Arch Ital Biol 125:135–141, 1987

141. Cordo P, Carlton L, Bevan L et al.: Proprioceptive coordination of movement sequences: role of velocity and position information. J Neurophysiol 71:1848–1861, 1994

142. Lee WA, Buchanan TS, Rogers MW: Effects of arm acceleration and behavioral conditions on the organization of postural adjustments during arm flexion. Exp Brain Res 66:257–270, 1987

143. Schmidt RA, Sherwood DE, Walter CB: Rapid movements with reversals in direction. I. The control of movement time. Exp Brain Res 69:344–354, 1988

144. Sherwood DE, Schmidt RA, Walter CB: Rapid movements with reversals in direction. II. Control of movement amplitude and inertial load. Exp Brain Res 69:355–367, 1988

145. Bouisset S, Zattara M: A sequence of movements precedes voluntary movement. Neurosci Lett 22:263–270, 1981

146. Frank JS, Earl M: Coordination of posture and movement. Phys Ther 70:855–863, 1990

147. Gahéry Y, Massion J: Coordination between posture and movement. TINS 4:199–202, 1981

148. Kornecki S: Mechanism of muscular stabilization process in joints. J Biomechanics 25:235–245, 1992

149. Lee WA: Anticipatory control of postural and task muscles during rapid arm flexion. J Motor Behav 12:185–196, 1980

150. Bevan L, Cordo P, Carlton L, et al.: Proprioceptive coordination of movement sequences: discrimination of joint angle versus angular distance. J Neurophysiol 71:1862–1872, 1994

151. Johansson RS, Cole KJ: Sensory-motor coordination during grasping and manipulative actions. Curr Opin Neurobiol 2:815–823, 1992

152. Dernier van der Gon JJ, Coolen ACC, Erkelens CJ, et al.: Self-organizing neural mechanisms possibly responsible for muscle coordination. p. 335. In Winters JM, Woo SL-Y (eds): Multiple Muscle Systems: Biomechanics and Movement Organization. Springer Verlag, New York, 1990

153. Abdusamatov RM, Adamovich SV, Berkinblit MB et al.: Rapid one joint movements: a qualitative model and its experimental verification. p. 261. In Gurfinkel V, (ed): Stance and Motion: Facts and Concepts. Plenum Press, New York, 1988

154. Hall LA, McCloskey DI: Detections of movements imposed on finger, elbow, and shoulder joints. J Physiol 335:519–533, 1983

155. Taylor JL, McCloskey DI: Detection of slow movements imposed at the elbow joint during active flexion in man. J Physiol Lond 457:503–513, 1992

156. Loeb GE: Strategies for the control of studies of voluntary movements with one degree of freedom (comment). Behav Brain Sci 12:227, 1990

157. Loeb GE, Levine WS: Linking musculoskeletal mechanics to sensorimotor neurophysiology. p. 165. In Winters JM, Woo SL-Y (eds): Multiple Muscle Systems: Biomechanics and Movement Organization. Springer-Verlag, New York, 1990

158. Dietz V: Human neuronal control of automatic functional movements: interaction between central programs and afferent input. Physiol Rev 72:33–69, 1992

159. Lacquinti F: Automatic control of limb movement and posture. Curr Opin Neurobiol 2:807–814, 1992

160. Massion J: Postural control system. Curr Opin Neurobiol 4:877–887, 1994

161. Massion J: Movement, posture, and equilibrium: interaction and coordination. Progr Neurobiol 38:35–56, 1992

162. Dietz V: Neuronal basis of stance regulation: interlimb coordination and antigravity receptor function. p. 167. In Swinnen SP, Massion J, Heuer H, et al. (eds): Academic Press, San Diego, 1995

163. Horak FB, Nashner LM: Central programming of postural movements: adaptations to altered support-surface configurations. J Neurophysiol 55:1369–1381, 1986

164. Dietz V, Horstmann G, Berger W: Involvement of different receptors in the regulation of human posture. Neurosci Lett 94:82–87, 1988

165. Mouchnino L, Aurenty R, Massion J, et al.: Coordination between equilibrium and head-trunk orientation during leg movement: a new strategy built up by training. J Neurophysiol 67:1587–1598, 1992

166. Winter DA, Patla AE, Frank JS: Assessment of balance control in humans. Med Prog Technol 16:31–51, 1990

167. Lacquinti F, Maioli C: Independant control of limb position and contact forces in cat posture. J Neurophysiol 72:1476–1495, 1994

168. Fung J, Macpherson JM: Determinants of pos-

tural orientation in quadrupedal stance. J Neurosci 15:1121–1131, 1995

169. Mackinnon CD, Winter DA: Control of whole body balance in the frontal plane during human walking. J Biomechanics 26:633–644, 1993

170. Mouchnino L, Aurenty R, Massion J, et al.: Is the trunk a reference frame for calculating leg position? Neuroreport 4:125–127, 1993

171. McCloskey DI: Kinesthetic sensibility. Physiol Rev 58:763–820, 1978

172. Jami L: Golgi tendon organs in mammalian skeletal muscle: functional properties and central actions. Physiol Rev 72:623–666, 1992

173. Crenna P, Frigo C, Massion J, et al.: Forward and backward axial synergies in man. Exp Brain Res 65:538–548, 1987

174. Crenna P, Frigo C, Massion J et al.: Forward and backward axial movements: two modes of central control. p. 145. In Gurfinkel VS, Massion J, Roll JP (eds): Stance and Motion: Facts and Concepts. Plenum Press, New York, 1986

175. Dietz V: Gating of reflexes in ankle muscles during human stance and gait. Prog Brain Res 97:181–188, 1993

176. Inglis K, Horak FB et al.: Importance of somatosensory information in triggering and scaling automatic postural responses in humans. Exp Brain Res 101:159–164, 1994

177. Keshner EA, Allum JHJ: Muscle patterns coordinating postural stability. p. 480. In Winters JM, Woo SL-Y (eds): Multiple Muscle Systems: Biomechanics and Movement Organization. Springer Verlag, New York, 1990

178. Rogers MW: Interaction of posture and locomotion during the initiation of protective stepping: implications for falls in older adults. Presented at Multisegmental Motor Control: Interfaces of Biomechanical, Neural, and Behavioral Approaches. New Hampshire, 1995

179. Macpherson JM: How flexible are muscle synergies? p. 33. In Humphrey DR, Freund H-J (eds): Motor Control: Concepts and Issues. John Wiley & Sons, New York, 1991

180. De Bono E: Creativity and quality. Quality Management in Health Care 2:1–4, 1994

181. Burleigh AL, Horak FB, Malouin F: Modification of postural responses and step initiation: evidence for goal directed postural interactions. J Neurophysiol 72:2892–2902, 1994

182. Allum JHJ, Honegger F, Schicks H: Vestibular and proprioceptive modulation of postural synergies in normal subjects. J Vestibular Res 3:59–85, 1993

183. Di Fabio RP, Graf B, Badke MB et al.: Effect of knee joint laxity on long-loop postural reflexes: evidence for a human capsular-hamstring reflex. Exp Brain Res 90:189–200, 1992

184. Johansson H, Sjölander P, Sojka P: Receptors in the knee joint ligaments and their role in the biomechanics of the joint. Crit Rev Biomed Eng 18:341–368, 1991

185. Bullock-Saxton JE: Local sensation changes and altered hip muscle function following severe ankle sprain. Phys Ther 74:17–31, 1994

186. Zätterström R, Fridén T, Lindstrand A, et al.: The effect of physiotherapy on standing balance in chronic anterior cruciate ligament insufficiency. Am J Sports Med 22:531–536, 1994

187. Shiavi R, Limbird T, Borra H, et al.: Electromyography profiles of knee joint musculature during pivoting: changes induced by anterior cruciate ligament deficiency. J Electromyogr Kinesiol 1:49–57, 1991

188. Hasan SS, Edmondstone MA, Limbird TJ et al.: Reaction force patterns of injured and uninjured knees during walking and pivoting. J Electromyogr Kinesiol 1:218–228, 1991

189. Nitz AJ, Dobner JJ, Kersey D: Nerve injury and grades II and III ankle sprains. Am J Sports Med 13:177–182, 1985

190. Horak FB, Diener HC, Nashner LM: Influence of central set of human postural responses. J Neurophysiol 62:841–853, 1989

191. Rogers MW, Pai Y-C: Dynamic transitions in stance support accompanying leg flexion movements in man. Exp Brain Res 81:398–402, 1990

192. Gottlieb GL, Agarwal GC: Coordination of posture and movement. p. 418. In Desmedt JE (ed): New Developments in Electromyography and Clinical Neurophysiology. Karger, Basel, 1973

193. Voight ML, Weider DL: Comparative reflex response times of vastus medialis obliquus and vastus lateralis in normal subjects and subjects with extensor mechanism dysfunction. Am J Sports Med 19:131–137, 1991

194. Grabiner MD, Koh TJ, Andrish JT: Decreased excitation of vastus medialis oblique and vastus lateralis in patellofemoral pain. Eur J Exp Muscu-loskel Res 1:33–39, 1992

195. Grabiner MD, Koh TJ, Draganich LF: Neuromechanics of the patellofemoral joint. Med Sci Sports Exer 26:10–21, 1994

196. Scovazzo ML, Browne A, Pink M et al.: The pain-

ful shoulder during freestyle swimming. An electromyographic and cinematographic analysis of twelve muscles. Am J Sports Med 19:577–582, 1991

197. Keshner EA: Controlling stability of a complex movement system. Phys Ther 70:844–854, 1990

198. Keshner EA, Woollacott MH, Debu B: Neck and trunk muscle responses during postural perturbations in humans. Exp Brain Res 71:455–466, 1988

199. Teasdale N, Bard C, Larue J, et al.: On the cognitive penetrability of posture control. Exp Aging Res 19:1–13, 1993

200. Maki BE: Biomechanical approach to quantifying anticipatory postural adjustments in the elderly. Med Biol Eng 31:355–362, 1993

201. Hutton RS, Atwater SW, Nelson DL: Do muscle sensory receptors compensate for or contribute to neuromuscular fatigue? Med Sports Sci 34:162–171, 1992

202. Thompson S, Gregory JE, Proske U: Errors in force estimation can be explained by tendon organ desensitization. Exp Brain Res 79:365–372, 1990

203. Evatt ML, Wolf SL, Segal RL: Modification of human spinal stretch reflexes: preliminary studies. Neurosci Lett 105:353–355, 1989

204. Gandevia SC, Burke D: Effects of training on voluntary activation of human fusimotor neurons. J Neurophysiol 54:1422–1429, 1985

205. Hutton RS, Atwater SW: Acute and chronic adaptations of muscle proprioceptors in response to increased use. Sports Med 14:406–421, 1992

206. Koceja DM, Burke JR, Kamen G: Organization of segmental reflexes in trained dancers. Int J Sports Med 12:285–289, 1991

207. Rochongar P, Dassonville J, Le Bars R: Modification of the Hoffmann reflex in function of athletic training. Eur J Appl Physiol 40:165–170, 1979

208. Casabona A, Polizzi MC, Perciavalle V: Differences in the H-reflex between athletes trained for explosive contractions and non-trained subjects. Eur J Appl Physiol 61:26–32, 1990

209. Nielsen J, Crone C, Hultborn H: H-reflexes are smaller in dancers from the Royal Danish Ballet than in well-trained athletes. Eur J Appl Physiol 66:116–121, 1993

210. Grabiner MD, Enoka RM: Changes in movement capabilities with aging. Exerc Sport Sci Rev 23:65–104, 1995

211. Gambetta V: Conditioning of the shoulder complex. p. 643. In Andrews JR The Athlete's Shoulder. Wilk KE (eds): Churchill Livingstone, New York, 1994

212. Ariel GB: Biomechanics. p. 271 In Teitz CC (ed): Scientific Foundations of Sports Medicine. B. C. Decker Inc., Toronto, 1989

213. Harris LR: Visual motion caused by movements of the eye, head and body. p. 397. In Smith AT, Snowder RJ: Visual Detection of Motion. Academic Press, London, 1994

214. Patla AE: The neural control of locomotion. In Spivak BS (ed): Evaluation and Management of Gait Disorders. Marcel Dekker, New York, 1995

215. Jonansson H, Magnusson M: Human postural dynamics. Crit Rev Biomed Eng 18:413–437, 1994

2

Neurosciences

ARTHUR J. NITZ

JOHN NYLAND

TONY BROSKY, JR.

DAVID CABORN

Knowledge of articular neurology is of primary importance in physical therapy. This knowledge can enhance the clinician's understanding of movement patterns and provide insight into the implementation of sensorimotor proprioception concepts within rehabilitation plans. The major role of joint proprioceptive systems is to convey and process the sensory signals of the mechanical stimuli generated by an organism's own actions.[1]

The neuromuscular system makes optimal use of the biomechanical structures and the organizational design of the skeleton, joints, and muscles as they relate to postural alignment, in order to meet the demands of the organism for mobility and maintenance of dynamic stability. This optimization includes the distribution of effort between osseous and ligamentous/capsular components of the joint, and the musculature that directly and indirectly acts at the joint. The relative contribution of each of these structures as stabilizers, or proprioceptors, is largely determined by the capability of the neighboring structures to perform these tasks. For example, the poor osseous stability and limited capsuloligamentous stability of the glenohumeral joint may necessitate increased proprioceptive and stabilizing contributions from the musculotendinous components.

Proprioceptive (reactive) and kinesthetic (conscious) position sense are largely instinctive skills that living systems possess. Rowinski[2] has defined *proprioception* as the cumulative neural input to the central nervous system (CNS) from mechanoreceptors in the joint capsules, ligaments, muscles, tendons, and skin. Garn and Newton,[3] have defined *kinesthesia* as the conscious awareness of joint position and movement resulting from proprioceptive input to the CNS. Muscle spindles are believed to be best suited for the responsibility of conveying conscious awareness of joint position sense, although the joint capsule may serve as a link between joint and muscle proprioceptive function in relation to the reflex coordination of muscle length and tone around a joint.[4] Following injury or relatively lesser perturbations to a component joint of a kinetic chain, normal protective (instinctive), and cognitive (e.g., motor planning) integrations of movement and position sense become increasingly important.

The term "joint injury" (peripheral or vertebral) underscores the interdependence of the *sensory* systems, which provide proprioceptive or kinesthetic information (i.e., skin, subcutaneous, capsuloligamentous, musculotendinous, periosteal). The involvement of the *motor* system following joint injury, in addition to the aberrant sensory feedback from injured articular receptors, serves as evidence for the contention that joint injury represents peripheral neurologic dysfunction caused by the sudden disruption of routine motor control signals within the peripheral and central nervous systems.[2] Researchers have concluded that altered sensory feedback from joint mechanoreceptors results in dysfunctions that are expressed in the form of compensatory changes in timing, sequencing, and duration of various kinematic, kinetic, and muscle activation parameters.[5] Rehabilitation must address the sensorimotor neurologic dysfunction associated with joint injury if recurrent episodes, chronic joint instability, and early degenerative changes are to be prevented.

The afferent neural network consists of multiple pathways that carry peripheral afferent input to central neural structures. This input and the way it is processed by the central neural structures have been referred to as *intersensory coordination*.[6] A broad distinction needs to be made between the afferent paths specifying the relative position of the body segments, and exteroception (primarily vision), which provides information about events that occur in extrapersonal space. Movements directed toward external objects are generally organized on the basis of several sensory signals. Repetitive active movements (both reactive and corrective) are crucial during motor learning. During repeated movements, minor kinematic, kinetic, and muscle activation compensations may occur normally to improve neuromuscular efficiency in the presence of fatigue.[7]

A correlation between proprioceptive and exteroceptive signals is required during the learning phase in order to induce the emergence of a unified sensory representation.[6] Perhaps this warrants consideration during the initial stages of rehabilitation as well. When vision and proprioception are experimentally dissociated during normal developmental stages, sensorimotor coordination is detrimentally affected.[8] Spatiotemporal aspects require consideration not only with regard to motor output and the way movements are executed, but also at the sensory level, as to how sensory inputs can induce a central representation of movements that actively reflect their dynamics.[6] Patients deprived of proprioceptive feedback are unable to effectively adjust their movements in the face of unexpected loads, and have difficulty attempting to maintain a steady joint angle without vision.[9,10] Ultimately, man, and presumably mammals, have the capacity to perceive limb position and movement in space without effective visual cues, and this proprioceptive sense greatly depends upon continuous input provided by structurally competent capsuloligamentous and musculotendinous joint mechanoreceptors.[11,12]

MULTIPLE INPUTS INTERACT FOR OVERALL SOMATOSENSORY ORGANIZATION

It is the task of the CNS to filter, organize, interpret, and utilize information from several sources simultaneously. The afferent system provides information on the condition of the limb segments to the CNS in order to modify and fine tune movement instructions. Joint afferent fibers converge on spinal cord interneurons, which modulate the threshold of the *musculotendinous responses* including intrinsic muscle stiffness and reflex motor neuron activation, facilitation, or inhibition. Central interneuronal mechanisms set activation threshold levels (bias and sensitivity). The result is that the peripheral system threshold for dynamic joint stability or movement is established.[13] This threshold can be greatly modulated by the patient's attentiveness to the demands of the task, therefore clinicians should choose tasks that are both challenging and of interest to the patient.[14,15]

Peripheral afference is integrated with visual and vestibular afference to provide dynamic postural balance. Joint and musculotendinous afference transmits some aspect of conscious (supraspinal) awareness of perceived body position and movement. In this fashion, the CNS is able to monitor the results of a movement, task, or perturbation with the expected results.

Joint Innervation

Extrinsic innervation of the joints constitutes a *dual* innervation. A specific articular nerve travels to a joint capsule, usually by way of articular blood vessels. Schutte et al.,[16] however, reported that the intraligamentous neural fibers of the human anterior cruciate ligament entered the knee joint capsule via an axon from adjacent connective tissue. Nonspecific, intramuscular branches of nerves to muscles that cross a joint are embedded in the interfascicular connective tissue. Joint innervation may also be provided by "twigs" from cutaneous or periosteal nerve branches. Therefore, synovial joints possess a dual pattern of innervation. This dual innervation arises from primary articular nerves, which are independent from larger peripheral nerves that (specifically supply the capsuloligamentous structures) and from accessory articular nerves that innervate the joint after having provided primary innervation to muscular or cutaneous tissues.[17,18] These primary and accessory articular nerves terminate in a wide variety of encapsulated and unencapsulated mechanoreceptors, which are sensitive to mechanical distortion associated with soft tissue stretching, relaxation, compression, and tension.

The observed pattern of innervation raises several clinically related questions such as: What is the functional significance of this dual innervation pattern? Does duality of innervation imply that primary and accessory nerves to the joint serve functionally distinct roles? What happens when injury occurs? Is joint movement or position sense more likely to be spared following joint injury because of this dual innervation pattern? Is this a form of designed redundancy to enable continued joint afference in the presence of injury to the system?

Functional Considerations

Joint protection occurs by sensorimotor integration providing information for optimally coordinated local muscle activation (under modulation control by the CNS) that prevents movement beyond a normal physiologic range. Joint instability and muscular imbalance have traditionally been reported to result in abnormal movement, musculoskeletal pain, tissue pathology, and disability.[11] Joint stability depends upon four primary factors: (1) the congruence

of the articular components, (2) the integrity of noncontractile periarticular connective tissues, (3) the function of muscles that exert their force across the joint to produce or inhibit motion, and (4) the function of distal synergistic muscles. Changes in joint function secondary to the disruption of any of these tissues can cause varying degrees of degenerative articular changes. Effective dynamic joint stability requires more than just adequate force generation via muscle tension. More importantly, the magnitude of these forces must be properly coordinated, beginning and ending at a precise range in the movement, with an exacting balance of agonistic and antagonistic contributions. The ability to learn and refine this type of skill requires proprioception, "the most important sensory modality participating in the control of human movement."[19]

Conscious perception of movement is greatly enhanced during active muscle contraction. When the CNS uses proprioceptive information to control ongoing movements, the dynamic resolution of joint angle, or angular distance, theoretically dictates the limits of accuracy with which movements can be performed in space and in time.[20] The results of microneurographic studies of human mechanoreceptor discharge suggest that joint angle resolution might differ between static and dynamic conditions because less than one-half of a muscle's spindle afferents have a background discharge in the resting limb.[21,22] Muscle spindle mechanoreceptors without a background discharge cannot provide information about joint position at rest. Therefore, it may be useful to compare the accuracy with which subjects perform a dynamic movement sequence task with previous tests of joint angle discrimination performed under static conditions.[20] Musculotendinous mechanoreceptors have a principle role with respect to "global" joint mechanoreception in the relaying of proprioceptive information.[23,24] Considerable evidence exists that supports man's capacity for consciously perceiving musculotendinous input and using it in a proprioceptive sense. Also, capsuloligamentous mechanoreceptors have been demonstrated to be incapable of adequately codifying all of the various possible angular positions of a joint.[12] Mechanoreceptive input is strictly dependent on the structural characteristics of the type of tissue in which it is situated and, in particular, on the potential for that tissue to generate tension of an adequate stimulus.[25]

Mechanoreception

Mechanoreceptors originating from any tissue act as transducers by converting the physical stimulus of tension into a specific neural signal. The strength of the stimulus changes the *frequency* of firing, but not the *amplitude* of the neural discharge regarding the position, motion, and angular acceleration of the joint from which information is derived. Mechanoreceptors also exhibit the property of either rapid or slow adaptability when neural excitation occurs over a protracted period of time.

Cutaneous Mechanoreceptors

Moberg[26] maintains that the role of cutaneous mechanoreceptors in proprioception has been largely overlooked. Lundberg et al.[27] established that low threshold electrical signals from cutaneous receptors were one of three excitatory influences converging upon Ib motoneurons, the others being low threshold joint afferents and input from cocontracting muscles. Joint rotation causes cutaneous tissue distortion, which is believed to contribute to joint position and/or movement sense.[28,29] However, Clark et al.[30] found that anesthetizing the skin had essentially no effect on the ability to detect slow joint rotation or return a displaced joint to its original position. By definition, cutaneous receptors are peripherally situated to provide input regarding tissue deformation, which may lead to improved dynamic stability through tension development in specialized connective tissue structures (e.g., Grayson's and Cleland's ligaments). At present, research (done primarily with human finger joints and electrical microstimulation) indicates that this contribution is probably a minor one, although with greater contributions when the skin is relatively "bound" to the joint as in the interphalangeal joints of the fingers.[31] Conceivably, the application of specific taping techniques[32] or protective garments[33] may enhance the capacity of the skin mechanoreceptors for contributing to overall joint proprioception.

Recent experimental evidence in a normal population suggests that ankle ligament anesthesia does not appreciably alter joint position sense.[28] The investigators concluded that intact afferent feedback from skin, muscle, and other joint receptors was sufficient to maintain joint positioning task accuracy in the presence of anesthetized anterior talofibular and calcaneofibular ligaments. Additionally, ankle orthosis application reduced joint position replication errors in these subjects, suggesting that such devices may provide benefit by increasing the afferent feedback from cutaneous receptors in the foot and leg, which, in turn, leads to improved dynamic ankle joint position sense.[28]

Musculotendinous Mechanoreceptors ("Kinesiologic Monitors")

Current research findings support the following basic observations:

1. Sensory afferent information from musculotendinous mechanoreceptors is integrated with information from cutaneous, subcutaneous, and capsuloligamentous structures to provide normal proprioceptive acuity.[23,24,26]

2. Large numbers of muscle afferents must be simultaneously excited to produce sensations of joint movement.[34]

3. Cocontracting muscles around a joint increases proprioceptive acuity by enhancing the stretch sensitivity of the muscle spindles in the activated muscles.[35]

4. Proprioceptive information originating in the golgi tendon organs are probably integrated in a complex fashion, with input from the musculotendinous spindles to help determine joint position.[24]

Further observations indicate that small muscles frequently act across joints in concert with larger, more powerful partners. For example, in man, the six deep hip external rotator muscles work in parallel with the comparatively massive gluteus maximus muscle to produce external rotation of the hip. In the upper extremity, the anconeus muscle extends the elbow in parallel with the large triceps brachii muscle. The small rotators brevis muscle of the spine is paralleled by the much larger multifidus and semispinalis muscles to produce vertebral rotation. Bastide et al.[36] have referred to these small muscles as the "active ligaments" of an articulation and propose that they serve a role as correctors or modifiers of major movements.

These functionally associated large and small muscles have also been referred to as "parallel muscle combinations" (PMCs).[37-39] In general, high muscle spindle densities characterize muscles that initiate fine skilled movements, maintain posture, possess slow contractile properties, or have many of their spindle units linked together in tandem or in compound arrangements.[40,41] Muscles with an extremely high spindle density coupled with a relatively low number of extrafusal fibers suggest a possibly greater role in sensory feedback. Nitz and Peck[38] have proposed that the small members of PMCs may function as "kinesiologic monitors," generating crucial proprioceptive or kinesthetic input to the CNS. The primary evidence for this proposal is that the smaller member of a PMC may have muscle spindle densities three times greater than their larger counterpart. This finding has been verified in human spinal and appendicular muscles.[38] This relationship has also been reported in other species.[37,42-44] Definitive studies have, as yet, not been conducted to determine whether the joint afferent fibers from small muscles surrounding a joint are the major contributors to the neurologic input from the joint. Clinical implications of this arrangement following joint injury will be discussed later.

Capsuloligamentous Mechanoreceptors

The joint capsule has traditionally been considered to be more highly endowed with mechanoreceptors than specific ligaments (Fig. 2-1, Table 2-1).[45] Investigations of the human anterior cruciate ligament (ACL), however, have revealed an extensive intraligamentous neural network, which is believed to provide the CNS with information about the ACL and its relationship with other important knee structures.[16,46]

Architecturally, these mechanoreceptors have been found near the surface and the distal end of the ACL, where they could be most sensitive to deforming forces.[47] Intraligamentous mechanoreceptors have also been reported in human vertebral ligaments.[48]

REGIONAL REVIEWS

The Upper Quarter

During upper extremity function, the mechanoreceptors in the connective tissue of the glenohumeral joint communicate vital proprioceptive information to the CNS. This information actuates the efferent system to properly regulate muscle spindle bias and sensitivity, effectively augmenting intrinsic muscle stiffness and viscosity, thereby enhancing its readiness for ensuing motor tasks and its capacity as a proprioceptor. Modulation of the mechanical behavior of a limb can reveal the strategies for the neural control of movement and posture.[49] Electrophysiologic studies have indicated that a primary action of joint afferent input is to provide continuous modulation of protective muscular responses, such as intrinsic stiffness and reflex activation. Consequently, overall limb stiffness is regulated by gamma motor neuron output, which provides motor input to the muscle spindles.[50-53] Multiple joint afferents appear to affect gamma efference at both the agonist and antagonist muscles, thereby encouraging a balancing effect on the muscle forces, which act at a joint.[51,52] Agonist and antagonist coactivation helps stabilize the joint so that forces are delivered at right angles to the joint surface, thereby diminishing damaging shear stresses. This arrangement neatly places joint mechanoreceptors into a feedback loop in which the loading history of the joint modulates intrinsic muscle stiffness and reflex sensitivity so that limb stiffness is ap-

TABLE 2-1 *Joint receptors*

RECEPTOR	LOCATION	DESCRIPTION	SENSITIVITY	DISTRIBUTION (OF RECEPTOR TYPE)	FUNCTIONAL CLASSIFICATION	PARENT AXON (FIBER DIAMETER, CONDUCTION VELOCITY)
Pacinian corpuscle	Fibrous layer of capsule, on capsule-synovium border, close to small blood vessels	Single terminal within lamellated encapsulation, appears in clusters of five or less (20–40 × 150–250 μm (cylindrical)	Sensitive to high-frequency vibration (>60 Hz), acceleration, and high-velocity changes in joint position; possible sensitivity to hemohydraulic, transient events and rapid contractile events of adjacent muscles	Found in all joints examined; sole corpuscular receptor in laryngeal and middle ear joints; greater density in distal than in proximal joints	Very rapidly adapting (RA); very low mechanical threshold	Group II (8–12 μm, 49 m/sec); terminal branch at 3–5 μm diameter
Golgi-Mazzoni corpuscles	Inner surface of joint capsule between fibrous layer and subcapsular fibroadipose tissue	Multiple terminating endings within thin encapsulation (30 × 200 μm cylindrical)	Sensitive to compression of joint capsule in plane perpendicular to its inner surface; insensitive to stretching of capsule	Knee joint and many others likely; may have very specific distribution within joint capsule	Slowly adapting (SA); response is linear function of compressive stress on capsule; low mechanical threshold	Group II–III (5–8 μm; estimate ≈ 30 m/sec)
Ruffini endings	Fibrous layer of capsule; few present in	Spray-type terminal endings within thin	Sensitive to stretching of joint capsule along either of its long axes	Few present in distal joints; greater density	Slowly adapting (SA); low mechanical	Group I–II (13–17 μm or 8–12 μm, 51 m/sec)

Receptor type	Location	Morphology	Sensitivity/Function	Distribution	Response	Afferent group
(continued)	extrinsic ligaments	encapsulation, having investment of collagen fibers (300 × 300–800 μm, two to six endings per axon)	within capsular plane; direction and speed of capsular stretch; intracapsular fluid pressure change; amplitude and velocity of joint-position change	in proximal joints; concentrated in capsular regions of most stress	threshold; response is linear function of axial components of capsular plane stress	Group I (13–17 μm; estimate ≈ 51 m/sec)
Golgi ligament endings (Golgi tendon organ-like)	Extrinsic and intrinsic ligaments, adjacent to bony attachments of ligaments	Thick encapsulation, profuse branching (100 × 600 μm total terminal spread)	Sensitive to tension or stretch on ligaments	Present in most joints with exception of cervical vertebral, laryngeal, and ossicular ligaments	Slowly adapting (SA); low-to-high mechanical threshold	
Free nerve endings (nociceptive and non-nociceptive)	Fibrous capsule, ligaments, subsynovial capsule, synovium, fat pads	Thin, bare nerve endings of small myelinated or unmyelinated axons, profuse branching	One type sensitive to nonnoxious mechanical stress; other type sensitive to noxious mechanical or biochemical stimuli	Present in all joints examined but density varies with particular joint component; most joints have relatively higher density in ligaments	Slowly adapting (SA); low-to-high mechanical threshold	Group III–IV (2–5 μm, <2 μm; 2.5–20 m/sec)

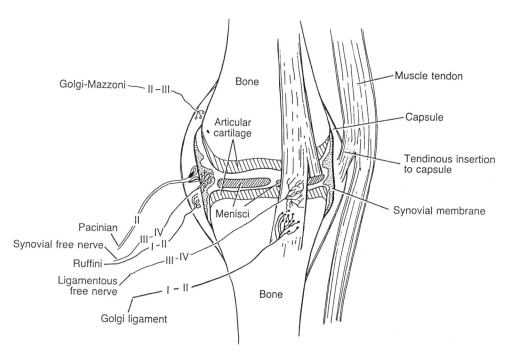

FIGURE 2-1 *Typical synovial joint receptor innervation pattern showing distribution of various receptor types. See references for Table 2-1 for sources of information on which this composite figure is based. (From Rowinski,[2] with permission.)*

propriate to the load applied to the involved structures.[50]

During task performance, mechanics may dictate the mode of interaction of a limb with the environment, serving as the interface between the neural commands and the environment.[53] During open kinetic chain functional tasks of the upper quarter, a proximal-to-distal sequential activation of musculotendinous structures to stabilize and mobilize contributing segments is evident. During closed kinetic chain tasks, the reverse is true.

Both types of functional tasks require effective kinesthesia and proprioception regarding scapulothoracic and scapulohumeral orientation for normal glenohumeral joint kinematics. Pacinian (fast movement sensitive) (type 2) mechanoreceptors are found in greater abundance at the glenohumeral than at the knee joint. They are located in the surroundings of the joint

capsule, rarely, in the intramuscular connective tissue.[54] Golgi-Mazzoni (type 1) mechanoreceptors are primarily found in contact with the periosteum of the bones participating in the composition of the glenohumeral joint and near muscular origins and insertions. In diminishing amounts, type 1 mechanoreceptors are located at the supraspinatus, infraspinatus, the short head of biceps brachii, coracobrachialis, teres minor, and the triceps brachii muscles.[55]

Musculotendinous mechanoreceptors are primarily located in the distal attachments of the supraspinatus, infraspinatus, and pectoralis minor, and in the proximal attachments of the biceps brachii, triceps brachii, coracobrachialis, and deltoid muscles. The number and development of these musculotendinous mechanoreceptors in general reveal differences between the "muscular species."[54] The supraspinatus, infraspinatus, and pectoralis minor muscles have smaller numbers of mechanoreceptors than do the brachial muscles, and these mechanoreceptors are believed to be developmentally inferior to those in the under-leg muscles.[54] In the glenohumeral muscles, especially in the supraspinatus and infraspinatus, mechanoreceptors are primarily located in the transitional musculotendinous tissue. In the long head of the biceps brachii, a rather large number of mechanoreceptors exist, descending from the glenoid labrum. These terminations are found in the loose connective tissue within the tendon, or in the synovial membrane that envelops the tendon.

Highly specialized musculotendinous junctions provide continuous monitoring of movement and tension parameters of muscle-tendon units and are prerequisite to coordinated movement.[56] In studying the palmaris longus and plantaris muscles, Jozsa et al.[56] reported that the sensitive, but relatively slower to adapt Ruffini (type 1) mechanoreceptors were located in equal numbers on the muscle and tendon sides of the junction, while the more rapidly adapting Pacini (type 2) mechanoreceptors were frequently found on the tendineal side, rarely on the muscular side. The opposite was true for the distribution of Golgi Tendon Organs (type 3). Further studies are necessary to determine functional explanations for these findings.

The concept that musculotendinous units are involved in position sense was proposed by Clark and Burgess[4] on the basis of their neurophysiologic studies of afferent units of the posterior articular nerve of the cat knee joint. Gandevia et al. reported that the ability to detect passive finger movements was reduced when the digital nerves (containing both joint and cutaneous afferent fibers) were blocked by local anesthesia.[35] This reduction in kinesthetic sense was less apparent with movements at higher angular velocities, when mechanoreceptors in both agonist and antagonist muscle groups could contribute to the detection and when active muscular tension was developed.[57] When intramuscular mechanoreceptors are unable to contribute to the detection of movements, kinesthetic acuity is substantially impaired compared with that obtained when intramuscular, capsuloligamentous, cutaneous, and periosteal mechanoreceptors each contribute to detection.[35,57] This performance impairment is greater when mechanoreceptors in both agonist and antagonist musculature are unable to contribute, compared to when those in the agonist contribute in isolation.[57] In assessing the human knee, Clark et al.[30] reported that both joint and intramuscular mechanoreceptors can contribute to kinesthetic perception, but relatively normal performance can be attained solely from intramuscular mechanoreceptor input when signals from joint mechanoreceptors are unavailable.

The Spinal Column

Most human facet joint capsules primarily contain two types of mechanoreceptors.[58] The vast majority of these receptors resemble large, encapsulated (type 2) endings as described by Freeman and Wyke.[59] Free nerve endings (type 4) are also evident in the capsular, synovial, and surrounding loose areolar tissue. The intrinsic neural surveillance provided by these structures is believed to be vital to the mediation of protective muscular responses that stabilize the cervical spine. Therefore, the loss of these mechanoreceptors because of iatrogenic denervation following surgical procedures at the cervical spine may have great clinical significance. Abnormal afferent signals from any class of spinal mechanoreceptor could alter proprioception. The lumbar spine has a similar mechanoreceptor structure which, presumably, performs the same functions.[60]

The small number of mechanoreceptors encountered in the cervical facet joint capsules suggests that they have a relatively large receptive field or that their individual functional contribution is of little importance.[58] Because these mechanoreceptors are relatively large, it is likely that their receptive fields are large and that one or two nerve endings may be sufficient to monitor the area of each individual facet capsule.[58] If this is the case, damage to even a small part of the capsule may substantially denervate the joint.

Low back pain is common in western society, affecting approximately 50–80 percent of the population.[61] Aging and cumulative trauma may also result in diminished proprioception.[62] Accumulated trauma has been described as a low grade injury that is not severe enough in any single event to produce a seemingly significant impairment, but prolonged or repetitive exposure produces observable effects.[63] Slowly conducting afferent units with relatively high thresholds are believed to serve a primarily nociceptive function (type 4), while the lower threshold afferent units (types 1–3) serve a proprioceptive function.[60] Yamashita et al.[64] have identified low to high threshold mechanosensitive afferent units in the lumbar facet joints of rabbits. The discovery of relatively high threshold mechanosensitive afferent units in the intervertebral disc (at the surface of the annulus fibrosus, and at the annulus fibrosus L5 and L6 insertions) leads to the hypothesis that they functioned at terminal range of motion, preceding tissue trauma.[64] Low to high threshold mechanosensitive afferent units were also discovered in the psoas muscle, probably providing a more important (mid-range) proprioceptive function at the lumbar region. Avramov et al.[65] reported the presence of three types of mechanosensitive receptors at the lumbar facet joints and surrounding tissues of rabbits. These included phasic-type mechanoreceptors, low threshold mechanoreceptors, and high threshold mechanoreceptors that only responded in the noxious range of loading. The units that demonstrated the phasic type of response were believed to serve as velocity detectors.[65] Low threshold, slowly adapting afferent units were believed to detect joint position changes by detecting changes in the mechanical strains in muscles and tendons.

The Pelvis and Hip

The extraordinarily strong hip joint ligaments (iliofemoral, ischiofemoral, and pubofemoral) allow for wide excursions and motions about three axes while also serving to restrict motion beyond the normal range.[66,67] Although the hip ligaments appear to predominantly serve as motion restraints, the muscle spindles of the multiple deep rotator muscles are believed to provide considerable proprioceptive input to the CNS.[68–70] This belief appears to be challenged by clinical observations of patients undergoing total hip replacement (THR), in which the standard of operative care involves detachment of these muscles from their insertion sites. Generally, the deep hip external rotator muscles are not reattached during this surgical procedure and patients seemingly maintain relatively normal hip joint position sense. Since the hip capsule is also divided and not preserved during the THR procedure, joint position sense following this operative intervention must be maintained by sources other than the standard capsuloligamentous receptors or deeply situated muscle spindles. Muscle spindles in the rectus femoris, psoas group, iliacus, sartorius, and gluteal muscles may provide adequate proprioceptive input for a joint with the inherent osseous/prosthetic stability of the human hip joint. The concept of joint specificity regarding the relative contributions of capsuloligamentous, musculotendinous and osseous joint stability and proprioception needs to be emphasized when evaluating both surgical and rehabilitation procedures. Generalizing information applied from basic science research of one joint to other joints is risky.

Rossi[12] has reported that specific capsuloligamentous cat hip mechanoreceptors are activated within a limited sector of the overall range of joint motion, according to the axis of rotation, which induces a given load upon these structures. Therefore, only in their limited sector of activation can capsuloligamentous joint mechanoreceptors codify with precise specificity both the axis of rotation and the expanse of joint movement.[66] The rotator muscles of the hip probably serve as the primary mid-range of motion proprioceptors.[68–70]

Grieve[71] contends that, not only the hip capsule, but the ligamentum teres as well, can produce powerful reflex effects upon the static and dynamic regulation of muscle activation, and upon postural awareness of joint position during both rest and movement. In addition, Grieve cites the work of Dee[72] to support his belief that subtle changes in muscle function during the early stages of hip arthrosis may result from disruption in the complex feedback loop from joint capsule mechanoreceptors and ligamentum teres.

The Knee

Cat[59,73–75] and monkey[76] knee mechanoreceptors have been studied extensively and tend to behave in a similar fashion, with their relative importance increasing as the joint approaches terminal flexion and extension range of motion. Human studies have also been performed that demonstrate similar characteristics.[77,78] Musculotendinous mechanoreceptors provide afferent input, which interacts with input from capsuloligamentous and cutaneous mechanoreceptors. Central neural processes ultimately control bias and sensitivity of muscle activation.[13] Since the knee functions as the relative mid-joint in the low quarter kinetic chain, it is greatly influenced by the musculature (both force-generating and proprioceptive contributions) that crosses it and the musculature that affects the position of each of its osseous components (some of which also act across the hip, ankle, and subtalar joints). Although traditional rehabilitative approaches have placed great emphasis on restoring normal thigh musculature function, recent reports have emphasized that the musculature of the lower leg (particularly the anterior tibialis and the gastrocnemius-soleus complex) and the hip may be particularly important in providing dynamic motion control to the knee, particularly when decelerating and changing direction quickly.[79–83]

The Ankle and Subtalar Joints—Universal Joint Tandem

While the ankle joint receives considerable proprioceptive input from the deltoid ligament (medially) and from the talofibular and calcaneofibular ligaments (laterally), it must be emphasized that the deltoid and the calcaneofibular ligaments provide extrinsic proprioceptive input at the subtalar joint in addition to the intrinsic input provided by the interosseous ligament.[84] Therefore, disruption of collateral ligaments at

either side of the ankle or at the distal tibiofibular syndesmosis[85] may affect stability and proprioception at the subtalar joint in addition to the ankle. Stephens and Sammarco,[84] using a cadaver model, found that the subtalar joint accounted for 50 percent or more of ankle/hindfoot inversion following ligament division with the ankle in the intermalleolar plane. These investigators identified contributions to subtalar stability from the inferior extensor retinaculum in both neutral and dorsiflexed positions, while the calcaneofibular, talofibular, talocalcaneal, cervical, posterior talocalcaneal, and interosseous ligament contributed to subtalar stability in all positions of the ankle.

In addition to the primary invertor musculature, the soleus muscle, through its insertional bias toward the medial aspect of the posterior calcaneus, and the tibialis anterior muscle, with its insertion upon the superior aspect of the tarsal navicular, can invert the subtalar joint, thereby dynamically assisting with eccentric muscular control of internal tibial rotation during the impact absorption phase of locomotion. Passive and dynamic control of the medial longitudinal arch could conceivably influence efficient internal rotation control of the leg. Eccentric activation of the tibialis anterior, gastrocnemius, soleus, and deep posterior calf musculature can both directly and indirectly affect subtalar joint control and proprioception. Concurrently, active dorsiflexion at the ankle enhances the preactivation of the gastrocnemius-soleus muscle complex, to increase the intrinsic stiffness and reflex potentiation sensitivity.[81] Eccentric peroneal muscle activation primarily provides dynamic subtalar control of excessive inversion from initial impact through the midstance phase of locomotion before concentrically assisting with the propulsive thrust before toe-off.[86] Muscle spindles in the peroneal muscles also assist with joint position sense at both the ankle and subtalar joints.

Foot Intrinsics

The contributions of the intrinsic musculature on the plantar aspect of the foot to subtalar, ankle, and even knee joint stabilization warrants consideration during rehabilitation planning and research investigations.[87] The contribution this musculature makes to multiplanar dynamic control of the longitudinal and transverse arches of the foot has a direct effect at the subtalar joint and may thereby have an indirect effect on tibiofibular rotatory force attenuation. Tasks that enhance the strength of these muscles may enable improved impact attenuation and ensuing propulsions[87,88] through the subtalar, ankle, and knee joints.

Organizational Concepts

THE INTEGRATION OF DYNAMIC INPUT

Chapter One reviewed the biomechanical concepts of stiffness, uni- and biarticular muscles, and problems associated with multijoint movements. One of the key variables in this equation is the selection of muscle functions from the available choices by the CNS. This involves choosing the set of muscle activations that allows a particular organization of movement to produce the power and control the mechanics of a moving segment so that a purposeful behavior is produced without affecting the equilibrium of the entire body. The muscle contractions must be sequenced and graded appropriately to provide for the generation and flow of power throughout the moving limb.[82] The control of movement is not dominated by one type of muscle contraction (i.e., eccentric or isometric). Rather, the selection of control features is determined by the task at hand and the goal of the movement.[83,89]

From Distal to Proximal—Impact Load Absorption/Eccentric Bias

During the weight acceptance phase of normal locomotion there is a sequential progression of forefoot abduction, subtalar eversion, ankle dorsiflexion, tibiofibular internal rotation, knee flexion, femoral internal rotation and adduction, posterior pelvic rotation, posterior pelvic tilt, and trunk flexion. During this progression, primarily eccentric activation of the musculature of the lower quarter and trunk acts to control, decelerate, and coordinate each segmental component for efficient three-dimensional deceleration. During this phase, kinetic energy is absorbed and stored.

From Proximal to Distal—Propulsion/Concentric Bias

The propulsion phase of normal locomotion is characterized by a sequential progression of trunk extension, anterior pelvic tilt, anterior pelvic rotation, femoral external rotation and abduction, knee extension, tibiofibular external rotation, ankle plantar flexion, subtalar inversion, and forefoot adduction. During this progression, primarily concentric activation of the musculature of the trunk and lower quarter acts to control, accelerate, and coordinate each segmental component for efficient three-dimensional acceleration. During this phase, kinetic energy is generated and released.

From Lumbopelvic/Scapulothoracic to the Extremities

Reports by Gracovetsky[90–92] and others[62,93] have emphasized the importance of the lumbopelvic region of the body for the generation and absorption of energy during locomotion and athletic performance. Optimal functional integrity of the static and dynamic tissues that cross this region is vital to the effective performance of maneuvers as diverse as pitching a baseball and rising from a chair. In addition to the intrinsic musculature of this region, components of the knee extensors and flexors, hip flexors, extensors, adductors, abductors, internal rotators, external rotators and elevators, glenohumeral extensors, adductors, and internal rotators contribute to the efficient function of this region. The postural dynamics of lumbopelvic and scapulothoracic linkages can greatly influence upper back/upper extremity and lower extremity function, respectively. The effect of subtle changes in proper scapulothoracic orientation and dynamic interaction with the glenohumeral joint among throwing athletes has recently been emphasized,[94] however, this phenomenon traditionally has been appreciated among other populations.[95] Rehabilitation of this region with consideration for normal scapulothoracic orientation and the attachments of muscles that act upon it should incorporate the lumbopelvic region. Just as lumbopelvic postural alignment is the foundation of lower extremity function, scapulothoracic alignment is the foundation of upper extremity postural alignment. Activities that evoke combined upper quarter and lower quarter activation must interface in a coordinated manner at the lumbopelvic and scapulothoracic "articulation." Deficiencies in strength or length of intrinsic and extrinsic musculature at the scapulothoracic articulation create an environment of less than optimal function at and throughout the entire upper extremity system.

Proprioceptive Triggering—The Applied Total Body System Approach

The application of the principle stated above is the use of an applied total body system approach to functional activities. Postural mechanisms are active both preceding and during activity of the limbs.[96] This implies that we must address the lumbopelvis during upper extremity activities and the scapulothoracic interface during lower extremity movements.

Throwing is an example of a discrete movement sequence in which two overlapping movements (acceleration and releasing) must be precisely coordinated for a thrown object to hit a target.[97] The shoulder, elbow, and wrist rotations overlap in this activity. Proprioceptive information from one joint rotation could potentially be used to trigger other joint rotations in the movement sequence, thereby providing the spatial and temporal coordination necessary for the accurate execution of the throwing task.[97] An important consideration when predicting performance is that the transmission and processing of proprioceptive information takes a finite amount of time. Proprioceptive triggering in movement sequences requires a mechanism that is distinctly different from servoregulation sen-

sorimotor control models.[97,98] Although servoregulation could adjust the amplitude and duration of joint rotations via "analog" control of movement parameters in both a spatial and a temporal sense, proprioceptive triggering within a movement sequence is essentially a digital process, arbitrarily changing between two states (movement or no movement) at a discrete moment in time.[97] Therefore, proprioceptive triggering in movement sequences and servoregulation are quite different types of neural control mechanisms that use proprioceptive input.

Movement sequences as diverse as locomotion, reaching and grasping, playing musical instruments, and throwing are all possible because of the effective higher center integration of proprioceptive input. The learning required to use proprioceptive input to accurately trigger joint rotations in movement sequences may be most evident in the reduction of error variability with repeated trials at progressively faster speeds.[97] Proprioceptive triggering appears to be readily available for the coordination of novel movement sequences as well as those that are highly practiced.

An example of an applied total body system activity is a diagonal two-armed ball toss. The exercise is divided into two main phases, loading and propulsion.

LOADING. Before a medicine ball is caught (or before initiation of the first throw), the anticipatory stages of the loading process are already well underway as the CNS prepares for the arrival of the medicine ball from a rebound source (wall, partner, mini-trampoline, etc.). As the ball is caught, the body responds in a cephalocaudal order. As an example of a possible sequential loading strategy, the dominant wrist extends; the elbow flexes and pronates; the shoulder adducts, externally rotates, and horizontally abducts; and the torso and pelvis rotate over the dominant hip, inducing internal rotation. The dominant knee flexes, the tibiofibular component internally rotates, the ankle dorsiflexes, and the subtalar joint and forefoot evert and abduct, respectively (pronation). The nondominant leg undergoes more of a supinatory motion.[99] During this phase, the

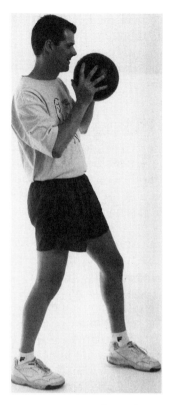

FIGURE 2-2 *Loading phase.*

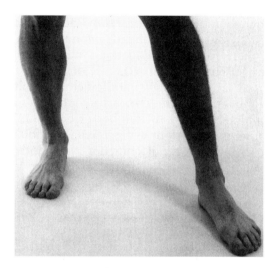

FIGURE 2-3 *Foot/subtalar joint orientation during loading phase.*

forces of impact are absorbed, and partially stored to be utilized during the next phase (Fig. 2-2, 2-3).

PROPULSION. As the medicine ball is propelled back at the rebound source, the energy stored during the loading phase is sequentially released with the ensuing concentric activations. During this phase, the body responds in a caudocephalad order. Sequentially, the forefoot and subtalar joint of the dominant leg adduct and invert, respectively; the ankle plantar flexes; the knee extends and the tibiofibular component externally rotates; the torso and pelvis rotate over the dominant hip, inducing external rotation; the shoulder abducts, internally rotates, and horizontally adducts; the elbow extends and pronates; and the wrist flexes as the ball is released. During this phase, the forces of propulsion are generated and released (Fig. 2-4, 2-5). The nondominant

leg undergoes a loading response in preparation for transition to the next catching and loading phase of the activity.

FUNCTIONAL SUMMARY

Multiple segment interaction greatly depends upon the capacity of biarticular muscles to transfer proprioceptive input and joint moments from one joint to the next to optimize coordinated performance within the relative restrictions of the desired functional outcome.[89,100-102] The medicine ball movement pattern presented here is intended to demonstrate the progressive interaction of body segments through the lumbopelvic and scapulothoracic regions. Different subjects may perform this task with differing biodynamic techniques based on anthropometric and training factors, postural orientation, the relative weight and velocity of the approaching ball, and the subject's readiness, interest, and attentiveness. The example presented here demonstrates a sagittal movement plane emphasis. When the task demands of catching the medicine ball require greater transverse plane movement, greater long axis rotational energy is stored throughout the entire body system (Fig. 2-6) with dominant side foot/subtalar orientation present-

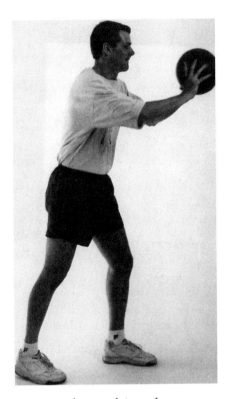

FIGURE 2-4 *Initial propulsion phase.*

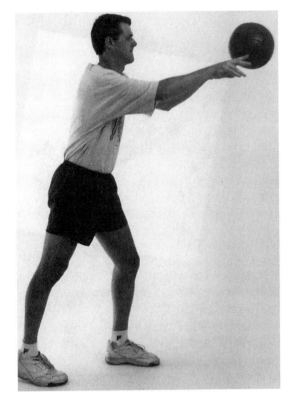

FIGURE 2-5 *Late propulsion/ball release phase.*

ing greater rigidity, through forefoot adduction and subtalar inversion (supinated) (Fig. 2-7). We believe that the more efficient energy storage (winding up) demonstrated during the loading phase of this primarily transverse plane type of movement necessitates this foot/subtalar joint orientation and optimizes its readiness for the ensuing propulsion phase.

THE EFFECT OF INJURY ON THE TOTAL JOINT NEUROLOGIC SYSTEM

Since all joints are supplied by neural structures that convey information from the periphery to the CNS, it could be argued that all joint injuries, to one extent or another, represent a neurologic dysfunction.[103,104] Patients who have sustained a joint injury must be carefully examined to determine what effect the neurologic dysfunction may have on the overall functional capacity of both the involved and the presumably normal or uninvolved extremity. Several investigators have identified nerve-related abnormalities in both the involved and the contralateral normal extremity following joint injury or surgery.[103,105–107]

Small-diameter afferents from articular tissues convey information from free nerve ending receptors regarding forceful joint rotations into the extreme limits of motion (so-called "noxious rotations").[108] These afferents are particularly sensitive to painful joint movements. Furthermore, chronic joint inflammation actually sensitizes these proprioceptive nociceptors so that afferents that were unexcitable in a normal joint now develop lower activation thresholds, becoming responsive to lessened mechanical stimuli following inflammation, and embellishing the painful response.[109] This dysfunctional joint information lacks the directional specificity that is normally only present with extreme, potentially

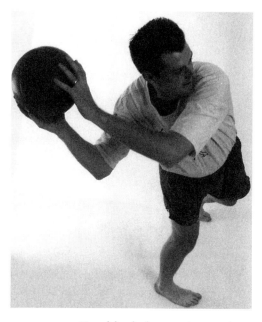

FIGURE 2-6 *Total body long axis rotation.*

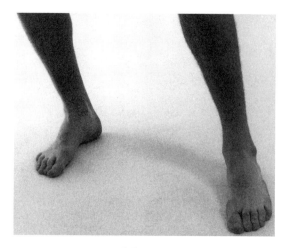

FIGURE 2-7 *Supinated foot.*

joint-damaging, end-range movements. Recent investigations regarding the plasticity of mechanoreceptors (functioning as nociceptors) in the presence of repetitious joint pathomechanics may implicate these components of the total joint neurologic system as prime players in the development of reflex sympathetic dystrophy.[110,111] Both afferent and efferent actions of the neurologic system may be impaired, with effects that can alter the behavior of the entire limb and spine-extremity junction (lumbopelvis or scaupulothorax) containing the damaged structure.

Joint De-"A"fferentation

The term articular *de-"A"fferentation* has gained wide acceptance following its introduction by Freeman et al.[112] to indicate the mechanism that they believed to be the cause of functional ankle instability. This term has come to include articular afferent impulse transmission disturbances and interference of the afferent neural code that is conveyed to the CNS. Diminished reflex excitation of motor neurons may re-

sult from either or both of the following events: (1) decreased proprioceptive input to the CNS, and (2) increased activation of inhibitory interneurons within the spinal cord.

Kennedy et al.[113] hypothesized that the failure of mechanoreceptor feedback resulting from knee ligamentous injury (laxity) led to the loss of reflex muscular splinting, rendering the joint vulnerable to repetitive major and minor injuries, and ultimately to progressive joint instability. This phenomenon could conceivably occur with any injured synovial joint (Fig. 2-8). However, it is difficult to completely validate such hypotheses with clinical studies alone. Animal studies provide much needed scientific data to clarify the nature of complex anatomic and physiologic events in cases such as these.

A series of reports by O'Connor et al.[114,115] have recently established the link between joint afference and the functional use of proprioceptive information in an animal model. They studied how articular afference serves to protect the joint in the event of injury and instability. These investigators found that joint de-"A"fferentation by neurectomy or dorsal root ganglionectomy does not solely lead to locomotor difficulties or the development of histologic evidence of articular cartilage disruption. Likewise, isolated ligament disruption and consequent joint instability, while producing some movement and cartilage

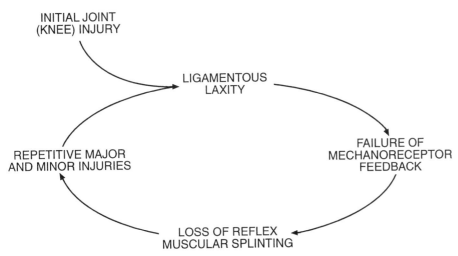

FIGURE 2-8 *Hypothesized role of mechanoreceptor failure in joint (knee) instability development. It is not known whether a similar sequence of events occurs following spinal joint injury. (From Kennedy JC,[113] with permission.)*

dysfunction does not lead to rampant joint changes either. However, joint de-"A"fferentation with concurrent ligament disruption (unstable joint) results in joint instability, severe limping, and gross evidence of osteoarthritic articular cartilage destruction.[114,115]

From the work of O'Connor et al., it is clear that animals use proprioceptive information from articular mechanoreceptors to maintain joint integrity. However, it is noted that both mechanical instability (ligament disruption) and loss of normal joint afference are required before functional instability. This suggests that some measure of adaptability in the presence of injury is built into the system. Proprioceptive input from one source or another enables the animal with an unstable joint to develop movement strategies that lessen tissue stress and minimize otherwise undampened joint forces. Proprioceptive tasks may prove to be the most beneficial rehabilitation component for patients who have sustained joint injury.

Following injury, or with aging, a certain number of joint afferent neurons are required to be reduced below a critical level before neurologic deficits are detectable.[50] This threshold may be determined by the ability of the surviving aged neurons to increase transmitter synthesis[116,117] and sprout additional new terminal axons[118] in order to compensate for the death of adjacent neurons.[119,120] Depending on the degree to which surviving joint afferents are able to functionally compensate for this loss, the protective muscular responses may be retained, thereby protecting the articular cartilage against overloading despite the age-related loss of a major proportion of the joint dorsal root ganglia. Salo and Tatton[50] reported that aging mice had a rate of knee joint dorsal root ganglia loss that was about twice the rate of loss of dorsal root ganglia that innervated other hindlimb tissue, such as muscle and skin. Losses in joint mechanoreceptor input less severe than Charcot arthropathy may provoke the progression of more common forms of degenerative osteoarthritis.[114,115,121,122] Unfortunately, the threshold level of dorsal root ganglion degeneration that produces detectable levels of neurologic deficits is unknown. The degree to which the surviving joint afferents are able to functionally compensate for joint afferent death determines the protective muscular responses that may be retained, sparing the articular cartilage against overloading despite the age-related loss of joint afferents.

The role of musculotendinous structures as agents of proprioception may become increasingly important with aging and injury.

De-"A"fferentation can disrupt the temporal precision with which muscles are sequentially activated during rapid single and multijoint force impulses.[123,124] Both visual and proprioceptive inputs are known to survey information about the state and configuration of the limb needed to program movements[125] and both can be used to correct errors introduced by externally applied perturbations. In addition to providing temporal information during the course of movements, proprioceptive input may allow calibration and updating of an internal model of the limb. Such a model could then be used to modify output commands during developing limb movements.[126]

Joint De-"E"fferentation

Neural control signals during multijoint movements integrate input from the variable effects of gravity and limb inertia as well as from the mechanical interactions that occur between limb segments.[125] Thus, the production of spatially accurate multijoint movements requires temporally precise patterns of muscle activity. Factors other than the isolated loss of joint afference contribute to the observed deficits associated with joint instability. One likely factor is muscle denervation (de-"E"fferentation), for which research evidence is now emerging.[105–107,127]

Muscle atrophy following joint injury or surgery is a ubiquitous observation that has historically been attributed to disuse. However, the rate at which the atrophy ensues following injury strongly suggests a neurologic explanation rather than simple disuse.[128] Electrophysiologic testing has documented evidence of such motor denervation following severe ankle sprain,[127] anterior cruciate ligament reconstruction undertaken without use of the pneumatic tourniquet,[105] shoulder injury or surgery,[129] and following open reduction internal fixation for femoral neck fracture.[130]

In addition to the muscle atrophy and electromyographic evidence of denervation, other clinically relevant deficits such as loss of active range of motion and strength are noted among patients with joint injury. The precise cause of this motor denervation is not known, but there is evidence to indicate that the best explanation is *neurogenic inflammation*. Direct trauma to the nerve, though occasionally observed, is clearly not the cause of this commonly observed muscle denervation. Levine et al.[131] have shown in an animal model that soft tissue inflammation in the periphery leads to spatially remote inflammatory responses, which affects the joints. This tissue response has been linked experimentally to the development of arthritis and is believed to be mediated by biogenic amines (histamine) or a host of other possible potent neurotransmitters such as substance P, vasoactive intestinal polypeptide (VIP), and calcitonin gene-related peptide (CGRP). In sufficient quantities following injury, these biochemical substances may have a denervating effect on the motor end-plate. We believe that the profound muscle atrophy so often noted following joint injury or surgery and the documented evidence of denervation in patients may be partially explained by neurogenic inflammation. Motor denervation (de-"E"fferentation) further impacts the protective muscle responses and the voluntary muscle activations that might otherwise defend joint structures. Large caliber joint afferent nerve transmission can mediate reflex modulation of muscular activation, which protects joints against force-related damage.[51,132–136] The degenerative joint changes associated with aging occur, in part, because a loss of mechanoreceptor afferent input diminishes protective motor responses, resulting in abnormal cartilage loading and consequent damage.[135,137] Age-related decreases in mechanoreceptor numbers have been reported for a variety of neuronal populations in a variety of mammalian species.[138]

Rehabilitation Implications

The observation that fluid distention of a joint produces muscle inhibition is believed to be indicative of the presence of an inhibitory reflexive mechanism involving joint mechanorecep-tors.[138] The importance of minimizing joint edema for maintaining normal joint afference was identified by Spencer et al.,[140] who found that as little as 20 ml of knee joint effusion resulted in afferent signal inhibition. Such joint effusion may cause persistent capsular distention which, itself, may lead to further neural inhibition even after the intra-articular fluid pressure has largely resolved. Early intervention with appropriate compression may reduce this capsular distention by compacting the periarticular soft tissues and translocating the edema proximally.

Chronic joint distention may also result from hypertrophy of synovial tissue on the inner layer of the capsule. Focal compression may reduce the potential for the development of posttraumatic synovial hypertrophy and fibrosis, by enhancing the resolution of edema and minimizing the potential space created by capsular distention.[141] A chronic inflammatory response may adversely affect protective neuromuscular function by increasing afferent nociceptive impulses, thereby altering the integration of other afferent input within the spinal cord. The correlation and possible interrelationships of various factors was proposed by Wilkerson and Nitz[104] and is noted in Figure 2-9.

FUNCTIONAL TRAINING CONCEPTS

Stretch-Shortening Cycles

Effective, functionally applicable training should utilize sequential eccentric-concentric-eccentric muscle activations if the desired outcome is to improve locomotor maneuvers such as running, jumping, or cutting in addition to events such as throwing. Optimal functional training of these maneuvers should attempt to increase the efficient use of the kinetic energy stored during eccentric loading or impact absorption for the ensuing concentric propulsion. Studies have demonstrated that the efficient use of this stored elastic energy increases the intensity of the ensuing concentric muscle activation during running or jumping maneuvers[142,143]; however, upper extremity data is lacking.

Specificity of Training

The use of sport-specific, and even player position-specific movement patterns can provide the repetitious training necessary to improve the motor plan organization for skilled performances. This type of training enables the clinician to replicate the sequential order of multiple joint interactions, coordinated muscle activations, and event timing that closely mimics actual sport performance. The use of varying temporal parameters regarding duration, cadence and frequency, as well as distance and playing surface parameters enables a controlled progression. Developing training tasks that are both physically and mentally challenging and of perceived importance to the patient is recommended to obtain an optimized training effect.

"Synergists at a Distance"

Effective upper extremity function is dependent upon other components of the entire kinetic chain. For example, the baseball pitcher may greatly benefit from the activation of the muscles that effectively adduct the foot, invert the subtalar joint, and plantar flex the ankle for forward propulsion, while the proprioceptive input from eccentric activation of stance hip external rotators and isometric activation of stance hip abductors and adductors maintains an effective platform for proper torso alignment. Concurrently, the coordinated activation of trained abdominal and low back musculature can enhance the efficient lower extremity to upper extremity transfer of momentum. *Movement pattern evaluation* should consider the structural integrity of each segmental component that contributes to the final outcome event. Clinicians should remember that each segment is an isolated component of an integrated system when evaluating movement dysfunction following injury.[144] Poor performance and/or injury generally occur when one or more of these component segments is deficient. When the weak segment has been identified, the therapeutic intervention should include sport-specific activities and movement patterns initially modified to bias (or assist) and later re-

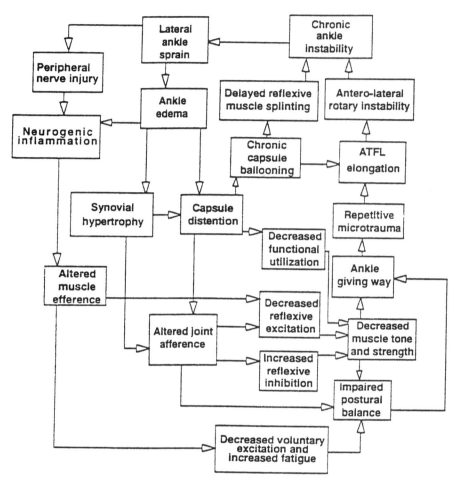

FIGURE 2-9 *Proposed relationships among many factors associated with chronic ankle instability. It is possible that similar factors play an important role in development of joint instability at sites other than the ankle. (From Wilkerson GB, and Nitz AJ,[104] with permission.)*

sist (motion return before strength return), with particular emphasis placed on the dominant plane(s) of movement. For example, the throwing motion, which has been likened to the winding and unwinding of a spring, is dominated by movement patterns that occur primarily in the transverse and sagittal planes of motion. During the loading or winding phase, the dominant side external rotators and extensors of the hip, the abdominal external oblique, and the scapular protractors elongate (prestretch eccentric activation). Contralaterally, the scapular retractors,

posterior deltoid, abdominal internal oblique, and hip flexor muscles also elongate.

Throwing athletes are believed to experience a high incidence of rotator cuff pathology because of "eccentric overload" during the terminal phase of unloading, or follow-through deceleration.[145,146] During this phase, the scapular retractors, humeral external rotators, dominant side internal obliques, and nondominant external obliques act synergistically to control deceleration of the trunk and arm. The concept of muscular synergies at a distance should be recognized in the treatment approach to shoulder dysfunction. When designing a rehabilitative or conditioning environment, the interrelationship of the trunk musculature as controllers of upper and lower quarter momentum warrants consideration. Therapeutic intervention with an appropriately designed medicine ball program enables coordinated strengthening of the trunk—lower quarter and upper quarter—within sport-specific movement patterns.[144–146]

During rehabilitation, it is important to remember that the primary area of injury or symptoms may not be the primary site of dysfunction. Injury often occurs at sites of precarious stability and structural orientation because of strength, tissue extensibility, or coordination deficiencies elsewhere in the kinetic system. This reinforces global assessment of synergistic structures during evaluation.

Normal and Abnormal Distributions of Effort

Although certain kinematic, kinetic, and muscle activation compensations may initially enable continued performance, it must be emphasized that they generally represent short-term solutions at best.[147,148] Any time the normal structural and proprioceptive integrity of a given segment is lacking, adjacent segments will attempt to replace their contributions. Whenever the normal kinematics, joint kinetics, and muscle activation parameters of a given segment are compromised; continued, prolonged use or more correctly, "misuse" of that component will ultimately be to the detriment of that segment and may initiate degenerative processes at contiguous segments.

REHABILITATION MODIFICATIONS FOR DE-"A"FFERENTATION AND DE-"E"FFERENTATION

Present therapeutic interventions cannot cause the nerve sprouting necessary for sensory and motor nerve recovery. This process proceeds at a predetermined rate. Part of early rehabilitation efforts must focus on strategies designed to recover motion and motor unit recruitment without deleteriously affecting this sensitive nerve regrowth. Improved peripheral nerve regeneration with low intensity magnetic fields[149–152] and tissue healing with low intensity ultrasound[153,154] have been reported using animal models. Eventually, these devices may show promise in augmenting regeneration of these sensory nerve terminations in addition to the neural axon in humans.

De-"A"fferentation

Rehabilitation of patients who demonstrate signs of de-"A"fferentation should progress gradually and cautiously, as motor and sensory nerve sprouting requires 3–12 months to make functional connections with appropriate target organs. Proprioceptive and balance deficits have been observed in the majority of patients following ankle sprain.[112,155] Peroneal muscle reaction times are also known to be altered[156,157] and recently, hip muscle function has also been shown to be adversely effected by previous severe ankle sprain.[103] Patients who have sustained lower extremity fractures and joint surgery (total knee replacement) may have delayed reaction and coordination times that can contribute to or be the result of their orthopedic condition. Although neuromuscular reaction tends to decrease with age, it tends to be more activity-than age-dependent, and can often be improved with simple rehabilitation exercises.[158,159]

Reports indicate that patients with postural or proprioceptive deficits following ankle injuries[160] as well as uninjured individuals[161] can improve ankle proprioception by training with an ankle disk system. Cocontraction of muscles acting across an injured joint have also been shown to temporarily improve joint proprioception.[162] Numerous studies have emphasized the importance of proprioceptive training following ACL reconstruction.[162–164] Protective neuromuscular responses for the hamstrings,[77,163–166] gastrocnemius-soleus complex,[167–169] and anterior tibialis[79,148] have all been reported as being vital to normal function following ACL injury or reconstruction.

De-"E"fferentation

Rehabilitation efforts for de-"E"fferentation may include high amplitude neuromuscular electrical stimulation to augment muscle volume and directly stimulate type 2 muscle fibers[170–173] and electromyographic biofeedback to promote physiological motor unit recruitment capabilities.[174] Since denervated muscle is readily fatigable, rehabilitation bouts of long duration should be minimized or eliminated. Early rehabilitation efforts may be enhanced by unloading the joint through the use of aquatic exercises, assistive devices, or controlled weight-bearing devices. Multiple, brief, and intense bouts of exercise should be undertaken that do not exceed the patient's fatigue resistance capabilities.[175] Clinicians should be alert for unwanted joint reactions during rehabilitation (e.g., inflammation), onset of fatigue (deterioration in performance), diminished kinesthesia or proprioception, or signs of soft tissue breakdown (e.g., patellar tendinitis with postoperative ACL rehabilitation), especially when denervation has promoted significant muscle compromise.

De-"A"fferentation and De-"E"fferentation Summary

Managed, functionally correct repetition is a major shaping force in the sensorimotor nervous system.[176] Joint usage patterns are known to affect the function of mechanoreceptors.[23] Short duration ankle platform training has produced objective improvements in ankle proprioception and corresponding decreases in reinjury rate.[168]

Continuing Development of Neuromuscular Control and Functional Movement Quantification

Of continual concern to the clinician is the dilemma that exists between measurement and function. Effective measurement implies both reliability and validity. Although certain devices may provide effective and somewhat valid measurements, they often (because of controlled isolation) may not provide the clinician with the functional insight they seek. Although functional movement pattern evaluations often provide this insight, they may not provide the measurement reliability, validity, and sensitivity that exists with more conventional systems, or information regarding the specific involvement of different contributing segments of the functional movement. What neuromuscular control measurement systems may lack in direct applicability to functional performance, they generally make up for through their reliability and sensitivity. New generations of relatively "high-tech" and "low-tech" methods of neuromuscular control and functional movement measurement are available to clinicians. Both types can be of value. Although manufacturers generally describe their particular device as providing a dynamic evaluation, for purposes of comparison, we have divided different evaluation methods into two groups: (1) relatively static (S) neuromuscular control measurement systems, and (2) relatively dynamic (D), more global functional movement evaluation systems. Although much work needs to be performed regarding their validity, reliability, durability, and clinical applicability, several of the more interesting systems are mentioned below.

1. High technology (functional movement measurement systems): Cybex Fastex, Cybex International, Ronkonkoma, NY (D or S); F-Scan System (Instrumented Insoles), Tekscan Inc., Boston, MA (D or S); Pedar System (Instrumented Insoles), Novel Electronics Inc., Minneapolis, MN (D or S).

2. High technology neuromuscular control (proprioceptive) Measurement systems: Biodex Stability System, Biodex Medial Systems, Inc., Shirley, NY (S); Chattanooga Balance System, Chattanooga Group, Inc., Hixson, TN (S); Neurocom Balance Master, Neurocom International, Inc., Clackamas, OR (S); Star Station, Spectrum Therapy Products, Jasper, MI (S).

These devices generally enable the assessment of closed kinetic chain joint proprioception through the subjects' ability to respond to visual cues and postural sway perturbations in a controlled manner. These devices generally demonstrate reasonable test reliability,[178] although their cost may be prohibitive to some clinics. Deficiencies noted during these tests are often attributed to the site of injury or surgical intervention; however, adaptations within the proprioceptive structures throughout the system can influence the final outcome measure. Also, the more complex the test task, the more likely a longer learning period is needed to attain adequate test reliability. None of these systems has built-in kinematic sampling capability. It is the responsibility of the clinician to evaluate the quality of task performance in regards to the strategy used by the subject.

3. Low technology relatively low cost, practical alternatives: Grid Systems, EFI Medical Systems, San Diego, CA (D); Single Leg Distance or Timed Hopping (D); Single Leg Vertical Jump (Vertex), Sports Imports, Columbus, OH (D); Dot Drills (D); Cone-Shuttle or Figure 8 Drills (D); Biomechanical Ankle Platform System (BAPS), Camp International, Jackson, MI (S); Kinesthetic Ability Trainer (KAT), Breg International, Vista, CA (S).

Through the use of instrumented timers, handheld stop watches, tape measures, and cadence cues such as metronomes, these methods (when used by trained clinicians and with task-specific criteria) can demonstrate reasonable measurement reliability.[178–180] These methods may be better suited to gross functional capability assessments (of which neuromuscular control, proprioception is a component) rather than proprioception proper.

Even with the promising systems that presently exist, clinicians are encouraged to experiment with exteroceptive denial, varying cadence responses, and performance following concentric and eccentric fatiguing episodes.[148] Applications such as these may further enhance the generalization of clinical test measurement results to environments that are relevant for each subject.

SUMMARY OF SYSTEMS

Neuromuscular control and functional movement measurement systems are still in the early stages of development. Clinicians must be encouraged to supplement and challenge traditional evaluative methods (seated isokinetics) with potentially more meaningful, three-dimensional methods that consider the cognitive processes/affect of the subject. Emphasis should also be placed on the quality of functional movement patterns within their predominant motion planes,[144] and the establishment of a series of reliable relatively low tech neuromuscular control and functional movement measurements that are valid to the performance of the client in a relevant environment.

References

1. Matthews P: Proprioceptors and their contribution to somatosensory mapping: complex messages require complex processing. Can J Physiol Pharmacol 66:430–438, 1988
2. Rowinski MJ: Afferent neurobiology of the joint. p. 49. In Gould JA (ed): Orthopedic and Sports Physical Therapy. C.V. Mosby, St. Louis, 1990
3. Garn S, Newton R: Kinesthetic awareness in subjects with multiple ankle sprains. Phys Ther 68:1667–1671, 1988
4. Clark F, Burgess P: Slowly adapting receptors in the cat knee joint: Can they signal joint angle? J Neurophysiol 38:1448–1463, 1975
5. Lorentzon R, Elmqvist L, Sjostrom M et al: Thigh musculature in relation to chronic anterior cruciate ligament tear: muscle size, morphology, and mechanical output before reconstruction. Am J Sports Med 17:423–429, 1989
6. Coiton Y, Gilhodes J, Velay J et al: A neural network model for the intersensory coordination involved in goal directed movements. Biol Cybern 66:167–176, 1991
7. Gambetta V: Rebuilding the completely . . .

Building the Complete Athlete. Optimum Sports Training: 1991

8. Held R, Hein A: Movement produced stimulation in the development of visually guided behaviour. J Comp Physiol Psychol 56:872–876, 1963

9. Rothwell J, Traub M, Day B et al: Manual motor performance in a deafferented man. Brain 105:515–542, 1982

10. Sanes J, Mauritz K, Dalakas M et al: Motor control in humans with large-fiber sensory neuropathy. Hum Neurobiol 4:101–114, 1985

11. Nyland J, Brosky T, Currier D et al: Review of the afferent neural system of the knee and its contribution to motor learning. J Orthop Sports Phys Ther 19:2–11, 1994

12. Rossi A: Joint receptors—kinesthesia and position sense a role as yet undefined. Rivista Di Neurobiologia 29:42–49, 1983

13. Prochazka A: Sensorimotor gain control: a basic strategy of motor systems? Prog Neurobiol 33:281–307, 1989

14. Llewellyn M, Yang JF, Prochazka A: Human H-reflexes are smaller in difficult beam walking than in normal walking. Exp Brain Res 83:22–28, 1990

15. Evarts EV, Shinoda Y, Wise SP: p. 189 Neurophysiological Approaches to Higher Brain Functions. John Wiley and Sons, New York, 1984

16. Schutte M, Dabezies E, Zimmy M et al: Neural anatomy of the human anterior cruciate ligament. J Bone Joint Surg 69A:243–247, 1987

17. Gardiner E: The innervation of the knee joint. Anat Rec 101:109–130, 1948

18. Wyke BD: Articular neurology: a review. Physiother 58:94–99, 1972

19. Brooks V: Motor control: how posture and movements are governed. Phys Ther 63:664–673, 1983

20. Bevan L, Cordo P, Carlton L et al: Proprioceptive coordination of movement sequences: discrimination of joint angle versus angular distance. J Neurophysiol 71:1862–1872, 1994

21. Al-Falahev N, Nagaoka M, Vallbo A: Response profiles of human muscle afferents during active finger movements. Brain 113:325–346, 1990

22. Edin B, Vallbo A: Dynamic response of human muscle spindle afferents to stretch. J Neurophysiol 63:1297–1306, 1990

23. Hutton R, Atwater S: Acute and chronic adaptations of muscle proprioceptors in response to increased use. Sports Med 14:406–421, 1992

24. Moore J: The golgi tendon organ: a review and update. Am J Occup Ther 38:227–236, 1984

25. Fukami Y, Wilkinson R: Responses of isolated golgi tendon organs of the cat. J Physiol 265:673–689, 1977

26. Moberg E: The role of cutaneous afferents in position sense, kinesthesia and motor function of the hand. Brain 106:1–19, 1983

27. Lundberg A, Malmgren K, Schomburg ED: Convergence from Ib, cutaneous and joint afferents in reflex pathways to motoneurones. Brain Res 87:81–84, 1975

28. Feurbach JW, Grabiner MD, Koh TJ et al: Effect of an ankle orthosis and ankle ligament anesthesia on ankle joint proprioception. Am J Sports Med 22:223–229, 1994

29. Nicholas J, Melvin M, Saraniti A: Neurophysiologic inhibition of strength following tactile stimulation of the skin. Am J Sports Med 8:181–186, 1980

30. Clark F, Horch K, Bach S et al: Contributions of cutaneous and joint receptors to static knee-position sense in man. J Neurophysiol 42:877–888, 1979

31. Clark FJ, Burgess RC, Chapin JW: Proprioception with the proximal interphalangeal joint of the index finger: evidence for a movement sense without a static-position sense. Brain 109:1195–1208, 1986

32. McConnell J: The management of chondromalacia patella: a long term solution. Aust J Physiother 32:215–223, 1986

33. Perlau R, Frank C, Fick G: The effect of elastic bandages on human knee proprioception in the uninjured population. Am J Sports Med 23:251–255, 1995

34. Macefield G, Gandevia SC, Burke D: Perceptual responses to microstimulation of single afferents innervating joints, muscles, and skin of the human hand. J Physiol (Lond) 429:113–129, 1990

35. Gandevia S, McCloskey D: Joint sense, muscle sense, and their combination as position sense, measured at the distal interphalangeal joint of the middle finger. J Physiol 260:387–407, 1976

36. Bastide G, Zadeh J, Lefebvre D: Are the "little muscles" what we think they are? Surg Radio Anat 11:255–256, 1989

37. Buxton D, Peck D: Neuromuscular spindles relative to joint movement complexities. Clin Anat 2:211–224, 1989

38. Nitz AJ, Peck D: Comparison of muscle spindle concentrations in large and small human epaxial muscles acting in parallel combinations. Am Surg 52:273–277, 1986

39. Peck D, Buxton D, Nitz A: A comparison of spindle concentrations in large and small muscles acting in parallel combinations. J Morphol 180: 243–252, 1984

40. Peck D, Buxton D, Nitz A: A proposed mechanoreceptor role for the small redundant muscles which act in parallel with large primemovers. p. 377. In Hnik P, Soukup T, Vejsada R et al (eds): Mechanoreceptors. Plenum, New York 1988

41. Barker D, Banks R: The muscle spindle. p. 309. In Engel A, Banker B (eds): Myology. McGraw-Hill, New York, 1986

42. Kjaersgaard P: M. articularis coxae: a possible receptor organ. Zbl Vet Med C Anat Histol Embryol 9:21–28, 1980

43. Lalatta-Costerbosa G, Barazzoni A, Clavenzani P et al: Histochemical profile of articularis humeri muscle in the horse. Boll Soc It Biol Sprt 66: 767–769, 1990

44. Rosser B, George J: An exceptionally high density of muscle spindles in a slow-tonic pigeon muscle. Anat Rec 212:118–122, 1985

45. Heppleman B, Heuss C, Schmidt RF: Fiber size distribution of myelinated and unmyelinated axons in the medial and posterior articular nerves of the cat's knee joint. Somatosensory Res 5:273–281, 1988

46. Zimny M, Schutte M, Dabezies E: Mechanoreceptors in the human cruciate ligament. Anat Rec 214:204–209, 1986

47. Schultz R, Miller D, Kerr C et al: Mechanoreceptors in human cruciate ligaments. J Bone Joint Surg 66A:1072–1076, 1984

48. Yahia LH, Newman NM, Rivard CH: Neurohistology of lumbar spine ligaments. Acta Orthop Scan 59:26–30, 1988

49. Agarwal GC, Gottlieb GL: Mathematical modeling and simulation of the postural control loop. Part III. CRC Crit Rev Biomed Eng 12:49–93, 1984

50. Salo P, Tatton W: Age-related loss of knee joint afferents in mice. J Neurosci Res 35:664–677, 1993

51. Johansson H, Sjolander P, Sojka P: Actions on gamma motoneurons elicited by electrical stimulation of joint afferent fibers in the hind limb of the cat. J Physiol 375:137–152, 1986

52. Johansson H, Sjolander P, Sojka P: Activity in receptor afferents from the anterior cruciate ligament evokes reflex effects on fusimotor neurones. Neurosci Res 8:54–59, 1990

53. Lacquainti F, Carrozzo M, Borghese N: Time-varying mechanical behavior of multijointed arm in man. J Neurophysiol 69:1443–1464, 1993

54. Shimoda F: Innervation, especially sensory innervation of the knee-joint and the motor organs around it in early stage of human embryo. Arch Histol Jap 9:91–108, 1955

55. Kikuchi T: Histological studies on the sensory innervation of the shoulder joint. J Iwate Med Assoc 20:554–567, 1968

56. Jozsa L, Balint J, Kannus P et al: Mechanoreceptors in human myotendinous junction. Musc Nerve 16:453–457, 1993

57. Gandevia SC, Hall LA, McClosky DI, Potter EK: Proprioceptive sensation at the terminal joint of the middle finger. J Physiol (Lond) 335:507–517, 1983

58. McClain R: Mechanoreceptor endings in human cervical facet joints. Spine 19:495–501, 1994

59. Freeman M, Wyke B: The innervation of the knee joint. An anatomical and histological study in the cat. J Anat 101:505–532, 1967

60. Yamashita T, Cavanaugh JM, El-Bohy AA et al: Mechanosensitive afferent units in the lumbar facet joint. J Bone Joint Surg 72A:865–870, 1990

61. Waddell G: A new clinical model for the treatment of low back pain. Spine 2:632–644, 1987

62. Skinner HB, Barrack SD, Cook SD et al: Joint position sense in total knee arthroplasty. J Ortho Res 1:276–283, 1984

63. Parkhurst T, Burnett C: Injury and proprioception in the lower back. J Orthop Sports Phys Ther 19:282–295, 1994

64. Yamashita T, Minaki Y, Oota I et al: Mechanosensitive afferent units in the lumbar intervertebral disc and adjacent muscle. Spine 18: 2252–2256, 1993

65. Avramov A, Cavanaugh J, Ozaktay C: The effects of controlled mechanical loading on group-II, III, and IV afferent units from the lumbar facet joint and surrounding tissue. J Bone Joint Surg 74A:1464–1471, 1992

66. Fuss FK, Bacher A: New aspects of the morphology and function of the human hip joint ligaments. Am J Anat 192:1–13, 1991

67. Singleton MC, Leveau BF: The hip joint: structure, stability, and stress. Phys Ther 55:957–973, 1975

68. Carli G, Fontani G, Meuci M: Static characteristics of muscle afferents from gluteus medius muscle: comparison with joint afferents of hip in cats. J Neurophysiol 45:1085–1095, 1981

69. Rossi A, Grigg P: Characteristics of hip joint

mechanoreceptors in the cat. J Neurophysiol 47: 1029–1042, 1982

70. Voss H: Tabelle der absoluten und relativen muskelspindelzahlen der menschlichen skelett-muskulatur. Anat Anz 129:562–572, 1971

71. Grieve GP: The hip. Physiotherapy 57:212–219, 1971

72. Dee R: Structure and function of hip joint innervation. Ann Royal Coll Surg Engl 45:357–374, 1969

73. Sjolander P, Johansson H, Sojka P et al: Sensory nerve endings in the cat cruciate ligaments: a morphological investigation. Neurosci Lett 102: 33–38, 1989

74. Grigg P: Response of joint afferent neurons in cat medial articular nerve to active and passive movements of the knee. Brain Res 118:482–485, 1976

75. Grigg P, Hoffman A: Properties of Ruffini afferents revealed by stress analysis of isolated sections of cat knee capsule. J Neurophysiol 47: 41–54, 1982

76. Grigg P, Greenspan BJ: Response of primate joint afferent neurons to mechanical stimulation of knee joint. J Neurophysiol 40:1–8, 1977

77. Solomonow M, D'Ambrosia R: Neural reflex arcs and muscle control of knee stability and motion. p. 389. In Scott WN (ed): Ligament and Extensor Mechanisms of the Knee: Diagnosis and Treatment. C.V. Mosby, St. Louis, 1991

78. Beynnon BD, Johnson RJ, Fleming B et al: The measurement of elongation of anterior cruciate-ligament grafts in vivo. J Bone Joint Surg Am 76: 520–531, 1994

79. Ciccotti M, Kerlan R, Perry J et al: An electromyographic analysis of the knee during functional activities; II. The anterior cruciate ligament-deficient and -reconstructed profiles. Am J Sports Med 22:651–658, 1994

80. McNair P, Marshall R: Landing characteristics in subjects with normal and anterior cruciate ligament deficient knee joints. Arch Phys Med Rehab 75:584–589, 1994

81. Nyland J, Shapiro R, Stine R et al: Relationship of fatigue run-rapid stop to ground reaction forces, lower extremity kinematics, and muscle activation. J Orthop Sports Phys Ther 20: 132–137, 1994

82. Palmitier R, An K, Scott S et al: Kinetic chain exercise in knee rehabilitation. Sports Med 11: 402–413, 1991

83. Zajac F, Gordon M: Determining muscle's force and action in multi-articular movement. Ex Sports Sci Rev 17:187–230, 1989

84. Stephens MM, Sammarco GJ: The stabilizing role of the lateral ligament complex and the ankle and subtalar joints. Foot & Ankle 13: 130–136, 1992

85. Brosky T, Nyland J, Nitz A et al: The ankle ligaments: considerations of syndesmotic injury and implications for rehabilitation. J Orthop Sports Phys Ther 21:197–205, 1995

86. Perry J: Gait Analysis: Normal and Pathological Function. Slack, New York, 1992

87. Rogers M: Dynamic foot biomechanics. J Orthop Sports Phys Ther 21:306–316, 1995

88. Robbins SE, Hanna AM: Running-related injury prevention through barefoot adaptations. Med Sci Sports Exerc 19:148–156, 1987

89. Van Ingen Schnau G: From rotation to translation: constraints on multi-joint movements and the unique action of bi-articular muscles. Human Movement Sci 8:301–337, 1989

90. Gracovetsky S: An hypothesis for the role of the spine in human locomotion: a challenge to current thinking. J Biomed Eng 7:205–216, 1985

91. Gracovetsky S, Farfan H, Helleur C: The abdominal mechanism. Spine 10:317–324, 1985

92. Gracovetsky S, Iacono S: Energy transfers in the spinal engine. J Biomed Eng 9:99–114, 1987

93. Norris CM: Spinal stabilisation. Physiother 81: 61–79, 1995

94. Kibler WB: Role of the scapula in the overhead throwing motion. Contemp Orthop 22:525–532, 1991

95. Cailliet R: The Shoulder in Hemiplegia. F.A. Davis, Philadelphia, 1980

96. Bouisett S, Zattara M: Biomechanical study of the programming of anticipatory postural adjustments associated with voluntary movement. J Biomechanics 20:735–742, 1987

97. Cordo P, Carlton L, Bevan L et al: Proprioceptive coordination of movement sequences: role of velocity and position information. J Neurophysiol 71:1848–1861, 1994

98. Marsden C, Merton P, Morton H: Servo action of the human thumb. J Physiol Lond 257:1–44, 1976

99. Gray G: Lower Extremity Functional Profile. Wynn Marketing, Inc., Adrian, MI, 1994

100. Farley C, Blickhan R, Saito J et al: Hopping frequency in humans: a test of how springs set stride frequency in bouncing gaits. J Appl Physiol 71:2127–2132, 1991

101. Chapman A, Sanderson D: Muscular coordina-

tion in sporting skills. p. 608. In Winters, J and Woo, S (eds): Multiple Muscle Systems: Biomechanics and Movement Organization. Springer-Verlag, New York, 1990

102. Stauber W: Eccentric action of muscles: physiology, injury, and adaptation. p. 157. In Pandolf, K (ed): Exercise and Sport Sciences Reviews, American College of Sports Medicine Series Vol. 17. Williams and Wilkins, Baltimore, 1989

103. Bullock-Saxton JE: Local sensation changes and altered hip muscle function following severe ankle sprain. Phys Ther 74:17–31, 1994

104. Wilkerson G, Nitz A: Dynamic ankle stability. J Sport Rehab 3:43–57, 1994

105. Nitz AJ: Limb denervation following anterior cruciate (ACL) reconstruction without tourniquet application. Phys Ther 68:822, 1988

106. Kleinrensink GJ, Stoekart R, Meulstee J et al: Lowered motor conduction velocity of the peroneal nerve after inversion trauma. Med Sci Sports Exerc 26:877–883, 1994

107. Dobner JJ, Nitz AJ: Post-meniscectomy tourniquet palsy and functional sequelae. Am J Sports Med 10:211–214, 1982

108. Schiable H, Schmidt R: Activation of group III and IV sensory units in medial articular nerve by local mechanical stimulation of knee joint. J Neurophysiol 49:35–44, 1983

109. Grigg P, Hoffman AH, Fogarty KE: Properties of golgi-mazzoni afferents in cat knee capsule, as revealed by mechanical studies of isolated joint capsule. J Neurophysiol 47:31–40, 1986

110. Schwartzman RJ: Reflex sympathetic dystrophy. Curr Opin Neurol Neurosurg 6:531–536, 1993

111. Na HS, Leem JW, Chang JM: Abnormalities of mechanoreceptors in a rat model of neuropathic pain: possible involvement in mediating mechanical alldynia. J Neurophysiol 70:522–528, 1993

112. Freeman M, Dean M, Hanham I: The etiology and prevention of functional instability of the foot. J Bone Joint Surg 47B:678–685, 1965

113. Kennedy J, Alexander I, Hayes K: Nerve supply of the human knee and its functional importance. Am J Sports Med 10:329–335, 1982

114. O'Connor BL, Palmoski MJ, Brandt KD: Neurogenic acceleration of degenerative joint lesions. J Bone Joint Surg 67A:562–572, 1985

115. O'Connor B, Visco D, Brandt K et al: Neurogenic acceleration of osteoarthritis. J Bone Joint Surg 74A:367–376, 1992

116. Greenwood C, Tatton W, Seniuk N, Biddle F: In-creased dopamine synthesis in aging substanstia nigra neurons. Neurobiol Aging 12:557–565, 1991

117. Tatton WG, Greenwood CE, Verrier MC et al: Different rates of age-related loss for four murine monoaminergic neuronal populations. Neurobiol Aging 12:543–556, 1991

118. Tatton W, Greenwood C, Seniuk N et al: Interactions between MPTP-induced and age-related neuronal death in a murine model of Parkinson's disease. Can J Neurol Sci 19:124–133, 1992

119. Himes B, Tessler A: Death of some dorsal root ganglion neurons and plasticity of others following sciatic nerve section in adult and neonatal rats. J Comp Neurol 284:215–230, 1989

120. Rotskenker S: Multiple modes and sites for the induction of axonal growth. TINS 11:363–366, 1988

121. Cooke T: Pathogenic mechanisms in polyarticular osteoarthritis. Clin Rheum Dis 11:203–238, 1985

122. Farfan HF: On the nature of arthritis. J Rheumatol 10(suppl 9):103–104, 1983

123. Forget R, Lamarre Y: Rapid elbow flexion in the absence of proprioceptive and cutaneous feedback. Human Neurobiol 6:27–37, 1987

124. Gordon J, Iyer M, Ghez C: Impairment of motor programming and trajectory control. Soc Neurosci Abstr 13:352, 1987

125. Flanders M, Helms Tillery SI, Soechting JF: Early stages in a sensorimotor transformation. Brain Behav Sci 15:309–320, 1992

126. Sainburg RL, Poizner H, Ghez C: Loss of proprioception produces deficits in interjoint coordination. J Neurophysiol 76:2136–2147, 1993

127. Nitz AJ, Dobner JJ, Kersey D: Nerve injury and grades II and III ankle sprains. Am J Sports Med 13:177–182, 1985

128. Herbison GJ: Effect of electrical stimulation on denervated muscle of rat. Arch Phys Med Rehab 52:516, 1971

129. DeLaat E, Visser C, Coene L et al: Nerve lesions in primary shoulder dislocations and humeral neck fractures. J Bone Joint Surg 76B:381–383, 1994

130. Nitz A: In Preparation

131. Levine JD, Dardick SJ, Basbaum AI et al: Reflex neurogenic inflammation: I. Contribution of the peripheral nervous system to spatially remote inflammatory responses that follow injury. J Neurosciences 5:1380–1386, 1985

132. Baxendale R, Ferrell W: Effect of knee joint affer-

ent discharge on transmission in flexion reflex pathways in decerebrate cats. J Physiol Lond 315:231–242, 1981

133. Baxendale R, Ferrell W, Wood L: Responses of quadriceps motor units to mechanical stimulation of knee joint receptors in the decerebrate cat. Brain Res 453:150–156, 1988

134. Grigg P, Harrigan EP, Fogarty KE: Segmental reflexes mediated by joint afferent neurons in cat knee. J Neurophysiol (Bethesda) 41:9–14, 1978

135. Marshall K, Tatton W: Joint receptors modulate short and long latency muscle responses in the awake cat. Exp Brain Res 83:137–150, 1990

136. Schiable H, Schmidt R, Willis W: Responses of spinal cord neurons to stimulation of articular afferent fibers in the cat. J Physiol (London) 372:575–593, 1986

137. Resnick D: Neuroarthropathy. p. 3154. In Resnick D, Niwayama G (eds): Diagnosis of Bone and Joint Disorders. W.B. Saunders, Philadelphia, 1988

138. Flood D, Coleman P: Neuron numbers and sizes in aging brain: comparisons of human, monkey and rodent data. Neurobiol Aging 9:453–463, 1988

139. Newton RA: Joint receptor contributions to reflexive and kinesthetic responses. Phys Ther 62:22–29, 1982

140. Spencer J, Hayes K, Alexander I: Knee joint effusion and quadriceps reflex inhibition in man. Arch Phys Med Rehab 65:171–177, 1984

141. Wilkerson GB: Treatment of the inversion ankle sprain through synchronous application of focal compression and cold. J Athl Training (J NATA) 26:220–237, 1991

142. Bosco C, Komi P, Ito A: A prestretch potentiation of human skeletal muscle during ballistic movement. Acta Physiologica Scand 114:557–565, 1982

143. Komi P: The stretch-shortening cycle and human power output. p. 27. In Jones NL, McCartney N, McComas A (eds): Human Muscle Power. Human Kinetics Publishers, Champaign, IL, 1986

144. Gray G. Chain Reaction. Course Lecture Notes, Wynn Marketing, Inc., 1990

145. Albert M: Physiologic and clinical principles of eccentrics. p. 11. In Albert, M (ed): Eccentric Muscle Training in Sports and Orthopaedics. Churchill Livingstone, New York, 1991

146. Wilk K, Voight M, Keirns M et al: Stretch-shortening drills for the upper extremities: theory and clinical application. J Orthop Sports Phys Ther 17:225–239, 1993

147. Andriacchi TP: Dynamics of knee malalignment. Orthop Clin North Am 25:395–403, 1994

148. Nyland JA: The effect of quadriceps femoris, hamstring, and placebo eccentric fatigue on knee and ankle dynamics during crossover cutting. Doctoral Dissertation, University of Kentucky, 1995

149. Kanje M, Rusovan A, Sisken B et al: Pretreatment of rats with pulsed electromagnetic fields enhances regeneration of the sciatic nerve. Bioelectromagnetics 14:353–359, 1993

150. Walker JL, Evans JM, Resig P et al: Enhancement of functional recovery following a crush lesion to the rat sciatic nerve by exposure to pulsed electromagnetic fields. Exp Neurol 125:302–305, 1994

151. Aaron RK, Mck. Ciombor D: Therapeutic effects of electromagnetic fields in the stimulation of connective tissue repair. J Cell Biochem 52:42–46, 1993

152. Cane V, Botti P, Soana S: Pulsed magnetic fields improve osteoblast activity during the repair of an experimental osseous defect. J Orthop Res 11:664–670, 1993

153. Heckman J, Ryaby J, McCabe J et al: Acceleration of tibial fracture-healing by non-invasive, low-intensity pulsed ultrasound. J Bone Joint Surg 76A:26–34, 1994

154. Wang SJ, Lewallen D, Bolander M et al: Low intensity ultrasound treatment increases strength in a rat femoral fracture model. J Orthop Res 12:40–47, 1994

155. Ryan L: Mechanical stability, muscle strength and proprioception in the functionally unstable ankle. Australian Physiotherapy 40:41–47, 1994

156. Konradsen L, Ravn J: Ankle instability caused by prolonged peroneal reaction time. Acta Orthop Scand 61:388–390, 1990

157. Konradsen L, Ravn J: Prolonged peroneal reaction time in ankle instability. Int J Sports Med 12:290–292, 1991

158. Adelsberg S, Pittman M, Alexander H: Lower extremity fractures: relationship to reaction time and coordination time. Arch Phys Med Rehab 70:737–739, 1989

159. Spalding TJ, Kiss J, Kyberd P et al: Driver reaction times after total knee replacement. J Bone Joint Surg 76B:754–756, 1994

160. Gauffin H, Tropp H, Odenrick P: Effect of ankle disk training on postural control in patients with

functional instability of the ankle joint. Int J Sports Med 9:141–144, 1988

161. Hoffman M, Payne VG: The effects of proprioceptive ankle disk training on healthy subjects. J Orthop Sports Phys Ther 21:90–93, 1995

162. Curl W, Markey K, Mitchell W: Agility training following anterior cruciate ligament reconstruction. Clin Orthop 172:133–136, 1983

163. Tibone J, Antich T, Fanton G et al: Functional analysis of anterior cruciate ligament instability. Am J Sports Med 14:276–284, 1986

164. Ihara H, Nakayama A: Dynamic joint control training for knee ligament injuries. Am J Sports Med 14:309–315, 1986

165. Walla D, Albright J, McAuley E et al: Hamstring control and the unstable anterior cruciate ligament deficient knee. Am J Sports Med 13:34–39, 1985

166. Kaalund S, Sinkjaer T, Arendt-Nielsen L, Simonsen O: Altered timing of hamstring muscle action in anterior cruciate ligament deficient patients. Am J Sports Med 18:245–248, 1990

167. Gauffin H, Tropp H: Altered movement and muscular activation patterns during the one-legged jump in patients with an old anterior cruciate ligament rupture. Am J Sports Med 20:182–192, 1992

168. Tropp H, Ekstrand J, Gillquist J: Stabiliometry in functional instability of the ankle and its value in predicting injury. Med Sci Sports Exerc 16:64–66, 1984

169. Oeffinger DE: Proprioception in the normal and ACL reconstructed knee. Master's Thesis, University of Kentucky, 1995

170. Delitto A, McKowen J, McCarthy J et al: Electrically elicited co-contraction of thigh musculature after anterior cruciate ligament surgery. Phys Ther 68:45–50, 1988

171. Delitto A, Rose S, McKowen J et al: Electrical stimulation versus voluntary exercise in strengthening thigh musculature after anterior cruciate ligament surgery. Phys Ther 68:660–663, 1988

172. Lopriesti C, Kirkendall D, Street G et al: Quadriceps insufficiency following repair of the anterior cruciate ligament. J Orthop Sports Phys Ther 9:245–249, 1988

173. Sinacore D, Delitto A, King D et al: Type II fiber activation with electrical stimulation. A preliminary report. Phys Ther 70:416–422, 1990

174. Draper V: Electromyographic biofeedback and recovery of quadriceps femoris muscle function following anterior cruciate ligament reconstruction. Phys Ther 70:11–17, 1990

175. Bohannon RW, Gajdosik RL: Spinal nerve root compression—some clinical implications. Phys Ther 67:376–382, 1987

176. Kottke F, Halpern D, Easton J et al: The training of coordination. Arch Phys Med Rehab 59:567–572, 1978

177. Irrgang J, Whitney S, Cox E: Balance and proprioceptive training for rehabilitation of the lower extremity. J Sport Rehab 3:68–83, 1994

178. Bandy WD, Rusche KR, Tekulve FY: Reliability and limb symmetry for five unilateral functional tests of the lower extremities. Isokinetics and Exercise Science 4:108–111, 1994

179. Barber S, Noyes F, Mangine R et al: Quantitative assessment of functional limitations in normal and anterior cruciate deficient knee. Clin Orthop 255:204–214, 1990

180. Brosky T: Intrarater reliability of selected clinical outcome measures following ACL reconstruction. J Orthop Sports Phys Ther (submitted)

3

Functional Outcomes and Measuring Function

RUSSELL PAINE

BRUCE BROWNSTEIN

DAVID MACHA

Measuring treatment outcomes in medicine has become a watchword for the orthopaedic and sports medicine professions, both for the physician and therapist. In this time of reorganization of the manner in which medicine is delivered and paid for, outcomes are perceived to be a tool by which services may be justified as cost-effective interventions in the disease/injury process. In theory, it is easily argued that measurement of patient status before and after treatment will provide a rational manner in which to determine what treatments achieve the goals of improving a patient's functional and health status, as well as their quality of life.

Difficulties arise on a few different levels. First, the challenge of developing measurement tools has not yet been fully met. Second, no one tool is appropriate for all types of patients, injuries, and diseases. Third, some treatments (i.e., total joint arthroplasty, ligament reconstructions) may take years to determine whether either health or life quality has been improved. Fourth, in patient populations such as sports medicine, the injury affects performance of an activity or group of activities that contribute to the patient's lifestyle and quality of life, rather than the individual's ability to function in daily life.

This chapter presents the conceptual basis for measuring outcomes, identifies the factors that are at issue with measuring function and performance, and presents the different methods now available for measuring performance in sports medicine. Outcome measurement tools pertaining to the various areas covered by the following chapters will be included in the appropriate chapter.

Concepts Underlying Outcome Measurement

MANAGEMENT ISSUES

Outcome represents one piece of the quality puzzle. Measuring an outcome, from any aspect of the patient's condition (Fig. 3-1), provides the data by which quality of care decisions can be made. Goals of continuous improvement in outcome can be implemented, as long as realistic time frames are adopted and the patient, not merely the cost or number of treatments, remains the focus of the measurement of successful treatment.

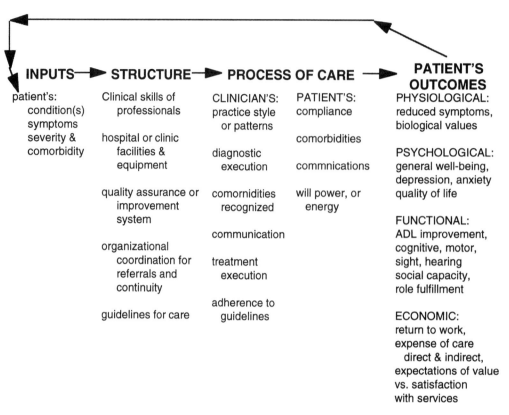

FIGURE 3-1 *Model for orthopaedic outcomes research. Similar factors apply to outpatient sports and orthopaedic physical therpay. Note that positive outcomes may occur in several aspects of function while other aspects may remain unchanged. Feedback between patient and clinician is essential. In the physical therapy model, interaction between other parties (physician, third-party payors, etc.) should be accounted for. (From Bradham DD,[6] with permission.)*

Certain aspects of care are relatively easy to evaluate. Broad measures of function such as return to work status can be easily measured, along with the cost associated with the care of those patients. Perhaps one of the reasons that costs are often the focus of outcomes is that they are relatively easy to measure. Cost is less subjective than function. Solomon et al.[1] measured the cost of treatment of injuries to dancers. In that study, they were able to track the participation (or lack thereof) of a company of professional dancers and the lost time as a result of injury. They showed that a well-trained injury management system that had the cooperation and participation of the dancers and health care providers was cost-effective. Savoie et al.[2] measured the cost and time associated with the return to work of individuals with work-related rotator cuff tears. They showed that the attention to injury provided by immediate diagnosis and care resulted in reduced cost and faster return to work than delayed treatment and diagnosis imposed by a gatekeeper system (Table 3-1). The finding that early treatment usually has better results is echoed by Di Fabio et al.[3] in their analysis of outcomes for patients with low back pain who

TABLE 3-1 *Comparison of costs and outcomes of workers' compensation patients with rotator cuff repair surgery in versus out of a gatekeeper system*

VARIABLE	PRIMARY REFERRAL	GATEKEEPER SYSTEM	COMBINED
Number	34	16	50
Medical cost	$13,512.62	$35,537.47	$20,683.50
Pay + Settlement	$12,358.02	$65,373.13	$29,618.75
Total cost	$25,870.64	$100,910.60	$50,302.26
Time to surgery	4 mo	10 mo	5 mo
Return to full work	6 mo	18 mo	10 mo

(Data from Savoie FH,[2] with permission.)

receive worker's compensation. They found that early intervention (less than 6 weeks) following injury resulted in better outcomes for patients, defined in terms of returning to work and extent of treatment. Patients with mechanical low back pain had better short-term outcomes and return to work percentages than patients with disk disease. In general, early treatment minimizes the physical and psychological effects of immobilization and deconditioning.

The traditional paradigm of a professional organization model emphasizes technical skill and individual responsibility. In this type of setting, outcome measurements are used to change the type of treatment that an individual uses, placing the responsibility for achieving "better" outcomes on the therapist. The therapist is evaluated, in part, on clinical skills and knowledge base. The organization (or insurance company) uses a quality assurance approach to retroactively evaluate performance, based upon relatively rigid expectations that change slowly.

Figure 3-2 lists the characteristics of a "traditional" organizational model versus a model based upon the "total quality management" model. Under a quality management paradigm, outcomes are used to monitor the performance of the therapist and the organization via a pro-

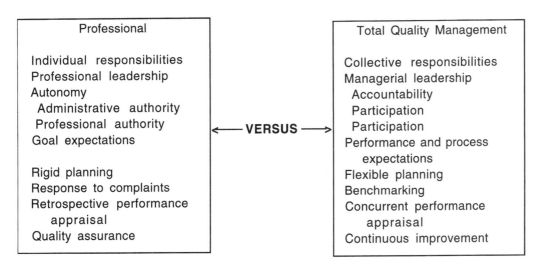

FIGURE 3-2 *Differences between two organizational models in health care: Professional and Total Quality Management. (From McLaughlin CP and Kaluzny AD,[32] with permission.)*

cess that includes participation, proactive planning, and involvement of all parties in the goal of improving outcomes. That means improving patient satisfaction with their treatment and the results of that treatment, provided at a reasonable cost.

Outcome research also helps to standardize care. A wide variation of treatments, some more effective or appropriate than others, can be used for a given diagnosis or injury.[4] Monitoring outcomes can identify a standard of care. The treatment approach with the best outcome should be available to all patients. Identification and dissemination of outcome information, coupled with strong clinical teaching, will improve the level of care in the physical therapy industry.

Outcome measurement is part of the new environment in which we now operate. This environment is highlighted by shifts in the organizational and service delivery focus, financial incentives, delivery orientation and accountability of the health care professions. These changes are summarized in Table 3-2. The use of outcome measures along with patient satisfaction is a way of tracking quality and accountability by shifting the focus towards patient-based results and optimal practice patterns and away from cost-based results, gross clinical measures (such as mortality, morbidity, complication rates, etc.) and measures of compliance.[5] The newer measures of satisfaction, effectiveness, return to work, and outcome are more in line with managed care-driven financial systems, which include capitation, contracted care, shared risk, and premiums for efficiency. Outcome measurement is our only mechanism for demonstrating the value of and receiving appropriate compensation for the work that is performed.

Bradham[6] identified the characteristics of a full blown medical outcome study (Fig. 3-1). Clearly, the health care management challenge is to identify that mix of structural, process, and outcome variables that will provide the best possible environment for achieving high quality, high satisfaction services, with outcomes that can be improved over time as new techniques and knowledge are incorporated into our care system. The model places equal weight on participation of the patient and skill of the provider.

TABLE 3-2 *Changing health care paradigms: description of changes in the way that certain aspects of health care management are evolving under the managed care model*

	OLD ENVIRONMENT	NEW ENVIRONMENT
Organization Focus	Hospitals	Networks
	Independent physician practices	Physician group contracting
	Independent provider services	Integrated delivery systems
Service delivery focus and style	Specialist physicians	Primary care providers
	Individual providers	Teams of providers
Financial Incentives	Fee for service with controls	Capitation and contracts
	Maximize care and revenue	Minimize/optimize care, cost
	Minimal risk to providers	Shared risk
	Revenue expands to cover cost	Efficiency and competitive premiums
Delivery Orientation	Clinically based	Clinical/functional outcomes, satisfaction
	Illness care	Illness prevention, healthy populations
	Illness episodes	Continuum of care
Accountability	Controls against overuse and abuse	Monitoring accessibility and underuse
	Individual providers	Networks, managed care organizations
	Insurers and third-party payors	Employers, government report cards, contractual accountability
	Regulation and accreditation	

(From Witter DM,[5] with permission.)

CLINICAL ISSUES

Berwick[7] identified four aspects for medical effectiveness research. They are:

1. Efficacy (what works in research settings)
2. Effectiveness (whether efficacious treatments work in the clinic)
3. Process of care delivery (does a delivery system enhance or reduce quality?)
4. Purpose of care (values of the clinician, patient, and society that underlie the care).

A fifth aspect should be added to this list. It is *appropriateness*—using effective treatments for the suitable patients and diagnoses.[4] The first two factors are most closely related to outcomes research, as it is used to measure orthopaedic and sports physical therapy. Outcomes tend to be specific to the medical condition.[6] Our challenge is to find the treatment techniques that produce the best results. This implies that we must be creative in our approaches to improving quality, constantly working to improve the processes that we use to deliver care and measure its effectiveness.[8,9]

The three major variables of outcome measurement are function, pain, and patient satisfaction.[10] Function can be measured in many different ways and is dependant on lifestyle. Athletes and other active individuals (either recreationally or occupationally) cannot always be measured using the same scale. Acceptable shoulder function is different for a bus driver than a tennis player. The scale used to measure function must be the appropriate one for the patient population. Acceptable criteria for measurement will vary depending upon the patient's lifestyle. Pain is relatively easy to measure using visual analogue scales or a similar instrument. Patient satisfaction is multifactorial and includes the above variables as well as cost and process. (Table 3-3) Small et al.[10] list additional outcomes upon which outcome measurement can be based. These include symptomatic relief, work status, sports activities and participation, and complications. This text is primarily interested in the measurement of function. The chapters on treatment are oriented towards the various functional scales available to the clinician.

A variable that is rarely examined in the course of physical therapy treatments is time. Time works both with and against physical therapy treatments. Time to heal and recover from injury is balanced against time lost as a result of injury. Function and goals can also be measured against this variable. Return to activities of daily living (ADL) generally occurs over a much shorter time span than return to full function and sports. The plasticity of the neuromuscular system is a powerful factor, but demands time to reorganize after injury,[8] (Fig. 3-3).

Measuring clinical performance via outcomes requires addressing whether effective care was rendered in an appropriate time frame in a safe environment resulting in an improvement that was as good as could be expected given the patient's condition and available resources.[11] Measures of clinical performance can be used to assess the impact of changes in the nature and style of delivery of care, demonstrate accountability for patient results, and provide guidelines for providers. To accomplish this task, the measurement tool must be sensitive and specific enough to detect the relationship between good care and good results, as well as identify whether those who had bad results were victims of bad care and not just poor prognoses.

Physical therapy, as well as most orthopaedic care, is directed toward recovering patient function. Unfortunately, function, like quality, is a naturally elusive quantity that is difficult to measure directly and objectively. Many diseases (e.g., diabetes or hypertension) can be monitored directly and the effectiveness of the treatment intervention can be defined by a quantified measure, blood sugar or blood pressure, and the time it took to achieve acceptable results. Orthopaedic and sports therapy is not blessed by such a simple measurement tool. We must make do with performance measures that may be limited in scope and are not standardized. The tool most often used in our field is the rating scale.

Clearly, an outcome is a relative value. Almost all rating scales are biased in one form or

TABLE 3-3 *Outcome variables for evaluating orthopedic procedures (example: arthroscopic menisectomy)*

PRINCIPAL OUTCOMES	
A. Pain	D. Occupational and avocational consequences
1. With activity	1. Work status
2. With rest	a. Employed
3. Location	b. Unemployed
4. Medication use	c. School
B. Functional status	2. Work consequences
1. Activities of daily living	a. Type of occupation
2. Functional independence	b. Off work
3. Occupational, social recreational activities	c. Impaired at work
C. Satisfaction	3. Housework
1. With symptom relief, functional improvement	4. Shopping
2. With process of care	5. Yard work
3. With costs of care	6. Sports
Additional outcomes:	a. Recreational
A. Health status	b. Nonrecreational with possible financial implications
1. Physical	c. Scholastic
2. Emotional	d. Collegiate
3. Social	e. Professional
B. Relief of disease-specific symptoms	7. Altered participation in appropriate sport
1. Swelling	a. Performance
2. Locking	b. Type of sport
3. Giving way	8. Dancing
4. Shifting	E. Complications
5. Catching	1. Hemarthrosis
6. Decreased strength	2. Thromboembolic disease
C. Improvement in disease-specific function	3. Infection
1. Squatting	i. Wound
2. Stair climbing and descending	ii. Joint
3. Gait disturbance	4. Artery of nerve damage
4. Ambulatory aids	5. Anesthetic complications
5. Running	6. Instrument breakage
6. Pivoting	7. Death
7. Jumping	
8. Endurance	
9. Transferring from low chair	
10. Transferring into and out of small automobiles	

(From Small NC,[10] with permission.)

another, either by the weighting given to certain aspects of function or by the patient population being measured.[12] Function is a difficult thing to measure, as all values assigned are subjective. Even scales that measure function on a yes/no basis (see ch. 4), show subjectivity in the selection of questions to be asked. Ideally, a rating scale will be independent of either patient diagnosis or activity level. Practically speaking, no such measurement scale meets that criteria. Also, a functional scale should be responsive and accurately reflect long-term changes in function level, not merely short-term improvement as a result of clinical or surgical intervention.[13] No matter the effort put into designing and validating a functional rating or evaluation scale, it is

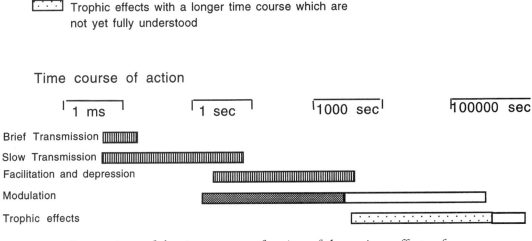

FIGURE 3-3 *Comparison of the time course of action of the various effects of physical therapy. A description of the characteristics of the response is shown in the lefthand column. Vertical shading shows action in the shorter term. (From Dale J and Kid G,[33] with permission.)*

not yet possible to reduce a person's ability to carry out everyday activities to a single number.

Despite that limitation, functional scales are valuable in judging relative improvements as a result of therapeutic intervention. Short-term results of treatment, however, are not predictors of long-term results. The need to prove efficacy and effectiveness of physical therapy treatment is being imposed from both within and without the medical profession. The most vital component of measuring outcomes is demonstrating how our treatment protocols can contribute to the most satisfactory recovery of the patient in terms of function and cost. Unfortunately, to date there is no standard of measure that is uniformly accepted as reproducible, reliable, and accurate. Moreover, the higher the preinjury level of activity, the more difficult it becomes to use standard functional tools to measure function. If a professional athlete is able to meet almost any standard of measurement but one, he or she cannot perform at the level demanded of them. Therefore, the concept of measuring performance subjectively was introduced into rating scales by Tibone and Bradley.[14]

Performance Measurement and Function Testing

Sports in particular demand some form of performance measurement. In a certain sense, the ability to successfully perform a sports activity can be easily answered in a yes/no fashion. Can you participate in your sport or athletic endeavor at the level you could before your injury without symptoms? In rehabilitation of sports injuries, we must have some mechanism by which progression can be determined as objectively as possible. In the early 1980s, Daniel et al.[15] showed us the importance of objective testing for the postoperative anterior cruciate ligament (ACL) patient population. In addition to isokinetic and KT-1000 testing, Daniel et al. required patients to undergo two simple, yet specific functional tests: the single leg hop for distance and a 40-yard shuttle run.[15]

Daniel et al. showed that these simple, functional tests can be valuable tools for postoperative ACL assessment. Functional testing is beginning to be included in the battery of tests for lower extremity function, along with isokinetic testing, which is still used to provide information regarding a patient's ability to participate in sports activities. Unfortunately, isokinetic testing and batteries of "functional" tests do not correlate strongly.[16,17] It still behooves us to perform some measure of isolated muscle capability along with tests of the entire kinetic chain.

In an unpublished study, Engle compared concentric and eccentric isokinetic testing of people with patella tendon ACL reconstruction to a series of functional tests (Fig. 3-4) including timed hop for distance, one-legged hop, and the shuttle run.[16] None of the tests correlated with the isokinetic data, except for a weak correlation between 60 degrees per second concentric testing and the one-legged hop. Barber et al.[18] also reported a correlation between the one-legged hop asymmetry and 60 degrees per second quadriceps deficits in ACL deficient patients. Greenberger and Paterno[17] found only a weak correlation between isokinetic testing at 240 degrees per second and a one-legged hop. They concluded that both types of test were necessary in evaluating the strength level of patients with knee problems.

Seto et al.[19] found a correlation between quadriceps and hamstring isokinetic testing and functional activity scores (Cincinnati knee scale and Lysholm) for patients with intra-articular, but not extra-articular, reconstruction. Anderson et al.[20] found a correlation between some measures of strength and three functional tests (agility run, 40-yard dash, and vertical jump). Eccentric measures were no better than concentric measures. Wilk et al.[21] found a correlation between isokinetic peak torque at 180 and 300 degrees/second subjective knee scores (Cincinnati knee scale). In all three above studies, the r value was never greater than .7, suggesting that other unmeasured factors were also involved. One of the studies reported finding significance between subjective knee rating, and functional testing with an r value of .31.[21]

An alternative to functional testing using hop and run tests is to identify proprioceptive deficiencies by measuring aspects of position sense. Impaired proprioception probably plays a role in the loss of functional performance. (Fig. 1-

12) The proprioceptive system may be damaged following a ligamentous injury.[22] Barrack[23] found a 25 percent variation in position sense in subjects who were ACL deficient. Proprioceptive losses have also been implicated in reaching and targeting the upper extremity.[24] Most proprioceptive and position sense studies of the lower extremity have been conducted in a nonfunctional position and require special equipment that is not readily available. Andersen et al.[25] compared open versus closed chain measurements of static joint position sense. They concluded that reproduction of knee joint position was superior in the closed chain position, probably as a result of increased muscle spindle and Golgi tendon organ activity.

Function testing is easier to perform in the lower extremity than in the upper. Functional tests and equipment for measuring lower extremity performance is more prevalent. Upper extremity isokinetic testing is reliable, but functional tests for the upper extremity are not as easily measured. A tennis player can either serve the ball accurately at 100 miles per hour or not. "Functional" treatment progressions have been developed for upper extremity pathologies, little equipment (other than research-related EMG and video) can be used to evaluate various aspects of function.

A major consideration in functional testing of the upper extremity is selected tasks that replicate the skills necessary for the upper extremity. The use of push-ups, modified push-ups, or arm spins[26] may offer information regarding symmetry of effort, or may demonstrate obvious stability problems, but does little in the way of defining arm function. Upper extremity function in sports occurs primarily in the open chain, involves reaching, placement, and tracking skills, and requires resistance of forces when contact occurs. Forwell and Carnahan[27] measured the difference in reaching tasks between subjects with anterior laxity and normals. They found that controlled reaching tasks were unaffected when normal vision conditions existed. This implies that kinesthetic deficits noted in the isolated condition by Smith and Brunoli[28] may not have functional consequences.

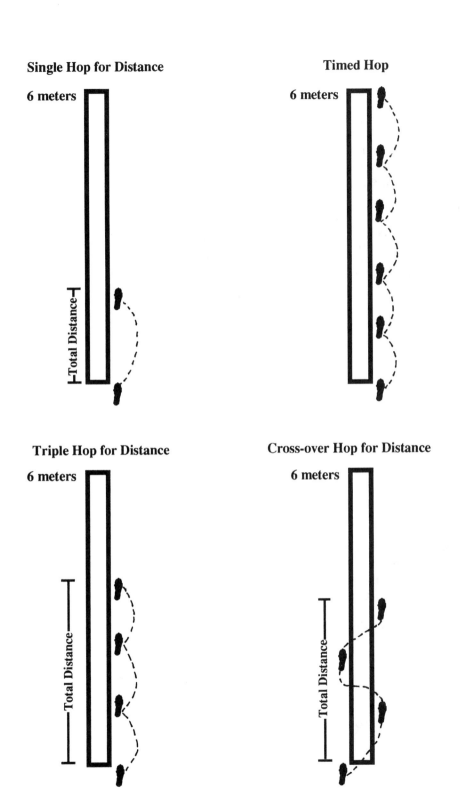

Single Hop for Distance

6 meters

Total Distance

Timed Hop

6 meters

Triple Hop for Distance

6 meters

Total Distance

Cross-over Hop for Distance

6 meters

Total Distance

The courses for the four fuction tests.

FIGURE 3-4 *Hop tests (From Barber SD,*[18] *with permission.)*

A successful outcome is achievement of a level of function that is equal to or greater than that which was present before injury, if possible. Our goal is to return the individual to their preinjury activities. Outcome studies that do not question or test the ability of a patient to resume full preinjury activity fall short in describing the outcome. Some insurance carriers believe that participation in athletic activities are not essential to everyday function. They believe that if a patient is able to walk and perform ADL, then full function has been achieved. The authors believe that obtaining the maximum amount of function and strength will lead to a greater long-term outcome with reduced reinjury rates. The burden is clearly on our profession to prove this aspect of effective physical therapy treatments.

Tools for Functional Testing of the Lower Extremity

At present, there are several systems that are used for grading outcomes following joint injury/surgery. These are reviewed in the chapters on regional function. They include the Cincinnati Knee Ligament system, Lysholm scale, Simple Shoulder Test (upper extremity), and Oswestry (lumbar) scores, among others. Rating scales offer some objectivity in evaluating activity level changes as a result of injury, but do not offer measures of performance.

Lephart et al.[29] has suggested "low-tech" alternatives to the "high-tech" computerized devices. His low-tech approach includes the timed hop for distance, the 40-yard obstacle course run, cocontraction lateral shuttles, the single leg hop test, and the vertical jump. Hopping and jumping tests are reviewed by Jenkins, Bronner, and Mangine in this volume.[30] Paine et al.[31] has established a "normal" figure-of-eight obstacle course time of 9.5 seconds for high school football players.

In short, almost any training drill or portion of a functional progression can be used as a functional "test." Proven validity and reliability of the movement skill being measured makes that measurement a useful testing tool. Continued research into testing and measurement procedures will contribute to the ability of physical therapists to justify our treatment protocols.

The need to develop functional testing and treatment protocols has led to the development of several commercially available devices. These new testing and training devices can be categorized into two groups: stable and unstable platform testing. The products that measure balance and proprioception with unstable platforms are the K.A.T., Biodex Stability System, and STAR Station. The stable platform testing systems are the Cybex Fastex and Neurocom Balance Master. Neurocom also makes systems that use an unstable platform as well.

Objective static balance testing devices have been introduced to quantify deficits and treat injuries that affect balance. Patients with balance and proprioceptive deficits may become at risk for injury as they participate in more strenuous activity. The interrelationship between neuromuscular factors and postural control makes it imperative to have specific and reproducible testing procedures to help identify at-risk patients.

The following is a review of currently available devices:

BREG K.A.T. The Breg Kinesthetic Activity Trainer (K.A.T.), (Fig. 3-5) is a device that utilizes all three systems that subserve balance and postural control—visual, proprioceptive, and vestibular. The primary system stressed is the proprioceptive. The K.A.T. 2000 offers the user a Windows-based system for measuring static and dynamic balance. Test data are described in terms of a "balance index" for both static and dynamic balance. The static balance index is calculated by the ability to maintain a centered position on the unstable platform. The system can also be used to match computer generated images to measure dynamic balance. The system offers visual feedback via these images, as well as protocols that can be used for specific balance deficits and injuries. The K.A.T. 2000 system offers handrails and a large circular grid with clearly marked foot positions, as well as charting

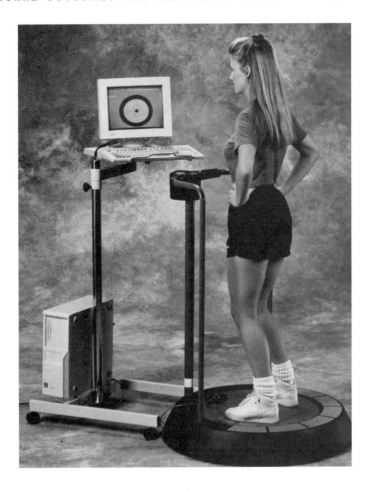

FIGURE 3-5 *Breg K.A.T.*

and note writing capability. The K.A.T. 1000 is a more basic system, which has a digital display that provides feedback by measuring relative pressure in a bladder placed under the balance platform. Objective assessment can be done with the K.A.T. 1000 balance measures. K.A.T. 2000 costs $5,995, and K.A.T. 1000, $1,395.

Advantages

- Cost
- Very short learning curve
- User friendly software (K.A.T. 2000)
- Reproducible testing protocols (K.A.T. 2000)
- Transportable with movable force sensors for individualized testing (K.A.T. 2000)

- Allows multiplane training
- Reliability studies have been performed with ongoing research funded by company

Disadvantages

- Testing and training may not carry over into dynamic, functional movement

CHATTANOOGA BALANCE SYSTEM. The Chattanooga Balance System (Fig. 3-6) measures and records a patient's "absolute" center of gravity utilizing a pair of patented foot plates. The plates each have four force transducers, which allow the user to locate the mean center of balance. The system allows testing in either sitting or standing positions, making it appropriate for a

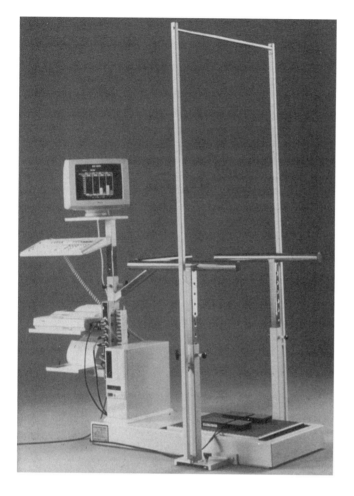

FIGURE 3-6 *Chattanooga Balance System.*

wide range of patients including orthopaedic, sports, and neurologic pathologies. The balance system can be used for proprioceptive exercises on either a stable or moving platform. Visual feedback can be added to the protocols. The software allows for documentation of sessions as well as comparative analysis over time. The cost is $25,000 for the base system.

Advantages

- Easy reproducibility of patient's stance and testing positions allows for more reliable testing
- Visual feedback for patient and tester
- Reliability studies already done

Disadvantages

- Single plane training and rehabilitation
- Long-term testing data not available

STAR STATION. The STAR (stability testing and rehabilitation) Station is designed for assessment, documentation, and rehabilitation of the closed chain. The system allows for triplane movement at the foot, ankle, knee, and hip joints. Weight-bearing ROM is quantified, as are mean balance and deviations. The STAR Station combines ROM, strength, and proprioceptive training during weight bearing. Visual feedback is provided. Progress reports, daily notes, and submissable insurance documentation are also available with the STAR Station. The cost is $26,259 for this base system.

Advantages

- Computer-assisted assessment
- Objective documentation
- Real-time animated rehabilitation

Disadvantages

- Difficult to reproduce original stance position
- Reliability studies needed

FASTEX. The Fastex (Fig. 3-7) is a series of force platforms that interface with a computer to provide balance, movement skills, and reaction time measurement and training. The system can be expanded and combined with a large screen television in order to provide realistic size, visual guidance, and feedback. The force platforms can be arranged in several formats, from two rows of four platforms (basic system) to four rows

(two of four, two of six). The Fastex measures static balance via the force and frequency of oscillations of the foot during stance. Dynamic movement skills are challenged by visual cuing regarding the next movement direction. Hopping and jumping skills also can be measured and trained. The system allows for a wide range of balance and movement testing that can be used in a variety of pathologies. The cost is $17,500 for the base system.

Advantages

- Functional movement patterns
- Allows plyometric and reaction time testing and measurement
- User-programmable patterns and test measurements
- Excellent visual feedback and patient response
- Company has experience in other testing/evaluation devices

Disadvantages

- Cost of full system
- Lack of reliability studies
- Space requirements, not portable

BIODEX STABILITY SYSTEM. The Biodex stability system (Fig. 3-8) is a platform that is similar to the Breg K.A.T. system. Neuromuscular control is assessed by measuring dynamic postural control on a surface of varying stability. The platform may be allowed to tilt up to 20 degrees. Data regarding the patient's ability to maintain a central position on the platform are expressed in a stability index. The results also provide information of percentage of time during the test spent in the four quadrants of the platform. The product allows the user to trace a pattern on the screen to provide training. The system can be interfaced with a computer for playing proprioception controlled games. The cost is $6,995.

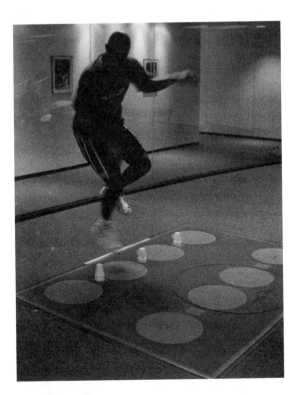

FIGURE 3-7 *Fastex.*

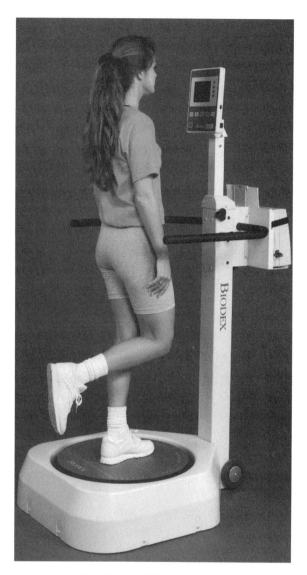

FIGURE 3-8 *Biodex Stability System.*

Advantages

- Quick, easy testing format
- Portable—device on wheels and can be moved around clinic
- Company supporting research on reliability and reproducibility
- Company has experience in other testing/evaluation devices

Disadvantage

- Interpretation of results
- No published reliability studies
- Use as a training device is limited for athletes beyond early rehabilitation phases

NEUROCOM BALANCE MASTER SYSTEMS. The purpose of the Neurocom (Fig. 3-9) balance master systems is to assess, quantify, and train persons with balance and mobility dysfunctions. The system uses predicted and unpredicted responses to movement in progressively more difficult tasks. Systems include a force plate of 18 inches, and a longer version, either stationary (Balance Master model) or moveable (Smart and Pro models). Tests can be performed to isolate visual, vestibular, and somatosensory function in the advanced models. Perturbations may be either expected or unexpected, requiring a wide range of postural adjustments. Real time feedback with graphic reports describe center of gravity movements. The cost is $12,000 for basic Balance Master, which is upgradable to other systems.

Advantages

- Well-documented body of literature regarding the test parameters
- Able to make distinctions between different contributory inputs to balance
- Reliability and validity demonstrated

Disadvantages

- Cost of full system
- Basic system cannot be used for testing
- Space requirements

Summary

Testing of function and performance is an exciting area. As products become available to measure a wide range of movement and proprioceptive skills, our ability to measure function

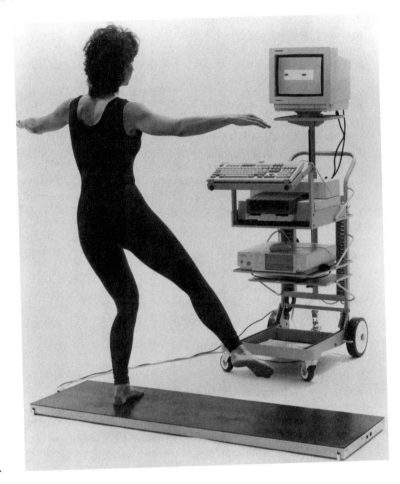

FIGURE 3-9 *Neurocom.*

improves. The questions remain: What do we need to measure? How do we interpret that data? Is the test meaningful? Is it reproducible and reliable? Great strides are being made in the clinic and by manufacturers to provide products in this area.

References

1. Solomon R, Micheli LJ, Solomon, J et al: The "cost" of injuries in a professional ballet company: anatomy of a season. Med Probl Art 10:3–10, 1995
2. Savoie FH, Field LD, Jenkins RN: Costs analysis of successful rotator cuff surgery: an outcome study. Comparison of gatekeeper system in surgical patients. Arthroscopy 11:672–676, 1995
3. Di Fabio RP, Mackey G, Holte JB: Physical therapy outcomes for patients receiving workers' compensation following treatment for herniated lumbar disc and mechanical low back pain. J. Orthop Sports Phys Ther 23:180–187, 1996
4. Keller RB: How outcomes research should be done. p. 487. In Matsen, FA, Fu FH, Hawkins RJ (eds): The Shoulder: A Balance of Mobility and Stability. AAOS, Rosemont, 1993
5. Witter DM: Transforming paradigms for provider information systems. Quality Management Health Care 4:7–13, 1996
6. Bradham DD: Outcomes research in orthopedics: history, perspective, concepts, and future. Arthroscopy 10:493–501, 1994
7. Berwick DM: Health services research and quality of care. Med Care 27:763–771, 1989
8. Murdock M: Creating, improving, and innovating. Quality Management in Health Care 2:56–61, 1994

9. de Bono E: Creativity and quality. Quality Management Health Care 2:1–4, 1994

10. Small NC, Sledge CB, Katz JN: A conceptual framework for outcomes research in arthroscopic meniscectomy: results of a group process. Arthroscopy 10:486–492, 1994

11. Palmer RH: Measuring clinical performance to provide information for quality improvement. Quality Management Health Care 4:1–6, 1996

12. Bulstrode CJK: Outcome measurements and their analysis. p. 1. In Pynsent P, Fairbank J, Carr A (eds): Outcome Measures in Orthopedics. Butterworth Heinemann, Oxford, 1993

13. Johanson NA, Charlson ME, Szatrowski TP, et al: A self-administered hip-rating questionnaire for the assessment of outcome after total hip replacement. J Bone Surg 74-A:587–597, 1992

14. Tibone JE, Bradley JP: Evaluation of treatment outcomes for the athlete's shoulder. p. 519. In Matsen FA, Fu FH, Hawkins RJ (eds): The Shoulder: A Balance of Mobility and Stability. AAOS, Rosemont, 1993

15. Daniel D, Malcolm L, Stone ML et al: Quantification of knee stability and function. Contemp Orthop 5:83–91, 1982

16. Engle RP: Comparison of isokinetic and functional tests. Unpublished data.

17. Greenberger HB, Paterno MV: Relationship of knee extensor strength and hopping test performance in the assessment of lower extremity function. J Orthop Sports Phys Ther 22:202–206, 1995

18. Barber SD, Noyes FR, Mangine RE et al: Quantitative assessment of functional limitations in normal and ACL knees. Clin Orth Rel Res 255:204–214, 1990

19. Seto JL, Orofino AS, Morrisey MC et al: Assessment of quadriceps/hamstring strength, knee ligament stability, functional and sports activity levels five years after anterior cruciate ligament reconstruction. AM J Sports Med 16:170–180, 1988

20. Anderson MA, Gieck JH, Perrin D et al: The relationships among isometric, isotonic, and isokinetic concentric and eccentric quadriceps and hamstring force and three components of athletic performance. J Orthop Sports Phys Ther 14:114–120, 1991

21. Wilk KE, Romaniello WT, Soscia SM et al: The relationship between subjective knee scores, isokinetic testing, and functional testing in the ACL-reconstructed knee. J Orthop Sports Phys Ther 20:61–73, 1994

22. Johansson H, Sjölander P, Sojka P: Receptors in the knee joint ligaments and their role in the biomechanics of the joint. Crit Rev Biomed Eng 18:341–368, 1991

23. Barrack RL, Skinner HB, Buckley SL: Proprioception in the anterior cruciate deficient knee. Am J Sports Med 17:1–6, 1989

24. Gordon J, Ghilardi MF, Ghez C: Impairments of reaching movements in patients without proprioception. I. Spatial errors. J Neurophysiol 73:347–360, 1995

25. Anderson SB, Terwilliger DM, Denegar CR: Comparison of open versus closed kinetic chain test positions for measuring joint position sense. J Sport Rehab 4:165–171, 1995

26. Tippett SR, Voight ML: Functional Progressions for Sport Rehabilitation. Human Kinetics, Champaign, 1995:39

27. Forwell LA, Carnahan H: Proprioception during manual aiming in individuals with shoulder instability and controls. J Orthop Sports Phys Ther 23:111–124, 1996

28. Smith RL, Brunoli J: Shoulder kinesthesia after glenohumeral joint dislocation. Phys Ther 70:507–513, 1990

29. Lephart SM, Perrin DH, Fu FH et al: Functional performance tests for the anterior cruciate ligament insufficient athlete. JNATA 26:44–51, 1991

30. Jenkins W, Bronner S, Mangine RE: Lower extremity functional evaluation and treatment concepts.

31. Paine R: "Normal" scores on a 40-yard figure of eight run in high school football players, unpublished study, 1994

32. McLaughlin CP, Kaluzny AD: Total quality management in health: making it work. Health Care Management Review 15:7–14, 1990

33. Dale J, Kidd G: Physiotherapy and the dimension of time. Physiotherapy 78:483–489, 1992

4

Evaluation and Treatment of the Shoulder

ANDREW R. EINHORN

MICHAEL MANDAS

MICHAEL SAWYER

BRUCE BROWNSTEIN

This chapter focuses on the functional shoulder and upper quarter examination. Once the dysfunction has been identified, comprehensive rehabilitation techniques are initiated, promoting the synchronous actions of the glenohumeral and scapulothoracic joints.

Emphasis will be placed on the scapulothoracic joint. This link system starts with proximal scapular stability and is influenced by upper extremity proprioception. The rotator cuff muscles steer and fine tune the humeral head in the glenoid fossa. These core elements help control upper extremity kinetic movement patterns.

Often, upper quarter postural deviations contribute to muscular imbalances about the shoulder girdle. These dysfunctions are frequently overlooked during shoulder treatment. Understanding their pathophysiology is the cornerstone to the evaluation and treatment of the shoulder.

Upper Extremity Movement

Kibler[1] has explained that to understand shoulder motion, it is necessary to review the entire kinetic chain. The shoulder relies on its position as a link to develop the forces necessary to complete overhead movement. Sequential involvement of each link combines ground reaction force and muscular activity of the large leg and trunk muscles to generate most of this force.[1] This ability to create rotational forces from various body segments is an important connection in the synchronization of joint movement from the lower extremities to the upper extremities. The propagation of power, starting from ground reaction forces and augmented by the activation of stretch-shortening cycles, sequentially moves up each body segment as power gradually cascades superiorly through the trunk and finally to the arm.[2] Lee,[2] presents the concept of stretch-shortening[3,4] as short bursts of end-range eccentric muscular contractions followed by quick full-range concentric contractions. During prestretching, energy potentials are stored in the elastic components of connective tissue and later released as kinetic energy during the concentric contraction.[3,4] A second mechanism describing this stretch-shortening cycle revolves around the concept of a prestretched, eccentrically contracted muscle performing within its physiologic limits, selectively exciting its muscle spindle to maximally facilitate the firing of agonistic and synergistic muscles fibers.[2] Lee concludes by reviewing the work of Albert[3] and states that eccentric contractions preceding concentric contractions result in greater magnitudes of contractile forces when compared with isolated concentric muscles contractions.

Accumulation of power is enhanced by muscle groups activating the stretch-shortening cycle at appropriate times through a timely coordination of segmental body and joint movement. Summation of forces is then passed distally, with contributions linking movements from the back, shoulder, elbow, and wrist joints. Kibler[1] suggests that the shoulder acts like a funnel. The funnel transfers, directs, and concentrates the delivered energy, adding force by concentration, with large developed forces passing through a small aperture. Forces developed in the proximal links (legs-trunk-back) are funneled through the shoulder to the hand by bony, capsuloligamentous, and muscular constraint systems of the shoulder joints. These movements and forces need to be dissipated, and require a sequential braking system of absorption (i.e., eccentric contractions). The absorption of forces by several joints is the best method of preventing shoulder and elbow injuries that commonly occur from repetitive overhead activity. If the constraint systems are working well, injury is minimized and mechanical efficiency of force transfer performance is maximized.[1] If the constraint systems are not effective, or are mechanically deficient, decreased performance and anatomic instability (clinical symptoms) may develop.[1]

SCAPULAR FUNCTION

Scapula movement contributes to the fine tuning of the upper extremity kinetic chain in several ways. It permits the glenoid fossa to move in synergy with the humeral head and shaft so that the instant center of humeral rotation is as close as possible to the same position throughout the extremes of overhead movement.[5] This concomitant movement of the glenoid and humeral head helps improve glenohumeral congruency by maintaining proper length-tension relationships

of the humeral head compressing muscle (supraspinatus) and humeral head-depressing muscles (subscapularis, infraspinatus, and teres minor). All anchor the humerus to the scapula.[6]

Scapular balancing muscles (serratus anterior and trapezius) assist scapular movement around the thorax, especially in conjunction with humeral elevation. These muscles contribute to optimal positioning of the scapula during overhead activities and serve an equally important function as stabilizing synergists for the deltoid acting at the glenohumeral joint.[7]

Morrison and Einhorn[8] have described the role of scapular movement around the thorax as a link in the absorption of tensile stresses placed upon the anterior capsuloligamentous structures as they relate to the throwing motion. Energy that has been stored up in the cocking phase of throwing (maximum abduction and external rotation) needs to be dissipated. This is accomplished by the mechanism of humeral deceleration and is fine-tuned through a system of scapular braking. As the humerus moves anteriorly during the acceleration and follow-through phases of throwing, eccentric control of the rhomboids helps to dissipate the forces that are being generated on the posterior rotator cuff muscles. This decreases the chances of tensile overload injury to the posterior capsule and rotator cuff muscles, which act eccentrically during the follow-through phase of throwing. During this phase of throwing, the humerus is adducted and internally rotated and the humeral head migrates into a posterior position. Failure to control these stresses can result in posterior subluxation. These stresses are dissipated by the bony stability of the protracted scapula and by the posterior shoulder capsule. Scapular protraction is a function that is often overlooked in the evaluation of posterior shoulder instability.[9]

POSTURAL CONSIDERATIONS

Postural deviations commonly found in the cervical and thoracic spine have been postulated to affect the normal function of the glenohumeral joint.[10,11] We know scapular movement contributes to normal function of the upper extremity.[1,3,12] The role of the scapula is extremely important in providing a stable base from which the glenohumeral joint must function.[1] The efficiency of muscle activity is dependent upon the optimal alignment of the scapula on the chest wall and the length tension relationships of the scapular stabilizers and rotator cuff muscles.[8,12] Without adequate neuromuscular control of the scapulothoracic articulation, the glenohumeral joint will not function around a stable base of support. Certain scapular balancing muscles can be adversely affected by the common postural deviations we observe in many of our patients. The importance of the scapular position and that alteration of normal positioning can lead to altered biomechanics of the shoulder. Scapular disassociation may be an end result of abnormal posturing, which, in most cases, includes repetitive and prolonged activities of daily living (ADLs). This malaligned positioning of the scapula may eventually contribute to a decrease in the subacromial space, resulting in a pathologic condition.

Greenfield et al.,[13] observed that forward head position was more common in individuals with shoulder overuse injuries, but no differences were noted in scapular position between subjects with overuse and healthy subjects. These results must be interpreted with total consideration of the multivariate nature of overuse syndromes. Overuse injuries are often a result of errors in training, conditioning, and performance, as opposed to having a true anatomic basis. Future research might duplicate the anatomic measurements used in the Greenfield et al study with a population of subjects with shoulder injuries more heavily influenced by the anatomy of the individual (i.e., multidirectional instability or primary impingement) than the activity they are undertaking.

EFFECTS OF CORRECT POSTURE

Good posture permits mechanically efficient function of the joints. Friction in the joints is minimized, tension of opposing ligaments is balanced, and pressures within the joints are equalized.[14] This allows a minimum of wear and tear on the joints. Aspects of good posture include a minimum of muscle force, a balance between antagonistic muscle groups, and sufficient flexibility.[14] It also includes adequate coordination, which implies good neuromuscular control and well-developed postural reflexes. It is noted that adjustments in posture can be made more readily by individuals who have a good kinesthetic awareness of postures they assume and of the degree of tension in their muscles.[14] Our treatment of postural deviations includes training to encourage proper neuromuscular control and education to improve postural awareness.

Scapular Disassociation

Disassociation of the prime scapular stabilizing muscles is caused by several contributing factors that include: derangement of the cervical spine, injury to the glenohumeral joint or muscles, upper extremity posture, or direct trauma to the scapular muscles (Feldman E, personal communication). These changes translate into inappropriate length-tension relationships of glenohumeral and scapulothoracic force couples.

Abnormal upper extremity movement is commonly associated with scapular dissociation, a term used by Feldman. Scapular dissociation is the inability of the scapula to maintain its normal stabilizing effect and association with the glenohumeral joint and related muscles. Trauma or abnormal posturing can contribute to scapular dissociation. These factors lead to a sequential change in upper extremity kinematics, and contribute to movement dysfunction, as noted in Table 4-1.

MOVEMENT DYSFUNCTION (HYPOMOBILITY)

One of the most common conditions treated in the clinic is adhesive capsulitis. Most cases of adhesive capsulitis develop scapular dissociation. Glenohumeral elevation and rotation is limited secondary to restricted capsular tightness. Stiffness at the glenohumeral joint is counteracted by compensatory movement at the scapulothoracic joint. This movement pattern is neces-

TABLE 4-1 *Upper extremity movement dysfunction*

	ETIOLOGY OF PAIN	POTENTIAL UNDERLYING FACTORS	ABNORMAL FINDINGS	TIME FACTORS	END RESULT
Hypermobility (excessive movement)	Poor mechanics during overhead activities Inefficient or poorly conditioned scapular balancing or rotator cuff muscles	Increased humeral head translation Positive laxity factors	Scapulothoracic Force Couple Decreased stability effect of scapular balancing muscles Scapular hypomobility Glenohumeral Force Couple Weakness of humeral head stabilizers Decreased humeral head mobility	Abnormal joint kinematics Dysfunctional pain cycle Inflammatory process	Overuse syndrome Impingement syndrome secondary to instability Rotator Cuff Tendonitis
Hypomobility (restricted movement)	Traumatic Atraumatic Cervical spine radiculopathy Acromial shape Other	Impingement Rotator Cuff Tendinitis	Scapulothoracic Force Couple Decreased stability, effect of the scapular balancing muscles Glenohumoral Force Couple Weakness of the humeral head stabilizers	Shortening of muscular and scapular structures	Adhesive capsulitis

sary to achieve elevation during ADLs. As the patient attempts to elevate, excessive scapular elevation (i.e., overuse of the upper trapezius muscles) occurs, as the lower trapezius remains hypoactive. Highly skilled activities are not obtainable during this period of abnormal kinetic movement patterning secondary to decreased functions of the glenohumeral/scapulothoracic force couples.

Evaluation of passive range of motion (ROM) reveals external rotation more limited than shoulder flexion or internal rotation. Joint mobility testing often uncovers decreased joint play. Static evaluation of the scapula reveals increased upward rotation and abduction positioning when compared to the uninvolved side. This objective finding indicates decreased stabilizing ability of the lower trapezius and both rhomboid muscles. Disuse atrophy of the supraspinatus and infraspinatus muscles may be visualized in patients that have symptoms for 6 months or longer. The atrophy may be mild or pronounced. A rotator cuff tear or suprascapular nerve palsy are additional causes of atrophy to this region. Rotator cuff strength testing with the arm at the side often reveals 4/5 level strength. Isolation of the supraspinatus is often difficult to evaluate when the patient presents limited active-passive ROM.

When moderate atrophy of the cuff muscles

is accompanied by moderate pain and weakness during manual muscle testing, a possible cuff tear should be suspected. Often the working diagnosis for the above case scenario is adhesive capsulitis. Treatment is initiated and the search for the actual cause of the condition begins. Most cases of adhesive capsulitis are idiopathic; others develop secondary to trauma. The shoulder hurts and the patient keeps the arm at the side. The actual problem heals during the period when the arm is held next to the patient's body. However, healing occurs with the capsular and muscular tissues in a shortened position. Pain is associated with patient attempts to move the extremity. Movement is avoided as the cycle of healing and shortening continues. Greater than 80% of the cases improve if motion is restored, although about half of the patients treated conservatively report mild stiffness and/or pain on an average of 7 years after onset and treatment.[15–17] Approximately 10% of patients report some functional limitation (overhead lifting, dressing, recreational activities), which does not correlate to motion loss.[17] Approximately 20% of the cases have pathology that requires more aggressive treatment. These cases may present with rotator cuff tendinitis, impingement syndrome, or full thickness cuff tearing, and may not respond to conservative care.

Treatment of adhesive capsulitis includes: glenohumeral joint mobilization, scapular stabilization, biofeedback, and postural awareness, emphasizing control of the rhomboids and lower trapezius. Pain control modalities can be used to supplement treatment. Initial treatment revolves around restoration of glenohumeral mobility and the stabilizing function of the above scapular muscles. After this has been accomplished, rotator cuff strengthening is directed to the humeral head depressing muscles. Aggressive strengthening when abnormal movement patterns exist usually do not result in improved muscle and joint function.[16]

MOVEMENT DYSFUNCTION (HYPERMOBILITY)

Excessive humeral head translation can also lead to abnormal joint kinematics and a dysfunctional pain cycle. Increased humeral head trans-

lation anteriorly, posteriorly, or inferiorly is a factor associated with impingement syndrome secondary to shoulder instability. Morrison and Einhorn[8] have described patients that exhibit specific findings associated with increased movement dysfunction. Physical examination reveals full to increased active glenohumeral movement, with uni- or multidirectional laxity. Neurologic scapular winging is usually absent. Patients may present with weakness, poor endurance, and inadequate control of the serratus anterior, upper trapezius, and lower trapezius. This worsens the problem of instability since these patients require the scapular stabilizers to function at a higher than normal level in order to minimize the chance of further overload of the rotator cuff. Electromyographic (EMG) investigation, however, shows that the exact opposite occurs.

The EMG activity of the rotator cuff, scapular rotators, and glenohumeral muscles has been investigated under varying conditions of instability, including anterior instability,[18–22] posterior dislocation,[23] and multidirectional instability.[21,23] All found that the timing and intensity of muscle activity was altered, especially in the rotator cuff and scapular muscles. Kronberg et al.[21] found that the supraspinatus and infraspinatus tended to be more active in patients with generalized laxity, and speculated that this was a stabilizing mechanism. In an earlier study by the same group, Broström et al.[19] noted similar results but also noted depressed subscapularis function until a dislocating event, when the subscapularis activity increased significantly to stabilize the joint. Howell and Kraft[20] found that the activity of the supraspinatus and infraspinatus was unchanged in patients with anterior instability. Their study used static analysis as opposed to dynamic contractions, which may account for the difference in results.

Pande et al.[23] studied voluntary posterior dislocators and noted sharp inhibition in the trapezius, infraspinatus, and serratus anterior muscles (ranging from a 60–100% reduction) during subluxation. This was accompanied by a 300–400% increase in activity of the muscles precipitating the event, either the posterior deltoid or biceps. The scapular stabilizers did not return to normal levels of contraction even after the joint was voluntarily relocated.

This selected patient population often presents with increased laxity factors such as passive movement of the thumb to the radial aspect of the forearm, hyperextension of the elbow, and metacarpophalangeal and distal interphalangeal joints of the hand. The clinical picture reveals classic objective findings that contribute to the excessive movement dysfunction.

Evaluation

SCAPULAR EVALUATION

Scapular position, stability, strength, and control is essential to proper shoulder rehabilitation. The anchoring position of the scapula can be estimated clinically by using the lateral scapula slide measurement test described by Kibler[5] and modified by Davies et al.[24] This test measures the ability of the posterior shoulder muscles to accomplish scapular stabilization and positioning. It also serves to provide a static measurement of scapular stability in three positions.

The lateral scapular slide test is illustrated in Figs. 4-1 to 4-3. These positions measure the ability of the scapular stabilizers to control the medial border of the scapula. Figure 4-1 denotes Position 1, with arms in a neutral position at the side. The spinous process of the seventh thoracic vertebrae is illustrated by a dot. The examiner has placed a dot on the inferior angle of the scapula. The examiner measures the distance between this position bilaterally and notes any differences. Measurements based on palpation technique can provide unreliable data.[25,26] However, in the hands of a skilled practitioner, this scapular evaluation maneuver will prove a higher degree of reliability.[26] It should be noted that assessing Position 1 requires very little skill to ensure reliability. Positions 2–3, which are discussed below, do require accurate palpation of bony landmarks. DiVeta et al.[27] also showed that a single tester can provide reliable measure-

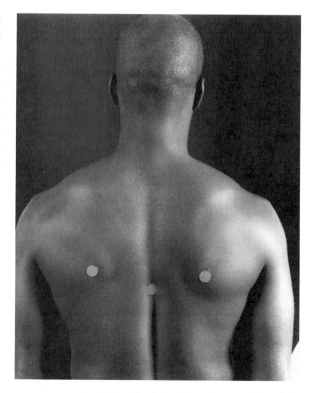

FIGURE 4-1 *Position 1 of the lateral scapular slide test. Arms are at the side, in "neutral." Dots have been placed on the spinous process of thoracic vertebrae seven (T7) and on each scapular inferior angle. The total distance is measured from T7 to inferior angle and compared to the uninvolved side.*

ment of scapula position, using vertebral and scapular landmarks.

Figure 4-2 illustrates Position 2 of the lateral scapular slide test. The patient places hands on the hips with thumbs pointing posteriorly. This position requires trapezius muscle activity. The distance is again measured as noted in Figure 4-1. This distance is greater than that seen in Position 1.

Figure 4-3 illustrates Position 3 of the lateral scapular slide test. Position 3 is one of maximum challenge to the scapular stabilizers. The humerus is abducted 90 degrees and internally rotated. Scapular stabilization requires muscular activity of the upper-lower trapezius and serratus anterior muscles. Bilateral measurements are again taken. In symptomatic individuals, differences of more than 1–2 cm in either Position 2 or Position 3 have been statistically proven to be associated with the onset of pain and decreased shoulder function.[24]

POSTURAL ASSESSMENT AND FINDINGS

Postural screening is important in a comprehensive evaluation of shoulder dysfunction. Our role as therapists is to identify any subtle abnormalities and begin working toward normalization of movement. Rarely will shoulder *pathology* be linked directly to postural deviations of the

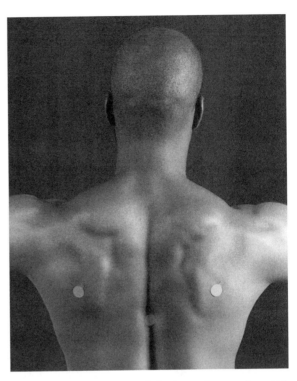

FIGURE 4-3 *Position 3 of the lateral scapular slide test. Distance between dots is again compared to the uninvolved side.*

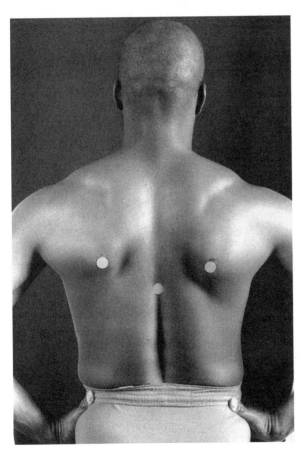

FIGURE 4-2 *Position 2 of the lateral scapular slide test. Hands are on hips. The total distance is greater than Position 1.*

upper quarter; however, shoulder rehabilitation must address postural changes as it relates to shoulder *dysfunction*. These postural deviations lead to shortening and tightening of certain muscle groups, and lengthening of other muscle groups.[28] This, through the course of time, leads to ultimate weakness and neuromuscular dysfunction. When assessing the glenohumeral joint, clinicians should not limit their assessment to the painful site about which the patient has complained. We must observe both static and dynamic posture. When we speak of normal posture, remember that it is theoretical and represents the most efficient use of energy. The "relative normal" is a function that, represents the most economical performance of an individual's own body. Any type of postural correction must aim at the best possible mechanical use of the individual.[29]

Postural assessment begins with observation

of static posture of the upper quarter and concludes with dynamic movement of the head and neck, shoulder and scapula, thoracic spine and finally, the lumbar spine. Our postural assessment takes into account the patient's daily activities, sport, or occupation. Abnormal posturing, which may contribute to the patient's current shoulder complaints, needs to be addressed. Through education and training, posture is altered or adapted to the patient's daily activities. Faulty posture involves heightened tension in muscles and requires excess muscular involvement for motion, which leads to fatigue and inefficient movement.[11] This may predispose the individual to injury.

The Scapular Balancing Index addresses posture as it is subjectively determined by the clinician (Table 4-2). The postural evaluation will assess the patient from an anterior, posterior, and lateral view. The clinician must consider whether the line of gravity in the individual represents his most economical functional position. Does the patient's posture lead to movement that is performed with minimum effort? Can movement take place in any direction with maximum ease and speed? Can movement be initiated with the minimum of preliminary adjustment of the body? What is observed by the clinician must be linked to the patient's daily activities, sport, or occupation. Findings are noted by the clinician and those determined to be abnormal and affecting shoulder function are treated without aggravation of current shoulder pain complaints. Postural deviations acquired by patients through habit can be reasonably changed or altered through training and education.[20] Posture, abnormal or normal, is a learned response. It is a neuromuscular reaction to proprioceptive stimuli from the periphery.[30]

SCAPULAR BALANCING INDEX

The 20-point Scapular Balancing Index, (Table 4-2) appraises the patient's upper quarter, combining results from the lateral scapular slide test, dynamic manual muscle evaluation, cervico thoracic posture, and joint mobility. This index includes six parts:

TABLE 4-2 *Scapular balancing index*

	LEFT SHOULDER	RIGHT SHOULDER
Part I: Lateral Scapular Slide		
Position One: 0–1 Pts.		
Position Two: 0–2 Pts.		
Position Three: 0–2 Pts.		
TOTAL SCORE: 0–5 Pts.		
Part II: Neuromuscular Evaluation		
Anterior Elevation: 0–1 Pts.		
Posterior Elevation: 0–1 Pts.		
Posterior Depression: 0–1 Pts.		
Scapular Adduction: 0–1 Pts.		
TOTAL SCORE: 0–4 Pts.		
Part III: Strength and Endurance		
Anterior Elevation: 0–1 Pts.		
Posterior Elevation: 0–1 Pts.		
Posterior Depression: 0–1 Pts.		
Scapular Adduction: 0–1 Pts.		
TOTAL SCORE: 0–4 Pts.		
Part IV: Cervical Posture		
Normal Cervical Alignment: 2 Pts.		
Mild Forward Head Position: 1 Pts.		
Forward Head Position: 0 Pts.		
TOTAL SCORE: 0–2 Pts.		
Part V: Thoracic Posture		
Normal Thoracic Alignment: 3 Pts.		
Mild Thoracic Kyphosis: 2 Pts.		
Moderate Kyphosis: 1 Pt.		
Severe Thoracic Kyphosis: 0 Pts.		
TOTAL SCORE: 0–3 Pts.		
Part VI: Thoracic Segmental Mobility		
Normal Thoracic Mobility: 2 Pts.		
Mild Decreased Mobility: 1 Pt.		
Hypomobility: 0 Pts.		
TOTAL SCORE: 0–2 Pts.		
TOTAL SCORE: PARTS I–VI RANGE (0–20 Pts.)		

Scapular Balancing Index Scores
0–10 pts.   Possible Neurologic Involvement
11–12 pts. Poor Scapular control
13–16 pts. Fair Scapular control
17–18 pts. Normal Scapular control
19–20 pts. Excellent Scapular control

- Part I (5 points) Static scapular positioning—lateral scapular slide test
- Part II (4 points) Neuromuscular control of the scapula
- Part III (4 points) Scapular strength and endurance
- Part IV (2 points) Cervical posture
- Part V (3 points) Thoracic posture
- Part VI (2 points) Thoracic segmental mobility

Each section of the index contains an evaluation scale. A high score is associated with a higher level of muscular performance or normalized postural position. For example, a zero point total identifies poor scapular muscle function during Part I–II of the Index, while the higher scoring levels are present with normal scapular function. A subjective score is determined by the examiner. A maximum index score of 20 points is possible when combining all six sections.

Evaluation and treatment of the scapulothoracic joint creates a real challenge for the rehabilitation team. The Scapular Balancing Index is a subjective and theoretical tool, which provides the examiner with beneficial standardized information that assists in the appraisal of the upper extremity kinetic chain. Many forms of evaluation and treatment begin as theory and are tested over time. The Scapular Balancing Index is currently under this type of scrutiny.

Scapular Balancing Index: Part I

Part I appraises the lateral slide test. Each segment of the lateral slide test receives between 0–1 points, with a total of 5 points at the completion of Part I. Position 1, the lateral scapular slide test, receives zero points for poor static scapular positioning or 1 point for normal scapular positioning. Positions 2 and 3 of the lateral scapular slide test have a 0–2 point scale on the Scapular Balancing Index. These positions require increased levels of muscular involvement and a higher grading scale. The greater point total allows for flexibility in evaluation of these three scapular positions. A 1-point score would indicate a performance less than normal, but not totally deficient. Two points are given if the difference is less than .5 cm, 1 point if the difference is greater than .5, but less than or equal to 1.5 cm, and zero points if the difference is greater than 1.5 cm.

Scapular Balancing Index: Part II

Part II evaluates the neuromuscular efficiency of the scapular platform. The movement patterns are modifications of Proprioceptive Neuromuscular Facilitation (PNF) developed by Kabat[31] and later popularized by Knott and Voss.[32] Engle and Canner[33] recommend specific movement patterns to help condition the scapular platform: anterior elevation, posterior elevation, and posterior depression. These stabilization techniques are conducted without appreciable movement of the glenohumeral joint, thereby avoiding stress to injured cuff muscles.

Figure 4-4 shows anterior elevation of the scapula. The patient is elevating his scapula in the direction of his nose as the therapist provides resistance. The therapist should avoid hand placement on the humeral head, as this can sublux the humeral head interiorly.

Figure 4-5 shows posterior elevation of the scapula. The patient elevates the scapula, using the trapezius muscles, as the therapist provides resistance. The patient tries to elevate the scapula toward the posterior region of the occiput. Manual resistance is applied as the patient elevates, depresses, and adducts the scapula. Emphasis is placed on scapular movement, control, and coordination during each pattern. The therapist applies a 0–1-point score for each individual pattern during the four tests, yielding an accumulative total of 4 points. This method is subjective, but proves the examiner with beneficial information on the patient's neuromuscular control during resisted pattern of scapular movement.

Scapular Balancing Index: Part III

Part III evaluates the strength and endurance component of scapular movement. Manual resistance is applied as the patient elevates, depresses, and adducts the scapula during a series

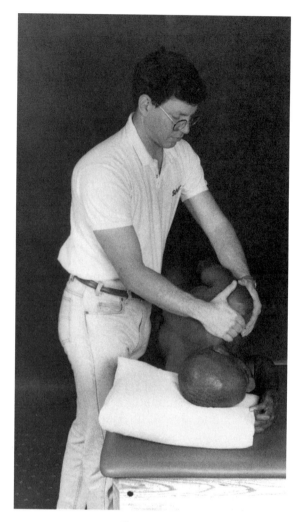

FIGURE 4-4 *Manually resisted anterior elevation of the scapula. Anterior elevation of the scapula can be used to test neuromuscular control, strength, and endurance of the serratus anterior muscle. This movement pattern can be used isometrically, concentrically, or eccentrically for scapular strengthening.*

of 10 repetitions. The therapist applies a 0–1-point score for each individual pattern during the four tests, yielding an accumulative total of 4 points. Movement patterns are scored as noted in Part II. A 1-point grade is given if the patient is able to complete the required repetitions with adequate control.

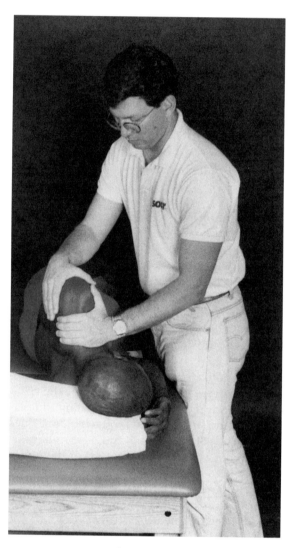

FIGURE 4-5 *Manual resistance is applied during posterior scapular elevation.*

Scapular Balancing Index: Part IV

Postural screening begins with the cervical spine. Observation of posture is quantified on a scale of 0–2 points. Normal cervical alignment is given 2 points. A tendency toward a forward head would be termed mild and is allotted 1 point. A forward head position would be given 0 points. It should be noted that a forward head posture graded zero points will likely be accompanied by an increase in the thoracic kyphosis.

Forward head posture commonly leads to subtle musculoskeletal deviations. The head moves forward causing backward bending of the cervical spine.[30] This leads to suboccipital muscle shortening, and a decrease of suboccipital mobility.[11] The cervical lordosis is increased and the tightness of the suboccipital structures inhibits the cervical flexors, which leads to their weakness.[30] As the head moves anteriorly, the posterior aspect of the occiput moves posteriorly-inferiorly. This may lead to shortening of the upper trapezius muscle and levator scapulae.[10,11] The end result is scapular elevation. As the midcervical lordosis is lost, there is a proportionate increase in thoracic kyphosis.[11] The increased thoracic convexity produces abduction of the scapula and may lengthen the rhomboid and lower trapezius muscles, while shortening the serratus anterior, latissimus dorsi, subscapularis, and teres major muscles.

Scapular Balancing Index: Part V

We again make a subjective examination of thoracic posture. If normal thoracic alignment is noted, 3 points are allotted. A mild increase in a patient's thoracic kyphosis is given 2 points. Moderate to severe thoracic kyphosis receives 1 and zero points respectively. Again, it should be noted that a forward head posture will most often accompany an increase in thoracic kyphosis. This most common combination of postural deviations creates a potential for multiple muscle imbalances in scapular musculature. The thoracic portions of the erector spinae and other extensors are elongated because of the increased convexity. The shoulder girdle is abducted and tilted laterally. Normally the scapula has a forward tilt in the sagittal plane.[34] This forward tilt has been found to increase as the slope of the thoracic spine is increased. The rhomboids and middle trapezius are elongated and the pectoralis minor and serratus anterior are shortened.[11] The pectoral fascia is likely to be tight. The glenohumeral joint becomes internally rotated.[11] Knowing that tight muscles inhibit their antagonists, these gradual changes create the potential for muscle imbalance throughout the scapular

region. We postulate that the increased kyphosis of the thoracic spine, which in turn, abducts the scapula, leads to tightening and weakening of certain muscle groups.[10,11] The anterior shoulder complex is also affected, as the pectoralis major and minor muscles are shortened, creating a pull of the scapula over the head of the humerus. The head of the humerus moves into internal rotation, which may shorten the glenohumeral ligament.[11]

A description of all possible outcomes of certain common postural deviations emphasizes the importance of addressing an oftentimes neglected component of our patient evaluation.

Scapular Balancing Index: Part VI

Thoracic mobility is commonly addressed in a gross assessment of mobility, unless pathology is known to be present. Thoracic mobility is affected by all the structures making up the thorax. The ribs, cartilages, sternum, and associated muscles and organs all affect thoracic spine mobility. The thoracic spine must be considered in its entire context. It is a component of the thorax, but the structures are so intimately united that it may be considered as a single structure. Thus, mobility is considered in this context. Loss of mobility in the thoracic spine will effect the outcome of postural adjustments. Limited mobility will also inhibit normal neuromuscular control. Segmental mobility deficits are compounded when they exist in the presence of the previously discussed postural deviations. Segmental mobility deficits in the presence of a normal postural alignment may have very little consequence in shoulder pathology.

The Scapular Balancing Index grades segmental thoracic mobility after observation of posture in standing. Spring tests or posterior-anterior glides can be used to assess and grade mobility. Techniques for testing mobility vary, and should be chosen on the basis of familiarity. Normal mobility will receive 2 points. A mild loss of mobility will receive 1 point and a severe loss of thoracic posterior-anterior gliding will receive zero points.

FUNCTIONAL SHOULDER EVALUATION AND OUTCOMES

The complete shoulder evaluation integrates range of motion, pain, glenohumeral-scapulothoracic strength, and shoulder stability, and is accompanied by functional assessment in a reproducible format. The patient usually begins therapy with a chief complaint of shoulder pain. The assessment of pain is subjective and difficult to quantify. What is mild pain to some patients, may be moderate or severe to others. When dealing with an active population, pain may be specific to athletic or occupational motions, without affecting other aspects of daily living. It is much easier and effective to measure the resulting impairment of shoulder function than the level of subjective pain.[35]

Shoulder function often correlates closely with the patient's chief complaint.[12] For example, the patient reports pain during overhead lifting, throwing a ball, or reaching behind the neck or back. The examiner should understand that certain aspects of the examination address different aspects of function. The range of motion parameters are less important to the patient than whether he or she can comb his or her hair, sleep on the affected side, or perform perianal care.

The patient's functional level is a critical issue to the payers of health care. Written documentation can confirm the benefits of treatment, and justify the cost to the individual or society. It is important, however, to select a functional tool that is applicable to the activity demands of the patient being treated.

RATING SCALES

Four relatively comprehensive numeric rating systems for shoulder outcomes include: the Rowe,[36,37] Neer,[38-40] UCLA,[41-43] and Hospital for Special Surgery[44] scales. Each system has strengths and weaknesses which reflects the patient population and range of problems they were designed to address. Each scale can be used for the general population, but the clinician should review the scale's history and select the one that matches the population being studied.

According to Gerber,[45] the ideal scoring system would precisely define terminology and methodology; include only parameters that relate to shoulder function; include and assess the most relevant parameters of function in the proper proportion; be accurate in describing shoulder function regardless of pathology; be reproducible; and be easy to administer. Clearly, given the range of demands placed on the shoulder complex, and the diverse pathologies that can arise, the ideal functional test has not yet been developed.

Rowe System

The Rowe system was designed to assess the outcome of anterior shoulder stabilization using a Bankart repair.[36] It evaluates stability, motion, and "function" via subjective and objective base questions. Strength is not addressed and pain is referred to only in the context of "function." There is some ambiguity about the test procedures and the scale is heavily weighted toward the absence of instability. The scale is designed to evaluate anterior stabilization in a population with moderate activity demands. A modified Rowe scale[37] was subsequently developed to address more active people, including higher activity demands and pain, but not strength (Table 4-3). This scale has been used by Montgomery and Jobe[46] to evaluate outcome following capsulolabral reconstruction of an unstable shoulder in athletes. Burkhead and Rockwood[47] used the modified Rowe scale to assess the results of an exercise program on patients with shoulder instability, regardless of direction or cause of the instability. In their series, 16 percent of patients with traumatic instability had good to excellent results, while 80 percent of the atraumatic sample had good to excellent results.

Neer Rating Scale

Neer's original scale evaluated the outcome of anterior shoulder acromioplasty by using a satisfactory/unsatisfactory rating system.[38] A similar system was used for total shoulder arthroplasty.[39] The criteria included assessment

TABLE 4-3 *Modified Rowe scale*

SCORING SYSTEM	UNITS	EXCELLENT (100–90)	GOOD (89–75)	FAIR (74–51)	GOOD (50 OR LESS)
Stability					
No recurrence or subluxation	50	No recurrences	No recurrences	No recurrences	Recurrence of dislocation or
Apprehension when placing arm in certain positions	30	No apprehension when placing arm in complete elevation and ER	Mild apprehension when placing arm in elevation and ER	Moderate apprehension during elevation and ER	Marked apprehension during elevation or extension
Subluxation (not requiring reduction)	10	No subluxation	No subluxation	No subluxation	
Recurrent dislocation	0				
Motion					
100% of normal ER, IR, and elevation	20	100% of normal ER, complete elevation and IR	75% of normal ER, complete elevation and IR	50% of normal ER, 75% of elevation and IR	No ER; 50% of elevation (can get hand only to face), 50% IR
75% of normal ER, normal elevation and IR	15				
50% of normal ER, 75% of normal elevation and IR	5				
50% of normal elevation and IR, no ER	0				
Function					
No limitation in work or sports; little or no discomfort	30	Performs all work and sports; no limitation in overhead activities; shoulder strong in lifting, swimming, tennis, throwing; no discomfort	Mild limitation in work and sports; shoulder strong; minimum discomfort	Moderate limitation doing overhead work and heavy lifting; unable to throw, serve hard in tennis, or swim; moderate disabling pain	Marked limitation; unable to perform overhead work and lifting; cannot throw, play tennis or swim; chronic discomfort
Mild limitation and minimum discomfort	25				
Moderate limitation and discomfort	10				
Marked limitation and pain	0				

Abbreviations: ER, external rotation; IR, internal rotation.
Total units possible 100
(From Rowe CR et al,[36] with permission.)

TABLE 4-4 *Neer shoulder assessment*

	PREOPERATIVE	POSTOPERATIVE EXAMINATION 1	POSTOPERATIVE EXAMINATION 2
I. Pain: 1 = none, 2 = slight, 3 = after unusual activity, 4 = moderate, 5 = marked			
II. Motion: (mark _____ if negative) Active elevation (sitting) Passive elevation (supine) External rotation at side External rotation at 90 degree abduction Internal Rotation at side (segment of posterior anatomy) Internal Rotation at 90 degree abduction			
III. Strength: 5 = normal, 4 = good, against resistance, 3 = fair: antigravity, 2 = poor: movement gravity eliminated, 1 = trace: contraction without motion, 0 = paralysis Anterior deltoid Middle deltoid External rotation			
IV. Function: 1 = normal, 2 = difficult, 3 = with aid, 4 = unable Use back pocket Perineal care Wash opposite axilla Eat with utensil Comb hair Use hand with arm at shoulder level Carry 10–15 lb with arm at side Dress Sleep on side Do usual work (if unable, specify change _____)			
V. Patient response: 1 = much better, 2 = better, 3 = same, 4 = worse			

From Neer CS II et al.,[40] with permission.

of pain, satisfaction, limitation of overhead motion, and 75 percent of "strength." Objective testing for strength, endurance, external rotation, and shoulder stability were not addressed.[38,39,48]

The system was later modified to include a graded examination of motion, strength, pain, and function (several ADLs)[40] (Table 4-4). Both systems were originally designed for an older population with lower activity demands than athletes—recreational or otherwise. The modified Neer scale is used to compare results from one evaluation to another, on the basis of individual variables, rather than produce a total score.[49] The Rowe score was also used to evaluate function in active, younger people with ante-

rior instability who had not been treated with either surgery or controlled rehabilitation. They found that there was no correlation between Rowe score, isokinetic torque, or ROM deficits to either the number or duration of the instability.

UCLA Shoulder Assessment

The UCLA shoulder assessment is another scale that has evolved. It originally evaluated pain, function, and muscle power using a 30-point scale.[41] The original scale assessed multiple ranges of motion (internal rotation and elevation) and strength in the same section. The scale was later modified[42] to divide strength and motion (Table 4-5). Active forward flexion is the only motion and muscle test measured. Patient satisfaction was included in the new version.

The UCLA assessment has been used for shoulder arthroplasty,[41] rotator cuff repair,[42] and subacromial decompression.[43] Preoperative scores are difficult to assess, since the 35-point scale includes patient satisfaction. Moreover, the 5-point subjective satisfaction score may bias the objectivity of the test. It does not address high performance demands, nor does it measure rotation motion or strength. It is independent of diagnosis.

Hospital for Special Surgery Scoring System

The Hospital for Special Surgery (HSS) system subjectively evaluates pain on motion, pain at rest, and functional limitations (five activities), and objectively considers range of motion and strength (Table 4-6).[50] The system was originally designed for total shoulder arthroplasty. This version of the HSS system is heavily weighted toward pain and motion in a low demand population.

Altchek et al.[44] modified the scoring system for use in a more active population following arthroscopic acromioplasty. They retained the evaluation of pain, functional limits, and ROM. Impingement tests and tenderness were included. Evaluation of sports was included in the pain and function sections. In his review of scoring systems, Tibone and Bradley[48] commented that this system did not evaluate strength, performance, or change in level of competition. The system is geared toward an athletic population following surgery for impingement syndrome.

The modified HSS shoulder score was used by Blevins et al.[51] to assess the results of arthroscopic assisted rotator cuff repair. The average score (out of 100) preoperatively was 44, postoperatively, 86. This change was significant at $P < .05$. In an attempt to address the concerns of Tibone noted above, strength and performance changes were measured along with the rating score. Instrumented testing of isometric eleva-

TABLE 4-5 *UCLA shoulder rating scale*

FUNCTIONAL/REACTION MEASURED	POINTS
Pain	
Present all of the time and unbearable; strong medication frequently	1
Present all of the time but bearable; strong mediation occasionally	2
None or little at rest, present during light activities; salicylates frequently	4
Present during heavy or particular activities only; salicylates occasionally	6
Occasional and slight	8
None	10
Function	
Unable to use limb	1
Only light activities possible	2
Able to do light housework or most of activities of daily living	4
Most housework, shopping, and driving possible; able to fix hair and dress and undress, including fastening brasiere	6
Slight restriction only; able to work above shoulder level	8
Normal activities	10
Active forward flexion	
150° or more	5
120° to 150°	4
90° to 120°	3
45° to 90°	2
30° to 45°	1
Less than 30°	0
Strength of forward flexion (MMT)	
Grade 5 (normal)	5
Grade 4 (good)	4
Grade 3 (fair)	3
Grade 2 (poor)	2
Grade 1 (muscle contraction)	1
Grade 0 (nothing)	0
Satisfaction of the patient	
Satisfied and better	5
Not satisfied and worse	0
Maximum score: 35 points	

(From Ellman H, et al,[42] with permission.)

TABLE 4-6 *HSS shoulder assessment*

	SCORE	PREOPERATIVE	6 MO	1 YR	≥2 YR
Pain on Motion (15 pts)					
None	15				
Mild: Occasional, no compromise in activity	10				
Moderate: Tolerable, makes concession, uses ASA	5				
Severe: Serious limitations, disabling, uses codeine	0				
Pain at Rest (15 pts)					
None: ignores	15				
Mild: occasional, no medication, no affect on sleep	10				
Moderate: uses ASA, night pain	5				
Severe: marked medication, stronger than ASA	0				
Function (20 pts)					
Comb hair	5				
Lie on shoulder	5				
Hook brassiere (back)	5				
Toilet	5				
Lift weight in pounds 1–10					
1 pt per pound—maximum 10 pts					
None					
Muscle Strength (15 pts—rate each)					
(normal = 3, Good = 2, Fair = 1, Poor = 0)					
Forward Flexion					
Abduction					
Adduction					
Internal Rotation					
External Rotation					
Range of Motion (25 pts)					
(1 pt per 20° of motion)					
Forward Flexion (maximum 3)					
Abduction (Maximum 7)					
Adduction (Maximum 2)					
Internal Rotation (Maximum 5)					
External Rotation (Maximum 3)					
Record Range of Motion (no pts)					
Backward Extension					
Glenohumeral Abduction (scapula fixed)					
Total Score possible: 100 pts					

(From Warren RF, et al,[50] *with permission.)*

tion and both rotations showed no significant differences between the surgical and nonsurgical sides. Analog pain scales were used to assess limitations with throwing, sports, reaching, and ADL. The average pain score (out of 5) was 2.8 preoperatively, and .8 postoperatively ($P < .05$). No correlation was found between size of rotator cuff tear and HSS shoulder scores.

ASES Shoulder Evaluation Form

The evaluation proposed by the American Shoulder and Elbow Surgeons Shoulder Society (ASES)[52] evolved from the Neer rating scale. The ASES system has five sections, including pain, motion, strength, stability, and function (Table 4-7). The ASES system is more applicable to the

TABLE 4-7 *ASES shoulder evaluation form*

I. PAIN: (5 = none, 4 = slight, 3 = after unusual activity, 2 = moderate, 1 = marked, 0 = complete disability, NA = not available)

II. MOTION:
   A. Patient sitting
      1. Active total elevation of the arm: _____ (in degrees)*
      2. Passive internal rotation:
         (Circle segment of posterior anatomy reached by thumb. Note if reach restricted by limited elbow flexion).

1 = Less than trochanter	5 = L5	9 = L1	13 = T9	17 = T5
2 = Trochanter	6 = L4	10 = T12	14 = T8	18 = T4
3 = Gluteal	7 = L3	11 = T11	15 = T7	19 = T3
4 = Sacrum	8 = L2	12 = T10	16 = T6	20 = T2

      3. Active external rotation with arm at side: _____ (in degrees)*
      4. Active external rotation at 90° abduction: _____ (in degrees)
   B. Patient supine
      1. Passive total elevation of arm: _____ (in degrees)*
      2. Passive external rotation with arm at side: _____ (in degrees)

III. STRENGTH: (5 = normal, 4 = good, 3 = fair, 2 = poor, 1 = trace, 0 = paralysis)
   A. Anterior deltoid _____   C. External rotation _____
   B. Middle deltoid _____   D. Internal rotation _____
   STABILITY: (5 = normal, 4 = apprehension, 3 = rare subluxation, 2 = recurrent subluxation, 1 = recurrent dislocation, 0 =
IV. fixed dislocation, NA = not available)
   A. Anterior _____
   B. Posterior _____
   C. Inferior _____

V. FUNCTION: (4 = normal, 3 = mild compromise, 2 = difficulty, 1 = with aid, 0 = unable, NA = not available)
   A. Use back pocket _____   I. Sleep on affected side _____
   B. Perineal care _____   J. Pulling _____
   C. Wash opposite axilla _____   K. Use hand overhead _____
   D. Eat with utensil _____   L. Throwing _____
   E. Comb hair _____   M. Lifting _____
   F. Use hand with arm at shoulder level _____   N. Do usual work _____
   G. Carry 10 to 15 lbs with arm at side _____   O. Do usual sport _____
   H. Dress _____

* Total elevation of the arm measured by viewing patient from the side and using a goniometer to determine the angle between the arm and the thorax.
(From Barrett WP et al,[52] with permission.)

general population than the Neer scale. The system is fairly easy to use accurately.

Pain criteria have not been clearly defined in this system, leaving room for interpretation between different evaluators. Passive and active motions are assessed during the movement of shoulder flexion, internal rotation, and external rotation. It should be noted that active motion measurements are used to test function, while passive testing is used as a diagnostic test to denote end feel.

Like the Neer form, the ASES system is designed to measure each section separately, rather than produce an overall rating number. The system is oriented towards a nonathletic population, although a modification has been used in active people with rotator cuff injuries.[53] The modified form, however, does not assess strength.

Strength is tested manually using (0–5) points for each muscle group tested. Muscle testing is limited to the anterior and middle deltoids.

Testing of internal and external rotators is part of the strength evaluation conducted with the arm at the side. No testing of the supraspinatus muscle is performed.

Anterior, posterior and inferior stability testing is evaluated. Five points are awarded for normal stability, 4 points with apprehension, 3 points on rare subluxation, 2 points on recurrent subluxation, 1 point for recurrent dislocation, and zero points for a fixed dislocation. Stability may or may not be related to functional loss; however, it is clinically important.

Function is assessed with a variety of active movements that represent ADLs. These include the 10 activities from Neer, plus four more to address overhead and throwing motions. The patient is given a point total of 4 points for normal movement, 3 points for mild compromise, 2 points for difficulty, 1 point with aid, and zero points if unable to perform the maneuver. The

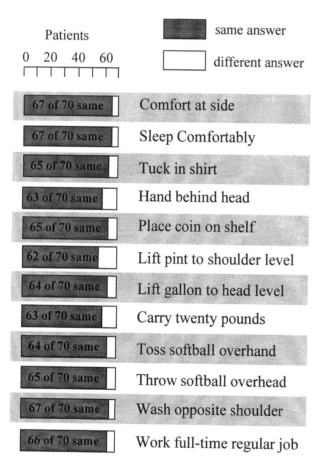

Test- retest Reproducibility of the SST

Patients

0 20 40 60

■ same answer
□ different answer

67 of 70 same	Comfort at side
67 of 70 same	Sleep Comfortably
65 of 70 same	Tuck in shirt
63 of 70 same	Hand behind head
65 of 70 same	Place coin on shelf
62 of 70 same	Lift pint to shoulder level
64 of 70 same	Lift gallon to head level
63 of 70 same	Carry twenty pounds
64 of 70 same	Toss softball overhand
65 of 70 same	Throw softball overhead
67 of 70 same	Wash opposite shoulder
66 of 70 same	Work full-time regular job

FIGURE 4-6 **(A)** *Reproducibility of the Simple Shoulder Test in 70 patients. Retests were administered between 5 and 30 (mean, 14 days) days after the first test was given. The chart shows the number of patients who gave the same answer to the SST questions. (Figure continues.)*

Normal Shoulders aged 60 to 70

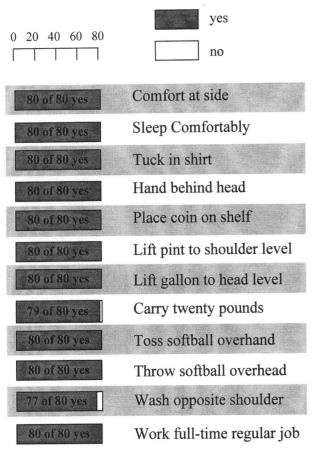

0 20 40 60 80

■ yes
□ no

80 of 80 yes — Comfort at side

80 of 80 yes — Sleep Comfortably

80 of 80 yes — Tuck in shirt

80 of 80 yes — Hand behind head

80 of 80 yes — Place coin on shelf

80 of 80 yes — Lift pint to shoulder level

80 of 80 yes — Lift gallon to head level

79 of 80 yes — Carry twenty pounds

80 of 80 yes — Toss softball overhand

80 of 80 yes — Throw softball overhead

77 of 80 yes — Wash opposite shoulder

80 of 80 yes — Work full-time regular job

FIGURE 4-6 *(Continued).* **(B)** *Results of SST on 80 normal subjects aged 60–70 years. Normal shoulders were determined by history, physical examination, and ultrasound to the rotator cuff. (From Matsen FA et al.,[12] with permission.)*

subjective nature of differentiating between "mild compromise" and "difficulty" is a drawback.

Simple Shoulder Test

The Simple Shoulder Test (SST) was designed as a function-based outcome assessment tool consisting of 12 questions that characterize abnormal function in patients with shoulder pathology.[12,35] The SST appears to be a promising tool for establishing outcomes of shoulder rehabilitation. The therapist can easily administer this test at the beginning and conclusion of treatment. This test is a quantitative tool that can be used to provide a practical outcome of treatment results. The 12 SST questions represent a quick, practical assessment of functional activities that can be administered inexpensively, assessing shoulder function (Table 4-8).

The SST is reproducible (Fig. 4-6 and 4-7) and addresses several levels of function. It is in-

TABLE 4-8 *Simple shoulder test*

1. Is your shoulder comfortable with your arm at rest by your side?	YES/NO
2. Does your shoulder allow you to sleep comfortably?	YES/NO
3. Can you reach the small of your back to tuck in your shirt with your hand?	YES/NO
4. Can you place your hand behind your head with the elbow straight out to the side?	YES/NO
5. Can you place a coin at the level of your shoulder without bending your elbow?	YES/NO
6. Can you lift one lb (a full pint container) to the level of your shoulder without bending your elbow?	YES/NO
7. Can you lift 8 lb (a full gallon container) to the level of your shoulder without bending your elbow?	YES/NO
8. Can you carry 20 lb at your side with the affected extremity?	YES/NO
9. Do you think you can toss a softball underhand 10 yards with the affected extremity?	YES/NO
10. Do you think you can toss a softball overhand 20 yards with the affected extremity?	YES/NO
11. Can you wash the back of your opposite shoulder with the affected extremity?	YES/NO
12. Would your shoulder allow you to work full-time at your regular job?	YES/NO

(From Lippitt SB, et al,[35] with permission.)

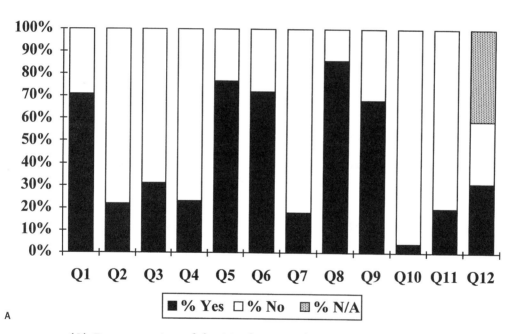

FIGURE 4-7 (A) *Representation of the SST functional outcome in a group of degenerative arthritis patients treated by total shoulder arthroplasty. The bar graph compares the group's preoperative function to their postoperative function at 3-month, 6-month, and 1 to 1.5-year follow-up intervals. (Figure continues.)*

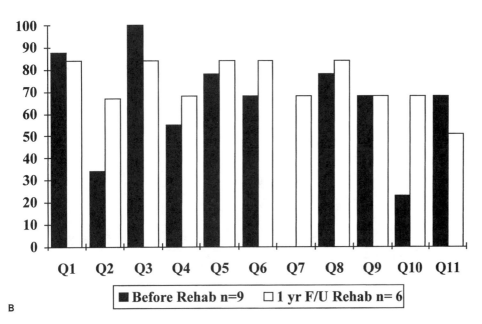

RCT: TREATMENT BY REHABILITATION

Before Rehab n=9   1 yr F/U Rehab n= 6

B

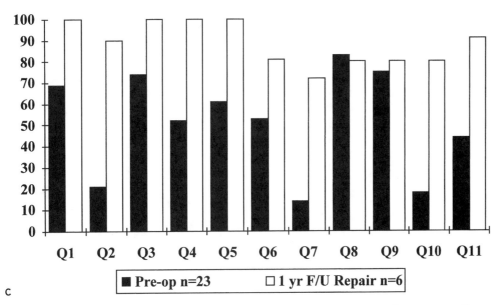

RCT: TREATMENT BY CUFF REPAIR

Pre-op n=23   1 yr F/U Repair n=6

C

FIGURE 4-7 *(Continued).* **(B)** *SST functional outcome in a group of rotator cuff tear patients before and one year after treatment by two different methods: treatment by rehabilitation (re-education, shoulder stretching/strengthening exercises) and* **(C)** *open acromioplasty and repair of rotator cuff tear. (Figure continues.)*

FROZEN SHOULDER

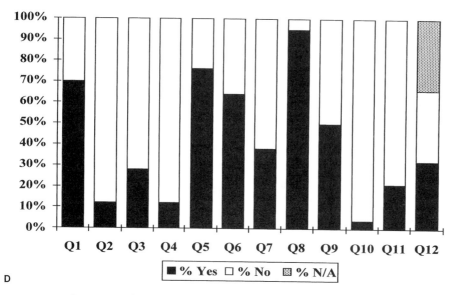

D

FIGURE 4-7 *(Continued).* **(D)** *SST evaluation of a group of patients with "frozen shoulder." (From Lippitt SB et al.,[35] with permission.)*

dependent of diagnosis. The SST is not a scoring system; rather, it is a true functional test. The test is also independent of patient satisfaction, which often rests with the surgeon, not with functional recovery. The test monitors a broad range of functional variables, but is insufficient for individuals with high performance demands.

Figure 4-7 includes sample data compiled with the SST 104.[12,35] Note the changes in SST responses as a result of treatment. One of the advantages of the SST is the graphic profile that it provides of patient function. If one compares the pretreatment profiles for the rehabilitation group versus the surgical group, it becomes apparent that the surgical group was less functional than the treatment group. The other trend is that despite a successful (seven questions had at least nominal, if not noticeable, improvement) comprehensive program, some functional indicators decreased in the rehabilitation group, underlining some of the progressive aspects of rotator cuff disease. The usefulness of this functional test in tracking progress is evident, but larger numbers are required for study. The authors do have some age-related normal values as well as diagnosis-specific data.[12]

Constant System

The Constant System[54] is designed to be used independent of diagnosis (Table 4-9). As such, it represents a pure functional scale that is oriented towards movement. Forty percent of the scoring system is made up of ROM assessment, including forward and lateral elevation, external rotation, and internal rotation. The rotation measures are not in degrees; rather they are based upon anatomic landmarks (similar to ASES and Neer). The Constant system may be the most valid[48] since it obtained assessments within 3 percent by independent observers, but it is not in use outside of Europe. Thirty five percent of the system is subjective, 65 percent objective.

TABLE 4-9 *Constant shoulder assessment*

Scoring for pain (maximum = 15)	None	15
	Mild	10
	Moderate	5
	Severe	0
Scoring for activities of daily living (maximum = 20)	Activity level: Full work	4
	Full recreation/sport	4
	Unaffected sleep	2
	Positioning: Up to the waist	2
	Up to xiphoid	4
	Up to neck	6
	Up to top of head	8
	Above head	10
Scoring for forward and lateral elevation (maximum = 20, 10 for each)	Elevation (in degrees)	Points
	0–30	0
	31–60	2
	61–90	4
	121–150	6
	91–120	8
	151–180	10
External rotation scoring (maximum = 10)	Hand position	Points
	Behind head, elbow forward	2
	Behind head, elbow back	2
	Top of head, elbow forward	2
	Top of head, elbow back	2
	Full elevation from top of head	2
Internal rotation scoring (maximum = 10)	Position dorsum hand	Points
	Lateral thigh	0
	Buttock	2
	Lumbosacral junction	4
	Waist (L3 vert)	6
	T12 vert	8
	Interscapular (T7 vert)	10
Scoring for individual parameters:		
Pain	15	
Activities of daily living	20	
Range of motion	40	
Power	25	
Total	100	

(From Constant CR and Murley AH,[54] with permission.)

Pain is defined relative to the worst pain the patient has experienced, which leaves some room for interpretation. The function testing is based upon subjective assessment of ability to work, sleep, perform recreational activities, and work at various levels of elevation. An unscored factor includes whether the patient is performing these activities at the desired level.[45]

Objectively, the system measures ROM in flexion, abduction, combined external rotation, and combined internal rotation. Points are awarded for available range without pain in flexion and abduction, and obtainable range for the other composite motions. The flexion score reflects the amount of flexion motion that the patient can actively use. The measured flexion is the range of active flexion without pain. If the arm can be lifted to 140 degrees with pain, but to 110 degrees without pain, the flexion retained in the score is 110 degrees; 0–10 points are allocated accordingly. External rotation is measured as functional external rotation, bringing the hand behind the head. Two points are accumulated for each of the five positions, 10 total points can be earned. It should be noted that confusion did exist in the interpretation of Constant's functional assessment of external rotation. Internal rotation is tested in combination with extension and adduction, with the idea that internal rotation serves to reach behind the body; 0–10 points are awarded. The amount of weight that can be lifted in the scapula plane (up to 25 pounds) makes up the remainder of the objective scoring (25% of the total score).

The Constant score is the first system that considers the effects of age and gender on shoulder function. Constant[54] studied 900 healthy individuals and determined normal functional scores for both age and gender categories.

Kerlan-Jobe Athletic Rating Scale

Individuals with high performance demands, particularly athletes, generally do not fit easily into functional rating systems designed for a more sedentary, older population. Issues of ROM, strength, and instability are overwhelmed by the need to perform. Traditional manual muscle and ROM tests are not as useful, since the functional loss may be one of effectiveness (i.e., throwing or serving accurately) rather than execution. High performance athletes are also concerned with the level of competition and their ability to maintain their performance over time (endurance). If one uses a scale designed for the general population, athletes may be unable to participate in their chosen sport at the desired level, but may still be considered as good to excellent.[48]

To address these and other special needs of athletes, particularly throwing athletes, an athletic shoulder rating scale was developed at the Kerlan-Jobe clinic.[48] The rating scale (Table 4-10) specifically scores intensity of competition and level of performance in addition to pain, strength/endurance, and ROM. Range of motion is considered as a loss of external rotation with normal elevation in the scapular plane. Any relative loss of elevation is severely penalized, whatever the external rotation. This scale reflects the somewhat skewed motion requirements of overhand athletes, who often have excessive external rotation at the glenohumeral joint with decreased internal rotation. The philosophy of the scale creators is that instability is the underlying problem for overhand athletes,[48] so 10 percent of the scale is devoted toward symptoms of instability during competition. The performance section accounts for 50 percent of the point total, while the intensity scale contributes an additional 10 percent.

SUMMARY

A variety of orthopaedic and athletic shoulder scoring systems have been reviewed. The results of these systems appear to be reproducible and can be administered without the use of sophisticated equipment. None of these systems has received universal acceptance, but future studies will need to justify the benefit to patient treatment. The patient's functional outcome has be-

TABLE 4-10 *Kerlan-Jobe athletic rating scale*

Type of Sport _____
Position Played _____
Years Played _____
Prior Injury _____

Activity Level
1) Professional (major league)
2) Professional (minor league)
3) College
4) High School
5) Recreational (full time)
6) Recreational (occasionally)

Diagnosis
1) Anterior instability
2) Posterior instability
3) Multidirectional instability
4) Recurrent dislocations
5) Impingement syndrome
6) Acromioclavicular separation
7) Acromioclavicular arthrosis
8) Rotator cuff repair (partial)
9) Rotator cuff repair (complete)
10) Biceps tendon rupture
11) Calcific tendinitis
12) Fracture

SUBJECTIVE (90 points)

I. PAIN	Points
No pain with competition	10
Pain after competition only	8
Pain while competing	6
Pain preventing competing	4
Pain with ADLs	2
Pain at rest	0

II. STRENGTH / ENDURANCE	
No weakness, normal competition fatigue	10
Weakness after competition, early competition fatigue	8
Weakness during competition, abnormal competition fatigue	6
Weakness or fatigue preventing competition	4
Weakness or fatigue with ADLs	2
Weakness or fatigue preventing ADLs	0

III. STABILITY	
No looseness during competition	10
Recurrent subluxations while competing	8
Dead-arm syndrome while competing	6
Recurrent subluxations prevent competition	4
Recurrent subluxations during ADLs	2
Dislocation	0

(Table Continues)

TABLE 4-10 *(Continued)*

IV. INTENSITY		
	Preinjury versus postinjury hours of competition (100%)	10
	Preinjury versus postinjury hours of competition (less than 75%)	8
	Preinjury versus postinjury hours of competition (less than 50%)	6
	Preinjury versus postinjury hours of competition (less than 25%)	4
	Preinjury and postinjury hours of ADLs (100%)	2
	Preinjury and postinjury of ADLs (less than 50%)	1
V. PERFORMANCE		
	At the same level, same proficiency	50
	At the same level, decreased proficiency	40
	At the same level, decreased proficiency, not acceptable to athlete	30
	Decreased level with acceptable proficiency at that level	20
	Decreased level, unacceptable proficiency	10
	Cannot compete, had to switch sport	0
OBJECTIVE (10 Points)		
VI. RANGE OF MOTION		
	Normal external rotation at 90°-90° position, normal elevation	10
	Less than 5° loss of external rotation, normal elevation	8
	Less than 10° loss of external rotation, normal elevation	6
	Less than 15° loss of external rotation, normal elevation	4
	Less than 20° loss of external rotation, normal elevation	2
	Greater than 20° loss of external rotation, or any loss of elevation	0

Overall Results:

Excellent	90 -100 pts.
Good	70-89 pts.
Fair	50-69 pts.
Poor	<50 pts.

(From Tibone JE, and Bradley JP,[48] with permission.)

come a critical issue for those who pay for therapeutic services. If the current trend continues, physical therapists must be able to confirm the benefits of their treatment methods before imposing additional costs on the individual or society.

ELBOW RATING SCALE

Evaluation schemes also exist for the elbow. Inglis and Pellicci[55] used the HSS elbow system to evaluate the results of total elbow replacement (Table 4-11). The scale provides an overall point total based upon pain (30 points), function (20 points), sagittal plane ROM (20 points), pronation ROM (4 points), supination ROM (4 points), flexion and extension contracture (6 points for each), and strength (10 points). The scale is clearly weighted toward an older population, among whom pain and loss of use are the main complaints of the degenerated joint. The scale could be adapted for other diagnoses,[49] as has been done with some of the shoulder scales.

TABLE 4-11 *Hospital of special surgery elbow assessment*

PAIN (30 Pts)	Points
No pain at any time	30
No pain when bending	15
Mild pain when bending	10
Moderate pain when bending	5
Severe pain when bending	0
No pain at rest	15
Mild pain at rest	10
Moderate pain at rest	5
Severe pain at rest	0
FUNCTION (20 Pts)	
Bending activities for 30 min	8
Bending activities for 15 min	6
Bending activities for 5 min	4
Cannot use elbow	0
Unlimited use of elbow	12
Limited only for recreation	10
Household and employment	8
Independent self-care	6
Invalid	0
Sagittal arc (20 Pts)	
One point for each 7 degrees arc of motion	
MUSCLE STRENGTH (10 Pts)	
Can lift 5 lbs. (2.3 kg) to 90 degrees	10
Can lift 2 lbs. (0.9 kg) to 90 degrees	8
Moves through arc of motion against gravity	5
Cannot move through arc of motion	0
FLEXION CONTRACTURE (6 Pts)	
Less than 15 degrees	6
Between 15 and 45 degrees	4
Between 45 and 90 degrees	2
Greater than 90 degrees	0
EXTENSION CONTRACTURE (6 Pts)	
Within 15 degrees of 135 degrees	6
Less than 125 degrees	4
Less than 100 degrees	2
Less than 80 degrees	0
PRONATION (4 Pts)	
Greater than 60 degrees	4
Greater than 30–60 degrees	3
Greater than 15–30 degrees	2
Less than 0 degrees	0
SUPINATION (4 points)	
Greater than 60 degrees	4
Greater than 45 to 60 degrees	3
Greater than 15 to 45 degrees	2
Less than 0 degrees	0

(From Inglis AE and Pellici PM,[55] with permission.)

PHYSICAL THERAPY FUNCTIONAL SHOULDER EVALUATION

This section will discuss the functional objective physical therapy shoulder evaluation. Our system has both subjective and objective measurements totaling 173 points (Table 4-12). A total of 83 points are allocated to the subjective questions, and 90 points are noted on the objective assessment. Points are assigned to individual parameters such as level of overhead activity (5 points), functional assessment (60 points), and pain patterns at rest, night, work/sports all receive 6 points each. Flexion in the scapular plane, external rotation from neutral and from 90 degrees of abduction are assessed with 5-point scores respectively. Internal rotation is evaluated as a functional movement, thumb to the highest spinal process level (5 points). These motions are also conducted using passive motions with a 5-point scoring system.

The shoulder evaluation system presented in this chapter does not utilize evaluation of glenohumeral abduction in the coronal plane for several reasons. First, Neer[56] has suggested that the highest upward excursion and the greatest ease and freedom for raising the arm is the scapular plane. This plane has been termed the "Plane of Maximum Elevation." Secondly, flexion in the scapular plane allows the highest degree of motion with the least amount of capsular tightness. Thirdly, this plane is used most often during ADLs (i.e., reaching for objects on a shelf or shaking hands). Most overhead sporting activities are conducted in this plane, such as a tennis serve or overhead throwing patterns. Our rehabilitation philosophy presented in this chapter includes passive shoulder ROM and strengthening (i.e., proprioceptive neuromuscular facilitation in the scapular plane). Abduction strictly in the coronal plane is a movement that has received far too much attention without any functional movement justification. In our experience, if full scapular elevation and external rotation are restored, abduction in the coronal plane returns. The exceptions to this model would include deltoid injury or nerve damage.

Glenohumeral and scapulothoracic strength

TABLE 4-12 *Physical therapy shoulder evaluation*

Left / Right   Left Handed / Right Handed
Date _____ Patient Name_____ Age_____
Dx _____DOS _____Date Of Injury_____
Occupation_____ Sport _____
Special Precautions_____

SUBJECTIVE:

GENERAL OBSERVATIONS:

Swelling _____ Wound Healing _____ Temperature _____ Sensation _____
Palpation:
Supraspinatus_____Infraspinatus_____TeresMinor_____Deltoid_____BicepsTendon____
AC Joint____Coracoacromial Ligament_____
Biceps Rupture: Yes - No / Cervical Pain: Yes - No / Spurling test (+) or (-)
Mental Attitude_____

Subjective Level of Overhead Activity (5 points)

Professional Athlete / Traumatic injury	5-points	Heavy Laborer / Traumatic injury
College Athlete or Regular Gym workouts	4-points	Moderate Laborer
High School Athlete	3-points	Mild Laborer / a lot of home ADL's
Recreational Athlete, occassionally competitive	2-points	Desk work, occasional overhead lifting at work, regular home ADL's
Weekend Athlete	1-point	Desk work, no overhead lifting
Completely Sedentary	0-points	Completely Sedentary

Total Points _____

Subjective Functional Assessment Questions: (60 points)

5-points = Normal shoulder usage
4-points = Mild shoulder compromise
3-points = Moderate compromise of shoulder usage
2-points = Needs assistance to complete activity
1-point = Inability to complete activity

1. Reach top of head	___	7. Carry 10 lbs.	___
2. Reach opposite axilla	___	8. Use hand at shoulder level	___
3. Reach back pocket	___	9. Do usual work	___

(Continues)

TABLE 4-12 *(Continued)*

4. Perineal care	___	10. Do usual sports ___
5. Dress self	___	11. Eat with utensils ___
6. Sleep on involved shoulder	___	12. Comb hair ___

Total Points _____

SUBJECTIVE PAIN PATTERNS: (18 points)
  a) **Rest**
  b) **Night**
  c) **Work / Sport**

1. Pain at Rest (6 points)

a) No Pain	6-points
b) Mild pain, no medication required	5-points
c) Mild pain, requires medication	4-points
d) Moderate pain, no medication	3-points
e) Severe pain, requires medical attention	2-points
f) Worst pain, ever experienced, requires medical attentions	1-point
g) Not applicable	0-points

Total points____

2. Pain at Night (6 points)

a) No Pain at night	6-points
b) Mild pain at night, does not affect sleeping	5-points
c) Mild pain, interrupts sleep	4-points
d) Mild pain, interrupts sleep unless taking medication	3-points
e) Moderate pain, interrupts sleep not release with medication and requires medical attention	2-points
f) Worst pain ever experienced and requires medial attention	1-point
g) Not applicable	0-points

Total points____

3. Pain during work / sports (6 points)

a) No pain during work or sports	6-points
b) Mild pain, no compromise in activity	5-points
c) Mild pain present during activity, but clears quickly	4-points
d) Moderate pain present, some concessions in activity	3-points
e) Severe pain present, marked limitations in activity	2-points
f) Severe pain, unable to work or participate in sports	1-point
g) Not applicable	0-points

Total points_____

RANGE OF MOTION:
  a) AROM
  b) PROM

1. ACTIVE RANGE OF MOTION: (20 points)
LEFT: Flexion ____ ER (Neutral & 90 Degrees) ____/____ IR _____
RIGHT: Flexion ____ ER (Neutral & 90 Degrees) ____/____ IR _____

(Continues)

TABLE 4-12 *(Continued)*

ACTIVE FLEXION IN THE PLANE OF THE SCAPULA (5 points)

150-above	5-points
120-150	4-points
90-120	3-points
60-90	2-points
50-60	1-points
<50	0-points

Total points _____

ACTIVE EXTERNAL ROTATION (SUPINE LYING) (10 points)

	NEUTRAL	90 DEGREES
Equal motion	5-points	5-points
Less than 10 degree loss of ER	4-points	4-points
Less than 15 degree loss of ER	3-points	3-points
Less than 20 degree loss of ER	2-points	2-points
Less than 25 degree loss of ER	1-point	1-point
> than 25 degrees loss of ER	0-points	0-points

Total points _____

ACTIVE INTERNAL ROTATION (5 points)

Thumb to spinous process level T-7 or above	5-points
Thumb to spinous process level T-8 / T-12	4-points
Thumb to spinous process level L-1 / L-4	3-points
Thumb to spinous process level L-5 / Sacrum	2-points
Thumb to Gluteal region	1-points
Thumb to greater trochanter	0-points

Total points _____

2. PASSIVE RANGE OF MOTION: (20 points)

LEFT: Flexion _____ ER (Neutral & 90 Degrees) _____/_____ IR _____
RIGHT: Flexion _____ ER (Neutral & 90 Degrees) _____/_____ IR _____

PASSIVE FLEXION IN THE PLANE OF THE SCAPULA (5 points)

160-180	5-points
140-160	4-points
120-140	3-points
100-120	2-points
80-100	1-point
< 80	0-points

Total points _____

PASSIVE EXTERNAL ROTATION (SUPINE LYING) (10 points)

	NEUTRAL	90 DEGREES
Equal motion	5-points	5-points
Less than 5 degree loss of ER	4-points	4-points
Less than 10 degree loss of ER	3-points	3-points

(Continues)

TABLE 4-12 *(Continued)*

Less than 15 degree loss of ER	2-points	2-points
Less than 20 degree loss of ER	1-points	1-points
Greater than 20 degrees loss of ER	0-points	0-points

Total points____

PASSIVE INTERNAL ROTATION (5 points)

Thumb to spinous process level T-5 or above	5-points
Thumb to spinous process level T-6 / T-9	4-points
Thumb to spinous process level T-9 / T-11	3-points
Thumb to spinous process level T-12 / L-2	2-points
Thumb to L-2 / L-5	1-points
Thumb to sacrum	0-points

Total points____

STRENGTH / PAIN WITH RESISTANCE? (50 points)

1. Anterior Deltoid	1 2 3 4 5 Y N	6. Supraspinatus
2. Posterior Deltoid	1 2 3 4 5 Y N	7. Scapula Anterior Elevation
3. Complete Deltoid	1 2 3 4 5 Y N	8. Scapula Posterior Elevation
4. Internal Rotation	1 2 3 4 5 Y N	9. Scapula Adduction
5. External Rotation	1 2 3 4 5 Y N	10. Scapula Posterior Depression

Total points____

Muscle Atrophy_____
Strength evaluation precluded due to pain: Yes ____ No ____

TESTS:
LEFT   IMPINGEMENT_____PLANE_____
RIGHT IMPINGEMENT_____PLANE_____

INSTABILITY
LEFT: Posterior   RIGHT: Posterior
          Anterior   Anterior
          Inferior   Inferior

APPREHENSION
LEFT   RIGHT

SPECIAL STABILITY TESTS
General Ligamentous Laxity Factors: Left ____ Right ____
Relocation Left____ Right____
          Left____Right____

OVERALL RESULTS:

EXCELLENT	155-173
GOOD	121-154
FAIR	86-120
POOR	< 86

is evaluated, using 50 points during the 10 tests. Manual muscle testing does create some discrepancies in muscle grades, but is still an important part of the shoulder evaluation. The inclusion of scapula muscle rating is a unique feature. Strength testing of the scapula motions may be even less accurate than those of the rotator cuff, but recognition of these muscle groups is important. Shoulder impingement and stability are also evaluated.

The rating system meets most of the criteria laid out by Gerber[45] for scoring systems. It is fairly explicit in its instructions, although there is the inevitable interpretation of mild versus moderate compromise in the subjective functional assessment. Only shoulder function parameters are used; there is no evaluation of "satisfaction." The scoring system allocates points in proportion to a perceived functional hierarchy: strength and ADL are the largest single blocks, but both are comprehensive sections. No single question is worth more than five percent of the total score. The system can be used for all diagnoses, but it is slightly weighted toward the normal, active person rather than the highly competitive athlete.

Rehabilitation Concepts

Proper and individualized shoulder rehabilitation will enhance the nonoperative and operative treatment of all shoulder disorders.[8,57] Treatment begins as early as possible following injury or surgery. The introduction of early treatment should assist rather than retard soft tissue healing. This will speed the return to activity and shorten the period of disability.

The central determinant of successful shoulder rehabilitation after injury or surgery lies in the restoration of motion.[58] Lack of motion (either passive or active) about the pectoral girdle can create a dyskinetic chain of events that may lead ultimately to clinical symptoms or functional loss.[58] For example, if the patient has a tight posterior capsule, this tight soft tissue structure can push the humeral head anteriorly or superiorly, causing stress to the anterior capsuloligamentous structures.[8] These increased coupled glenohumeral motions may lead to mechanical impingement of the rotator cuff. One could also theorize that this subtle translation of the humeral head could contribute to impingement secondary to instability.

Once full ROM has been obtained, the strengthening phase can begin in most cases. Patients that present with generalized increased laxity factors—as noted by laxity testing (passive movement of the thumb touching the forearm) or increased passive humeral head translation in either the anterior, posterior, or inferior directions—are the exception to this treatment concept. After functional ROM has been re-established in this patient, stability exercises are stressed and ROM exercises de-emphasized.

TRAINING THE SCAPULAR PLATFORM

The significance of the scapular rotators is frequently and erroneously overlooked.[9,59] The rehabilitation program presented in this chapter places considerable emphasis on retraining of the scapular muscles. Facilitation of the scapular platform is accomplished through manual proprioceptive neuromuscular facilitation (PNF). Smooth, coordinated linear and diagonal patterns of scapular facilitation can be maintained through combinations of concentric and eccentric techniques.[33] Figure 4-4 shows the movement of anterior scapular elevation. The patient is elevating his scapula using the serratus anterior muscle, in the direction of his nose as the therapist provides resistance. The therapist should avoid hand placement on the humeral head, as this can sublux the humeral head interiorly.

Figure 4-5 shows posterior elevation of the scapula. The patient elevates the scapula, using the trapezius muscles, as the therapist provides resistance. The patient tries to elevate the scapula toward the posterior region of the occiput.

The Scapular Stabilizer (Breg, Inc., Vista, CA), is another part of the rehabilitation armamentarium useful in the development of scapular strength and endurance. This device allows for selective scapular strengthening without appreciable movement or stress to the glenohumeral joint or injured cuff muscles. This permits early strengthening of the scapular muscles as the repaired shoulder capsular or rotator cuff is still healing. Exercise techniques using the stabilizer (Fig. 4-8–4-11) are described below. The listed muscle actions were tested using EMG surface electrodes to confirm muscle activity.[60]

TRAINING MOVEMENT

The transitional phase between restoring motion and focusing on full strengthening is the movement phase. During the passage from ROM to strength, the therapist focuses on ensuring that the timing and mechanics of basic movement patterns (i.e., PNF) are appropriate. The progression of muscular function during activities in which the hand is free (pointing, throwing) or is being positioned for a skilled function (catching, painting, striking/serving) is proximal to distal.[61,62]

One of the goals of upper extremity rehabilitation is increased function or return to a previous level of skill. Put another way, we are trying to minimize the errors that occur during activity by improving the strength, stability, and motor control of the injured extremity. Minimizing error during movement is accomplished by having a good central image of the activity, adequate sensory input (vision, proprioception, exproprioception, spindles, etc.) to identify the environmental factors and be aware of the orientation and position of the limb in space, and stable proximal joint support, including the glenohumeral joint, scapula, trunk, and lower extremities.

Achieving a stable scapula (see section on training the scapula platform) is a basic goal of most shoulder protocols. Yet the scapula is a freestanding bone with no proximal bony attachments. Its proximal attachments are muscular. Overuse and weakness of these muscles are often the causes of pain and functional loss associated with shoulder dysfunction.

Two solutions are available to the therapist when trying to increase joint stability. The first

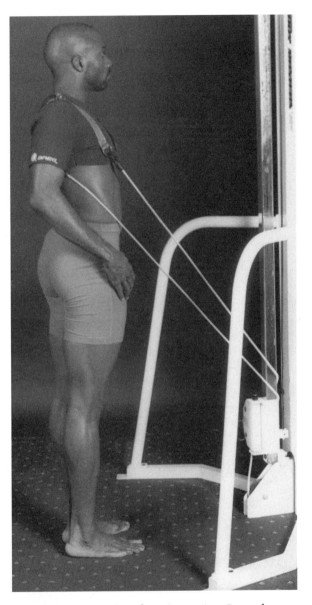

FIGURE 4-8 *Posterior elevation using Scapular Stabilizer in standing (primary muscles: upper trapezius and levator scapula). Additional tension can be added by stepping backward to increase resistance.*

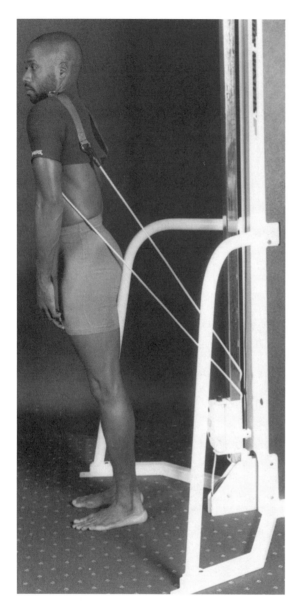

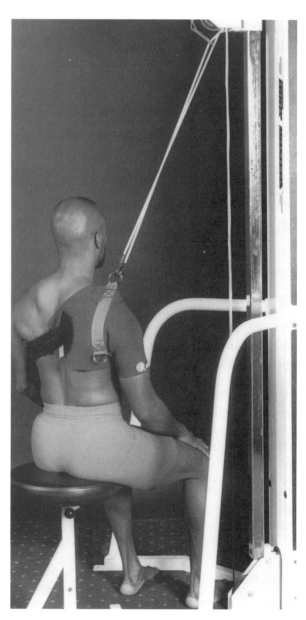

FIGURE 4-9 *Anterior elevation using the Scapular Stabilizer in standing (primary muscle: serratur anterior). Additional tension can be added by stepping forward to increase resistance.*

FIGURE 4-10 *Posterior depression (primary muscle, lower trapezius).*

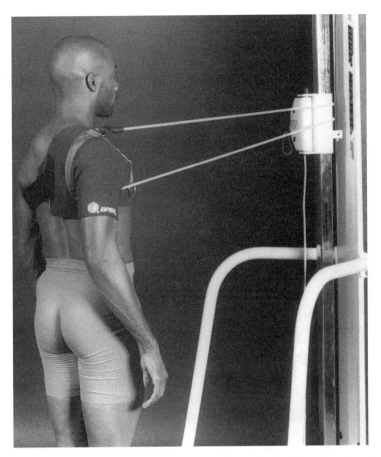

FIGURE 4-11 *Scapular adduction (primary muscles: rhomboids and middle trapezius).*

is to add joint compression and to stabilize using joint reaction force. This is the closed chain approach for the upper extremity. The second is to utilize input from other joints and muscles. The former may be an acceptable solution when the glenohumeral joint is lax and the scapula platform needs strengthening. Adding compression to the glenohumeral joint may improve the ability of the scapula and rotator cuff musculature to fire appropriately.[24] When the scapula itself is "unstable," this solution may not be effective. In this case, the therapist must select the latter option and use other muscles to add stability. The muscles available for this option are the paraspinal and contralateral scapular muscles. They can be recruited by locking the upper arms and

focusing the patient on scapular stabilization during elevation and movement patterns (Figs. 4-12, 4-13). Also, placing the hand in a closed chain environment does not necessarily foster upper extremity function.

Shoulder strengthening should place its emphasis on strengthening three main areas: scapular balancing muscles (upper and lower trapezius, serratus anterior, and rhomboids), humeral head depressors (subscapularis, infraspinatus, teres minor), and the prime humeral positioners (deltoid, pectoralis major, and latissimus dorsi). The supraspinatus is not routinely emphasized in the early phases of rehabilitation, especially in treatment of impingement syndrome. Review of the biomechanical function of this highly

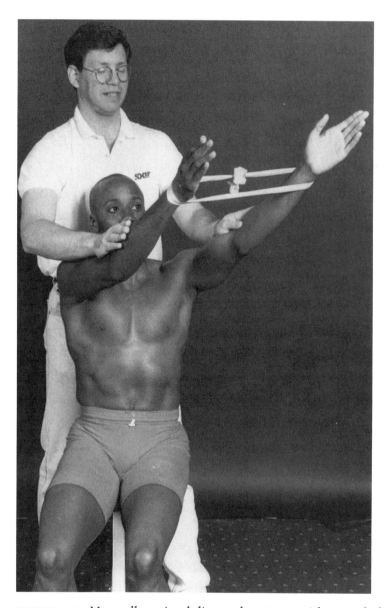

FIGURE 4-12 *Manually resisted diagonal patterns with scapula band for scapula stabilization.*

studied muscle reveals that it primarily acts in concert with the deltoid as a humeral elevator and secondarily assists with compression and stabilization of the humeral head in the glenoid.[63,92,94] Our rehabilitation program strengthens this muscle after the humeral depressing muscles have achieved full strength

(Figs. 4-14, 4-15). Supraspinatus strengthening is conducted with those patients that present shoulder instability.

The rehabilitation program should be progressive, cost-effective, and include specific exercises that address the dysfunction in an expedient manner. This program should promote

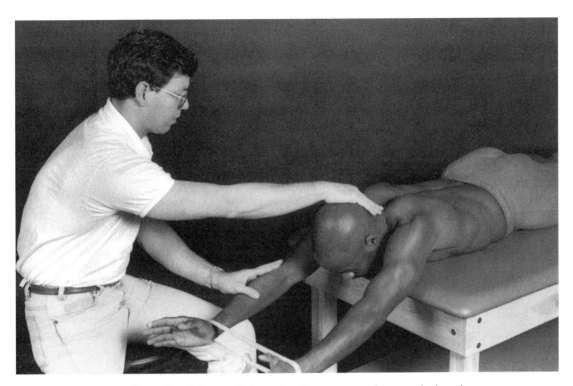

FIGURE 4-13 *Manually resisted forward elevation in prone with scapula band for scapula stabilization.*

principles of the soft tissue healing about the shoulder. The physician, therapist, and patient all have individual responsibilities during the rehabilitation process, and each should be advised of their respective roles.

For a detailed review of the muscle activity during exercise and various athletic activities, the reader is referred to the series of exercises from the lab of Jobe and Perry,[18,22,63–73] as well as other sources[19,21,74–76] (also see Ch. 7). These articles describe the timing and intensity of the scapula stabilizers, rotator cuff, and glenohumeral muscles during swimming, throwing, golfing, and rehabilitation. It is important to note the delicate interaction between the scapular rotators, stabilizers, rotator cuff, and deltoid muscles. Often, a recognizable pattern is present with repetitive activities such as swimming and throwing. The effect of pain and instability are noted by changes in muscle function. Concomitant effects on sensory inputs from the patho-logic as well as normal supporting structures must be taken into account.

SHOULDER PROPRIOCEPTION

Shoulder joint proprioception or kinesthesia appears to be an important part of shoulder rehabilitation. This section focuses on methods employed to improve joint position sense and kinesthesia. However, limited studies on this topic exist, and few provide the clinician with much practical and easy application.[77]

Davies and Malone[77] use a definition of kinesthesia based upon the work of Newton[78] as the ability to discriminate joint position, relative weight of body parts, and joint movement including direction, amplitude, and speed. In theory, retraining of proprioception should match the sports-specific stimulation of the joint and muscle receptors.[79]

Loss of shoulder proprioception following shoulder subluxation, dislocation, or rotator cuff injury is an area of controversy.[80–82] Lephart et al.[83] have attempted to provide normative data involving the measurement of shoulder proprioception. This data, coupled with future mechanoreceptor research, should assist the clinical assessment of joint sense in those patients that have suffered bouts of shoulder instability.

In a second study, Lephart et al.[84] investi-

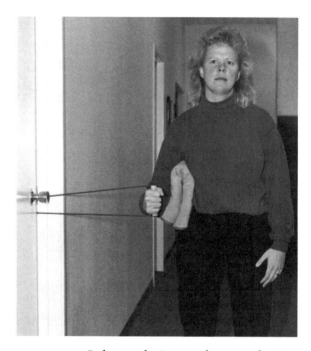

FIGURE 4-15 *Subscapularis muscle strengthening. Care is taken to avoid overloading of the cuff until inflammation is controlled. A small towel roll or bolster is placed between the humerus and body. In selective patients this has decreased pain during resisted internal rotation. One could theorize this reduction in pain by noting that the vascular supply of the supraspinatus may be improved by positioning the humerus in slight abduction. Positioning the humerus in slight abduction may improve the depressor effect of the subscapularis, providing another factor in the resultant decreased pain.*

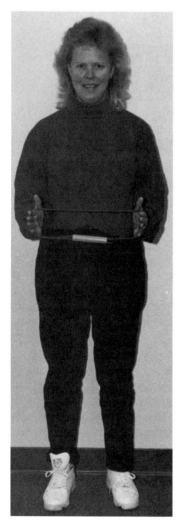

FIGURE 4-14 *Infraspinatus and teres minor muscles strengthening with resisted external rotation.*

gated proprioception by measuring kinesthesis and joint position sense in normal, unstable, and postcapsulolabral reconstructed shoulders. They concluded that proprioception of the shoulder is not related to shoulder dominance, diminishes following capsuloligamentous injury, and is restored following capsulolabral reconstruction for shoulder instability.

Jerosch et al.[85] evaluated proprioceptive function by placing the arm in different positions without visual control. Tests were performed on both dominant and nondominant extremities using volunteers. The results showed significant differences between the measurements with and without visual control. No differences between dominant and nondominant extremities or between male and female subjects were reported. This study did reveal a low variance of the proprioceptive function of the glenohumeral joint in healthy subjects.

Rotator cuff tears and joint position sense have also been investigated.[86] Subjects were blindfolded and asked to elevate the humerus in two positions. There was a significant correlation between the affected side (rotator cuff tear) and the control group at 45 degrees of shoulder abduction. No significant differences were noted at 90 degrees of shoulder abduction.

Speer et al.[58] has proposed that a reflex neurologic inhibition or "global dyskinetic" shutdown of shoulder muscles occurs following injury or surgery. Many patients present muscle spasm or guarding following injury or surgery. The described global dyskinetic shutdown theory may also contribute to the loss of normal movement patterns and reduction of upper extremity proprioception.

Speer et al.[58] recommended the use of aquatic therapy during treatment of the involved upper extremity. Aquatic therapy utilizes buoyancy-assisted, and-supported, and progresses to buoyancy-resisted levels of exercises.[87] Progression of exercise is based on the principles of soft tissue healing that have been used during land-based rehabilitation.[88] The increased shoulder hydrostatic pressures combined with the buoyancy effects of water, help stimulate skin proprioceptors, which aid in a biofeedback-like loop that helps to normalize movement and shoulder proprioception.[58,88]

Proper shoulder rehabilitation involves both open and closed kinematic chain training to facilitate joint proprioceptors to enhance stability and dynamic muscular control. Our position on shoulder rehabilitation is to provide proximal control of the scapulothoracic joint to facilitate stability of the glenohumeral joint. Townsend et al.[73] have identified a combination of four exercises that have been electromyographically shown to be a solid core of the rehab program.

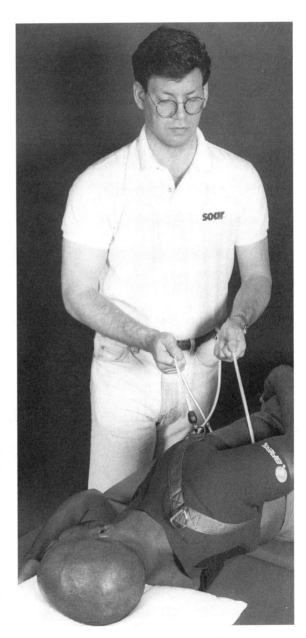

FIGURE 4-16 *Open chain posterior elevation is used early in the rehabilitation program as controlled resistance is applied by the therapist.*

These exercises include: scaption, rowing, push-ups with a plus, and press-ups. Exercises combine both open and closed chain shoulder rehabilitation techniques. However, proper soft tissue healing must be considered before implementing these "core" exercises.

Joint position information from joint, skin, and muscle receptors is also used to determine the orientation of joints and limbs in space.[89] In the upper extremity, many skills and functions are dependent upon hand placement. The placement of the hand in space is a determined by the action of the proximal joint musculature acting on directions from the central nervous system. The data from multiple sensory inputs (vision, proprioception, etc.) are transformed into knowledge of hand position and limb orientation in three-dimensional space. Loss of neuromechanical integrity of a joint not only causes increased tissue stress but also affects the afferent input from related structures. This may result in increased errors and decreased accuracy in placement of the distal segment.[89-92] In the upper extremity, this may result in problems with throwing, racquet sports, or control of golf clubs and baseball bats. All of these activities depend upon a combination of applied power with accuracy, which may be difficult to

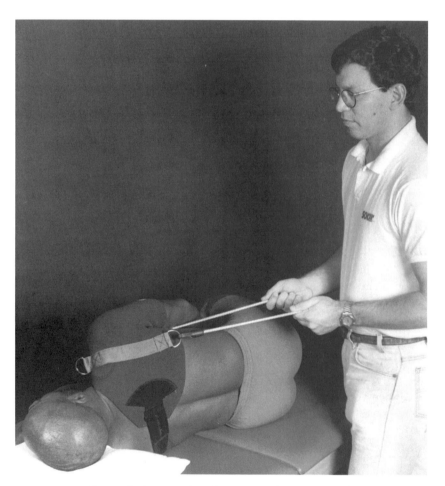

FIGURE 4-17 *Open chain anterior elevation. Therapist applies resistance during this movement pattern.*

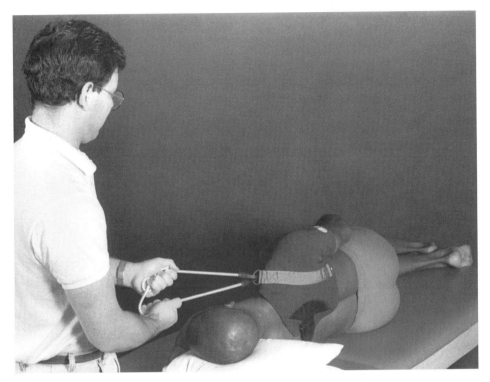

FIGURE 4-18 *Resisted posterior depression.*

achieve in the face of an altered neuromotor program.

Open/closed chain scapular proprioception exercises that we commonly use are reviewed in Figures 4-16 to 4-25. Initial open chain scapular exercises begin using either manual resistance or the Breg Scapular Stabilizer, conducted side-lying with resistant cords hooked to the front and back "D" rings (Fig. 4-16). The patient elevates the scapulothoracic joint to the posterior occiput region. The therapist applies and regulates proprioceptive input by adjusting tension in the resistance cords during movement.

Resistance cords are adjusted similar to flying a kite that requires directional adjustments by the controller to achieve the desired movement pattern. By adjusting tension via the resistance cords, the therapist can maintain the desired scapula movement pattern. If the patient deviates from the movement pattern, the therapist places additional resistance on the appropri-

ate cord (proprioceptive input), which moves the patient into the desired movement pattern. Figure 4-17 denotes a similar concept for anterior scapular elevation. Posterior scapular depression (Fig. 4-18) is trained as the resistant strap(s) are placed on the top "D" ring. The patient is advised to pull the shoulder blade toward midline and the elbow toward the ipsilateral posterior hip pocket. This particular exercise requires some teaching to achieve the desired movement pattern.

Lower trapezius, middle trapezius, rhomboids, and serratus anterior strengthening are noted in Figures 4-19 to 4-22. These exercises require normal function of the deltoid-rotator cuff force couple before attempting these movements.

Open chain glenohumeral proprioceptive training is the next area we will address. The most commonly used form of proprioceptive-kinesthetic shoulder training involves the use of rhythmic stabilization. Figure 4-23 shows this

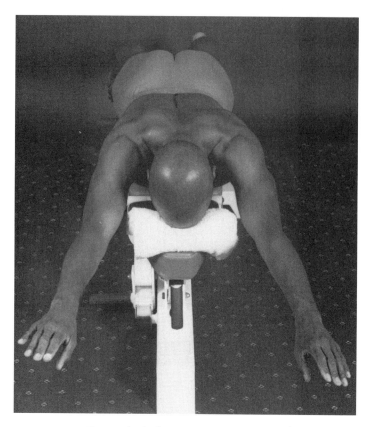

FIGURE 4-19 *Open chain lower trapezius strengthening with glenohumeral joint involvement.*

technique at 90 degrees of shoulder elevation in the plane of the scapula. The therapist applies resistance in a known direction as the patient applies resistance to stabilize movement. The next progression includes the same exercise conducted at 120 degrees of shoulder elevation in the plane of the scapula.[93] Precautions are needed during rhythmic stabilization at higher ranges of elevation. Glenohumeral stability should be a consideration at higher degrees of elevation.[94] Scapular stability and rotator cuff strength should also be considered during any progression of shoulder exercises.

Proprioceptive neuromuscular facilitation (PNF), developed by Kabat[31] and later popularized by Knott and Voss,[32] is introduced. These patterns of exercise are implemented for facilita-

tion of shoulder strength and kinesthesia.[95] These patterns are used during the final phases of shoulder rehabilitation. The reader is referred to the work of Kabat[31] and Knott and Voss[32] for further description of PNF patterns.

Closed chain scapulothoracic proprioceptive and strengthening exercises are commonly used in our clinic. Closed chain scapulothoracic exercises include the use of stabilization balls to strengthen the lower trapezius muscle (Fig. 4-24). Quadruped stabilization is another form of closed chain training. The patient focuses on controlling scapula movement during a weight-bearing position on all fours. Exercise is progressed to all threes using a known pattern and later an unknown applied resistance/movement produced by the therapist (Fig. 4-25).

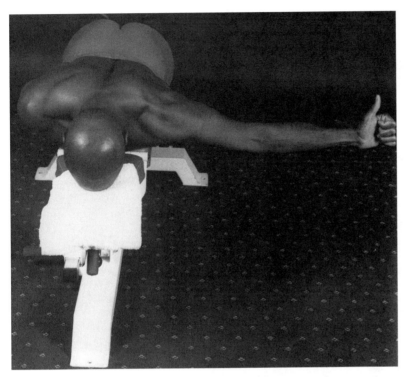

FIGURE 4-20 *Open chain middle trapezius strengthening with glenohumeral joint involvement.*

The final phase of neurophysiologic training includes the use of plyometrics. This form of training has been defined to provide a quick and powerful movement involving a prestretching of the muscle, thereby activating the stretch-shortening cycle.[4] This type of training has been shown to increase the excitability of the neurologic receptors for improved reactivity of the neuromuscular system.

POSTURAL CORRECTIONS

As we proceed with a treatment plan, we must remember that postural deviations have usually developed over many months, and even years. Assessment of posture will direct our attention to these deviations and the possible effects they have had on normal muscle function as it relates to the scapulothoracic and glenohumeral joints. The therapist should address shortening and

weakening caused as a result of certain postural deviations. Training and education will be a very important part of this aspect of care. Movement patterns must incorporate an understanding of correct posturing during work, play, and sport.

Treatment of Upper Quarter Postural Deficits

Therapeutic treatment of shoulder pathology must establish priorities in care. Identifying key events that contribute to the patient's current complaints is extremely important in reaching desired outcomes. An area of concern, often neglected, will be the patient's postural habits. Determination of involved muscle groups, likely to have shortened or weakened given the patient's postural deviations, will be noted upon examina-

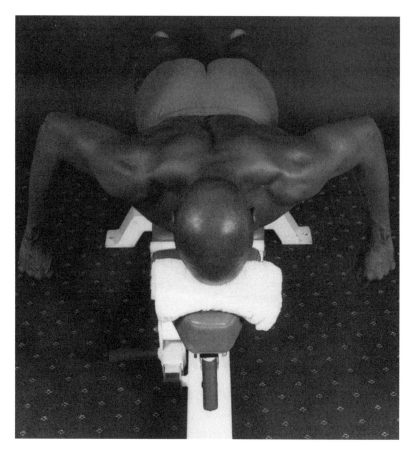

FIGURE 4-21 *Open chain rhomboid strengthening.*

tion. Prescribed postural activities will address issues that are related to months or even years of poor posturing and positioning. Therefore, any direction we take with postural deviations will produce results that are time-dependent. Effectiveness is achieved through education and patient compliance. The patient must understand the postural deviation, and take an active role in correcting the deviation through appropriate exercise and positioning. A patient's growing awareness of movement can greatly assist them in correcting current postural deviations as they perform their home program on a daily basis. Patients need to feel and understand movement that is performed with a minimum of effort. They must attempt to establish greater aware-

ness of movement, taking place in any direction, with maximum ease and efficiency. Finally, patients can learn again to initiate movement with a minimum of preliminary adjustments while performing daily activities.

Our care of postural conditions should include or consider four key components:

1. Mobilization of joints as necessary
2. Myofascial stretching of tight or shortened muscles
3. Strengthening of weakened muscles
4. Re-education of movement awareness

Postural corrections are best made when the patient understands movement awareness and can

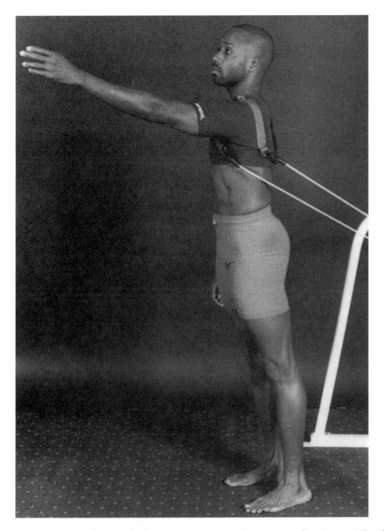

FIGURE 4-22 *Open chain serratus anterior strengthening with glenohumeral joint involvement.*

easily identify inappropriate postural positions.[14] Our ultimate goal in postural correction is to restore the postural muscles that have altered the scapulothoracic function. Thus, through restoration of neuromuscular control, scapular muscles can now dynamically position the glenoid fossa, correctly producing efficient glenohumeral movement.

Key elements of correcting postural deviations are first applying overcorrection, and then adding duration to the over-correction.[14] This can only be accomplished through a diligent home program performed by the patient. An example is a patient who presents with a forward head and rounded shoulder position. The patient is taught proper postural alignment and issued activities to reverse the effect of his current daily postural malalignment. Expected performance of postural exercises are to be completed hourly, and in some cases every quarter hour.

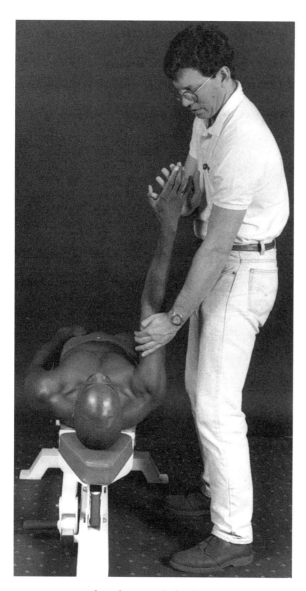

FIGURE 4-23 *Glenohumeral rhythmic stabilization is conducted as the patient controls movements generated by the therapist. The therapist changes directions providing both strengthening and proprioceptive-kinesthetic training.*

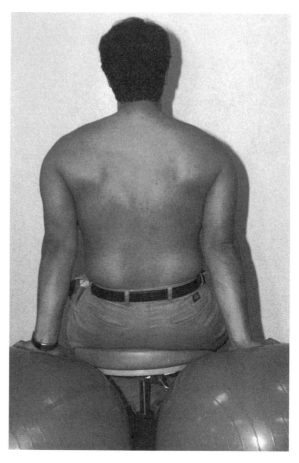

FIGURE 4-24 *Closed chain lower trapezius strengthening using stabilization balls as the patient depresses the shoulder girdle.*

Priority of care will address the acute signs and symptoms we find in our patient. However, we may choose familiar joint or soft tissue mobilization techniques to assist in the restoration of normal muscle function of the upper quarter. Myofascial changes can be evoked immediately with proper techniques. These selected techniques are used in preparation for range of motion and strengthening activities. It can be said there is nothing special about treatment protocols that address postural deviations. This is an area in which simplicity is the best choice and patient compliance is mandatory.

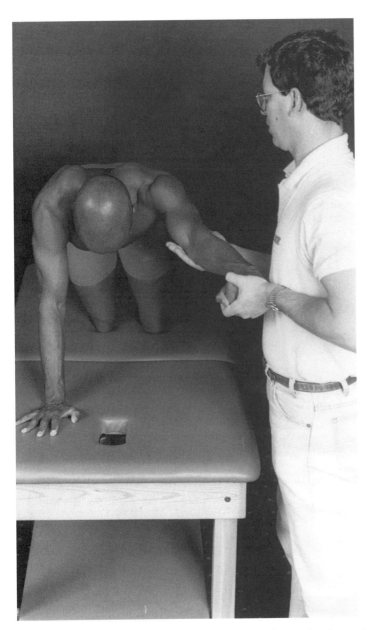

FIGURE 4-25 *The patient receives resistance from the therapist from the all-three position. Exercise begins as the therapist applies a pushing force to the left shoulder. The patient is forced to fire the lower trapezius muscle. Additional movements can be applied by the therapist in known directions, later progressing to unknown patterns.*

Acknowledgments

The authors would like to thank Karen Dobbins for her assistance in preparing this manuscript.

References

1. Kibler WB: Biomechanical analysis of the shoulder during tennis activities. Clin Sports Med 14: 79–85, 1995
2. Lee HWM: Mechanics of neck and shoulder injuries in tennis players. J Orthop Sports Phys Ther 21:28–37, 1995
3. Albert M: Eccentric Muscle Training in Sports and Orthopaedics. Churchill Livingstone, New York, 1991
4. Wilk KE, Voight ML, Keirns MA et al: Stretch-shortening drills for the upper extremities: theory and clinical application. J Orthop Sports Phys Ther 17:225–239, 1993
5. Kibler WB: Role of the scapula in overhead throwing motions. Contemporary Orthop 22:526–532, 1991
6. Luttgens K, Deutsch H, Hamilton N: Kinesiology Scientific Basis of Human Motion. 8th Ed. WCB Brown and Benchmark Publishers, Wisconsin, 1992
7. Norkin C, Levangie P: Joint structure and function: a comprehensive analysis. F.A. Davis, Philadelphia, 1983
8. Morrison DS, Einhorn AR: Rehabilitation of impingement syndrome. In Seitz WH (ed): Rehabilitation of the Shoulder C.V. Mosby, Churchill, Ill. (In publication)
9. Paine R, Voight M: The role of the scapula. J Orthop Sports Phys Ther 18:386–391, 1993
10. Janda V: Muscles and cervicogenic pain syndromes. p. 153. In Grant R (ed): Physical Therapy of the Cervical and Thoracic Spine. Churchill Livingstone, New York, 1988
11. Ayub E: Posture of the upper quarter. p. 81 In Donatelli R, (ed): Physical Therapy of the Shoulder. Churchill Livingstone, New York, 1987
12. Matsen FA, Lippitt SB, Sidles JA, et al: Practical Evaluation and Management of the Shoulder. W.B. Saunders, Philadelphia, 1994
13. Greenfield B, Catlin PA, Coats PW et al: Posture in patients with shoulder overuse injuries and healthy individuals. J Orthop Sports Phys Ther 21:287–295, 1995
14. Culham E, Peat M: Functional anatomy of the shoulder complex. J Orthop Sports Phys Ther 18: 342–363, 1993
15. Clarke GR, Willis LA, Fish WW, et al.: Preliminary studies in measuring range of motion in normal and painful stiff shoulders. Rheumatol Rehab 14: 39–46, 1975
16. Binder AI, Bulgen DY, Hazelman BL et al: Frozen shoulder: a long term prospective study. Ann Rheumatol Dis 43:288–292, 1984
17. Shaffer B, Tibone JE, Kerlan RK: Frozen shoulder. A long term follow-up. J Bone Joint Surg 74A: 738–746, 1992
18. Glousman R, Jobe F, Tibone J et al: Dynamic electromyographic analysis of the throwing shoulder with glenohumeral instability. J Bone Joint Surg 70A:220–226, 1988
19. Broström L-Å, Kronberg M, Nemeth G: Muscle activity during shoulder dislocation. Acta Orthop Scand 60:639–641, 1989
20. Howell SM, Kraft TA: The role of the supraspinatus and infraspinatus muscles in glenohumeral kinematics of anterior shoulder instability. Clin Orthop Rel Res 263:128–134, 1991
21. Kronberg M, Broström L-Å, Nemeth G: Differences in shoulder muscle activity between patients with generalized joint laxity and normal controls. Clin Orthop Rel Res 289:181–192, 1991
22. Glousman R: Electromyographic analysis and its role in the athletic shoulder. Clin Orthop Rel Res 288:27–34, 1973
23. Pande P, Hawkins R, Peat M: Electromyography in voluntary posterior instability of the shoulder. Am J Sports Med 17:644–648, 1989
24. Davies G, Dickoff-Hoffman S: Neuromuscular testing and rehabilitation of the shoulder complex. J Orthop Sports Phys Ther. 18:449–458, 1993
25. Neiers L, Worrel T: Assessment of scapular position. J Sport Rehab 2:20–25, 1993
26. Gibson MH, Goebel GV, Jorden TM et al: A reliability study of measurement techniques to determine static scapular position. J Orthop Sports Ther 21:100–106, 1995
27. DiVeta J, Walker ML, Skibinski B: Relationship between performance of selected scapular muscles and scapular abduction in standing subjects. Phys Ther 70:470–476, 1990
28. Ayub E, Glasheen-Wray M, Kraus S. Head posture: a case study of the effects on the rest position of the mandible. J Orthop Sports Phys Ther 5: 179–185, 1995

29. Paris S: Extremity Dysfunction and Mobilization. Course notes, 1979

30. Calliet R: Shoulder Pain. F.A. Davis, Philadelphia, 1991

31. Kabat H: Proprioceptive facilitation in therapeutic exercises. p. 327. In: Therapeutic Exercises. Waverly Press, Baltimore, MD, 1965

32. Knott M, Voss DE: Proprioceptive Neuromuscular Facilitation. Harper and Row, New York, 1968

33. Engle RP, Canner GC: Posterior shoulder instability: approach to rehabilitation. J Orthop Sports Phys Ther 10:488–494, 1989

34. Grieve GP: Mobilization of the Spine. Churchill Livingstone, Edinburgh, 1991

35. Lippitt SB, Harryman DT, Matsen FA: A practical tool for evaluating function: the simple shoulder test. In Matsen FA, Fu FH, Hawkins RJ (eds): The Shoulder: A Balance of Mobility and Stability. American Academy of Orthopaedic Surgeons, Rosemont, IL, 1992

36. Rowe CR, Patel D, Southmayd WW: The Bankart procedure: A long-term end-result study. J Bone Joint Surg 60A:1–16, 1978

37. Rowe CR, Zarins B: Recurrent transient subluxation of the shoulder. J Bone Joint Surg 63A:863–871, 1981

38. Neer CS II: Anterior acromioplasty for the chronic impingement syndrome in the shoulder: a preliminary report. J Bone Joint Surg 54A:41–50, 1972

39. Neer CS II: Replacement arthroplasty for glenohumeral osteoarthritis. J Bone Joint Surg 56A:1–13, 1974

40. Neer CS II, Watson KC, Stanton FJ: Recent experience in total shoulder replacement. J Bone Joint Surg 64A:319–337, 1982

41. Amstutz HC, Sew Hoy AL, Clarke IC: UCLA anatomic total shoulder arthroplasty. Clin Orthop Rel Res 155:7–20, 1981

42. Ellman H, Hanker G, Bayer M: Repair of the rotator cuff: end-result study of factors influencing reconstruction. J Bone Joint Surg 68A:1136–1144, 1986

43. Ellman H, Kay SP: Arthroscopic subacromial decompression for chronic impingement. J Bone Joint Surg 73B:395–398, 1991

44. Altchek DW, Warren RF, Wickiewicz TL et al: Arthroscopic acromioplasty: technique and results. J Bone Joint Surg 72A:1198–1207, 1990

45. Gerber C: Integrated scoring systems for the functional assessment of the shoulder. In Matsen FA, Fu FH, Hawkins RJ (eds): The Shoulder: A Balance of Mobility and Stability. American Academy of Orthopaedic Surgeons, Rosemont, IL, 1992

46. Montgomery WH, Jobe FW: Functional outcomes in athletes after modified anterior capsulolabral reconstruction. Am J Sports Med 22:352–358, 1994

47. Burkhead WZ, Rockwood CA: Treatment of instability of the shoulder with an exercise program. J Bone Joint Surg 74A:890–896, 1992

48. Tibone JE, Bradley JP: Evaluation of treatment outcomes for the athlete's shoulder. In Matsen FA, Fu FH, Hawkins RJ (eds): The Shoulder: A Balance of Mobility and Stability. American Academy of Orthopaedic Surgeons, Rosemont, IL, 1992

49. Pynset P, Fairbank J, Carr A: Outcome Measures in Orthopaedics. Butterworth Heinemann, Oxford, 1994

50. Warren RF, Ranawat CS, Inglis AE. Total shoulder replacement indications and results of the Neer nonconstrained prosthesis. pp. 56–57. In: Inglis AE (ed) The American Academy of Orthopaedic Surgeons: Symposium on Total Joint Replacement of the Upper Extremity. C.V. Mosby, St. Louis 1982

51. Blevins FT, Warren RF, Cavo C et al: Arthroscopic assisted rotator cuff repair: results a mini-open deltoid splitting approach. Arthroscopy 12:50–59, 1996

52. Barrett WP, Franklin JL, Jackins SE et al: Total shoulder arthroplasty. J Bone Joint Surg 69A:865–872, 1987

53. Gartsmann GM: Arthroscopic acromioplasty for lesions of the rotator cuff. J Bone Joint Surg 72A:169–175, 1990

54. Constant CR, Murley AH: A clinical method of functional assessment of the shoulder. Clin Ortho Rel Res 214:160–164, 1987

55. Inglis AE, Pellicci PM: Total elbow replacement. J Bone Joint Surg 62A:1252–1258, 1990

56. Neer CS: Shoulder Reconstruction. W.B. Saunders, New York, 1990

57. Einhorn AR, Jackson DW: Rehabilitation of shoulder. p. 103. In Jackson DW (ed): Shoulder Surgery in the Athlete. Aspen Systems, Maryland, 1985

58. Speer KP, Cavanaugh JT, Warren RF et al: A role for hydrotherapy in shoulder rehabilitation. Am J Sport Med 21:850–853, 1993

59. Pink M, Jobe F: Shoulder injuries in athletes. Clinical Management 11:39–47, 1991

60. Bradley D, Einhorn, A: Unpublished EMG Report, 1993

61. Chapman AE, Sanderson DJ: Muscular coordination in sporting skills. p. 609. In: Winters JM, Woo SL-Y (eds). Multiple Muscle Systems: Biomechanics and Movement Organization. Springer Verlag, New York, 1990

62. Putnam CA: Sequential motions of body segments in striking and throwing skills: descriptions and explanations. J Biomechanics 26(suppl 1): 125–135, 1993

63. Jobe FW, Moynes DR, Antonelli DJ: Rotator cuff function during a golf swing. Am J Sports Med 14:388–392, 1986

64. Jobe FW, Tibone JE, Perry J, Moynes D: An EMG analysis of the shoulder in throwing and pitching. A preliminary report. Am J Sports Med 11:3–5, 1983

65. Jobe FW, Moynes DR, Tibone JE, et al: An EMG analysis of the shoulder in pitching. A second report. Am J Sports Med 12:218–220, 1984

66. Jobe FW, Perry J, Pink M: Electromyographic shoulder activity in men and women professional golfers. Am J Sports Med 17:782–787, 1989

67. Gowan ID, Jobe FW, Tibone JE et al: A comparative electromyographic analysis of the shoulder in pitching. Professional vs amateur pitchers. Am J Sports Med 15:586–590, 1987

68. Mosely JB, Jobe FW, Pink M et al: EMG analysis of the scapula muscles during a shoulder rehabilitation program. Am J Sports Med 20:128–134, 1992

69. Nuber GW, Jobe FW, Perry J et al: Fine wire electromyography of the shoulder during swimming. Am J Sports Med 14:7–11, 1986

70. Pink M, Perry J, Browne A et al.: The normal shoulder during freestyle swimming. An electromyographic and cinematographic analysis of twelve muscles. Am J Sports Med 19:569–576, 1991

71. Ryu RKN, McCormick J, Jobe FW et al.: An electromyographic analysis of function in tennis players. Am J Sports Med 16:481–485, 1988

72. Scovazzo ML, Browne A, Pink M et al.: The painful shoulder during freestyle swimming: an electromyographic cinematographic analysis of twelve muscles. Am J Sports Med 19:577–587, 1991

73. Townsend H, Jobe FW, Pink M, et al.: Electromyographic analysis of the glenohumeral muscles during a baseball rehabilitation program. Am J Sports Med 19:264–272, 1991

74. Blackburn TA, McLeod WD, White B, et al.: EMG analysis of posterior rotator cuff exercises. Athletic Training 25:40–45, 1990

75. McCann PD, Wooten MP, Kadaba MP: A kinematic and electromyographic study of shoulder rehabilitation exercises. Clin Orthop Rel Res 288: 179–188, 1993

76. Warner JJP, Micheli LJ, Arslanian LE et al.: Patterns of flexibility, laxity, and strength in normal shoulders with instability and impingement. Am J Sports Med. 18:366–374, 1992

77. Davies GJ, Malone T: Open and closed kinetic chain exercises and their application to testing and rehabilitation. Presented at American Orthopaedic Society for Sports Medicine, Eighteenth Annual Meeting, San Diego, CA July 6–9, 1992

78. Newton RA: Joint receptor contributions to reflexive and kinesthetic responses. Phys Ther 62: 22–29, 1982

79. Allegrucci M, Whitney SL, Irrgang JJ: Clinical implications of secondary impingement of the shoulder in freestyle swimmers. J Orth Sports Ther 20: 307–318, 1994

80. Muller GF, et al.: Distribution and morphology of mechanoreceptors in the shoulder joint, abstracted. Shoulder and Elbow Surg, 4:S22, 1995

81. Blasier RB: Shoulder proprioception: effect of joint laxity, joint position, direction of motion, and muscle fatigue, abstracted. J Shoulder and Elbow Surg 4:S34, 1995

82. Tibone J, Fechter, J: Evaluation of shoulder proprioception in stable and unstable shoulder patients utilizing somatosensory evoked potentials. J Shoulder and Elbow Surg 4:S51, 1995

83. Lephart SM et al.: Normal shoulder proprioception measurements in college age individuals. Presented at the Eighteenth Annual Meeting, American Orthopaedic Society for Sports Medicine. San Diego, CA, July 6–9, 1992

84. Lephart SM et al.: Proprioception of the shoulder joint in normal, unstable and post capsulolabral reconstructed individuals, abstracted. J Shoulder and Elbow Surg 4:S2, 1995

85. Jerosch J: Proprioceptive function of the glenohumeral joint in healthy volunteers, abstracted. Shoulder and Elbow Surg 4:S21, 1995

86. Morisawa Y et al.: A study on the position sense of the shoulder joint in the cases of rotator cuff tears, abstracted. J Shoulder and Elbow Surg 4: S82, 1995

87. Marlier, L: Progressive Techniques for the Aquatic therapist. Presented at Integrating Aquatic Rehab

into Physical Therapy Programs and Progressive Techniques for the Aquatic Therapist. February 25–26, 1995, Richardson, TX

88. Einhorn, AR, Sawyer M: The problem knee soft tissue considerations. In Engle RP: Knee Ligament Rehabilitation. Churchill Livington New York, 1991

89. Soechting J, Flanders M: Sensorimotor representations for pointing to targets in three-dimensional space. J Neurophys 62:582–594, 1989

90. Gordon J, Ghilardi MF, Ghez C: Impairments of reaching movements in patients without proprioception. I. Spatial errors. J Neurophysiol 73:347–360, 1995

91. Ghez C, Gordon J, Ghilardi MF: Impairments of reaching movements in patients without proprioception. II. Effects of visual information on accuracy. J Neurophysiol 73:361–372, 1995

92. Perry J: Anatomy and biomechanics of the shoulder in throwing, swimming, gymnastics, and tennis. Clin Sports Med 2:247–270, 1983

93. Einhorn AR: Shoulder rehabilitation: equipment modifications. J Orthop Sports Phys Ther 6:247–253, 1985

94. Morrison DS, Frogameni AD, Woodworth P: Conservative management of impingement syndrome of the shoulder (in preparation)

95. Voss DE, Ionta MK, Myers BJ: Proprioceptive Neuromuscular Facilitation. Patterns and Techniques. 3rd Ed. Harper & Row, 1985, Philadelphia

5

Functional Rehabilitation of the Spine: The Lumbopelvis as a Key Point of Control

SHAW BRONNER

Traditional evaluation of the spine emphasizes gross and segmental spinal range of motion (ROM) in standing and gravity-eliminated positions. This is correlated with a neurologic workup of strength, reflexes, sensation, and neural tension tests. A structural tissue-specific diagnosis is then attempted. In subsequent treatment, the symptoms may be reduced or eliminated, structural ROM improved, and deconditioning and specific strengthening addressed. But many patients are still afraid to move for fear of pain or reinjury. Perhaps we continue to neglect the most important link: return to functional movement with its multiple degrees of freedom and richness of expression.

Common sense tells us that in standing, squatting, sitting, performing upper extremity (UE) gestures and tasks in any number of postures, the transition from one posture to another, running, walking, jumping, dancing, or skating—the lumbopelvic-hip segments are key points of control. Control of these segments determines whether we have enough proximal stabilization to execute movement in order to ac-

complish desired motor tasks. Evaluation and rehabilitation of the spine must address trunk-pelvic control and tolerances for the static and dynamic postures required in a patient's life. If a ballet dancer must achieve an arabesque with the leg at 90 degrees (Fig. 5-1), the task is to find a way to accomplish this with minimal stress to the injured area. When an individual cannot tolerate particular positions due to structural damage, alternative strategies must be incorporated into their movement vocabulary. Laying the groundwork of tissue healing and recovery of flexibility and strength is only part of the therapist's job. The crucial and often missing key is to provide the necessary neuromuscular learning experiences and feedback to achieve optimal, safe motor control of the lumbopelvic area.

Epidemiologists have found a 60–90 percent overall lifetime prevalence of low back pain (LBP).[1–3] The majority of episodes of LBP are benign and self-limiting, and symptoms of pain will spontaneously resolve within a 6-week timespan.[4] Ten percent of adults with LBP will not improve; these patients go on to chronic LBP

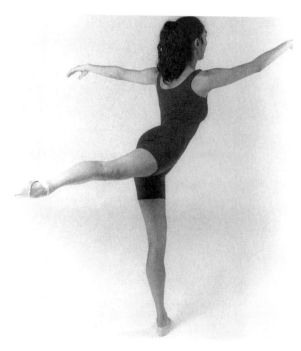

FIGURE 5-1 *Arabesque.*

(CLBP) and account for 90 percent of the health care and disability costs incurred in the treatment of LBP.[5] The United States has a higher lumbar surgery rate than any other industrialized Western nation, yet our spine recovery and disability rates are no better or are worse than those of other countries.[6–8] The incidence of LBP peaks in the 35–55 age group,[2,9] but decreases with further aging, even though degenerative changes continue to progress throughout the adult lifespan.[7] Controlled studies show little correlation between clinical symptoms and radiologic signs of degeneration.[4]

Medical practitioners have been fixated by the idea that there is one identifiable anatomic structure responsible for a patient's LBP, yet 80 percent of LBP complaints cannot be correlated with specific diagnoses.[3,10] Evaluation and treatment strategies must then focus on identification, protection, modification, and self-management of biomechanical factors that contribute to lumbopelvic dysfunction. This requires a team approach, with the patient an active participant on the team. In this chapter, mechanical low

back pain is defined as activity-related spinal disorders. Functional rehabilitation follows the SAID (specific adaptation of imposed demands) principle to prepare the body for the stresses it will encounter.

Problems of Diagnosis and Classification

In 1985, Nachemson[10] wrote that only 20 percent of patients with acute low back pain can be given a precise pathoanatomic diagnosis. In 1990, Haldeman,[11] as president of the American Spine Society, reiterated, "We do not know the cause of low back pain." Despite increasingly sophisticated evaluative tools: magnetic resonance imaging (MRI); computed tomography (CT) with locally injected contrast media; EMG (electromyography); reflex-, somatosensory-, and cortical motor-evoked responses; computerized assessment of posture, strength, and motion; and development of new treatment and surgical techniques—the overall incidence, cost, or disability of spinal disorders has not changed. Haldeman[11] stated that LBP does not fit into the classic pathology model of disease (Fig. 5-2). Increasing

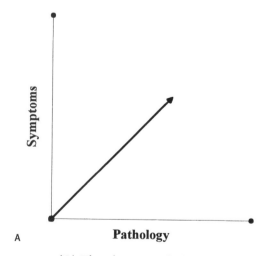

FIGURE 5-2 *(A) The classic pathology model relating increasing symptoms to increasing pathology.*

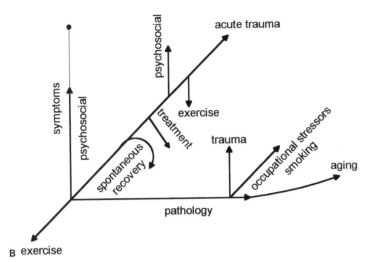

FIGURE 5-2 *Continued.* **(B)** *A composite of six factors contributing to low back pain. (From Haldeman S,[11] with permission.)*

symptoms do not necessarily correlate with increasing pathology. Haldeman cited six major factors that appear to contribute to the pathogenesis of back pain (Fig. 5-2b):

1. Acute trauma
2. Mechanical occupational stress (truck driving, heavy lifting, etc.)
3. General health (smoking, obesity, diabetes, etc.)
4. Exercise (as a decreaser of symptoms)
5. Psychosocial factors (job satisfaction, anticipation of compensation, etc)
6. Aging

It is interesting to note that spontaneous recovery does not return the patient to their initial starting point, in Haldeman's model. While symptoms may resolve, structure and motion remain altered.

Waddell[4] has done extensive investigation into the influence of psychosocial factors (e.g., coping skills, job satisfaction, support systems, anticipation of financial compensation) on LBP and has concluded that LBP disability should be approached as an illness rather than as a physi-cal disease. In his work, Waddell makes an important distinction between acute and chronic pain, which differ in characteristics as well as in time scale. Acute pain has more direct correlation to physical injury, while chronic pain becomes dissociated from physical cause and is self-sustaining. Bearing in mind the potential influence of psychosocial considerations, the interplay of Haldeman's six factors may hold a key to understanding the pathology, symptomatology, and disability of LBP.

Kirkaldy-Willis[12] defined mechanical LBP as pain due to pathoanatomy, pathophysiology, and pathomechanics. Using an osteoarticular system model, he divided the natural history of degenerative changes in the spinal unit into three phases.

1. Dysfunction—minor pathology resulting in abnormal function of the posterior joints and disc.
2. Instability—progressive degeneration due to repeated trauma, producing laxity of the posterior joints and annulus.
3. Stabilization—fibrosis of the posterior joints and capsule, loss of disc material, and formation of osteophytes render the segment stable, as movement is reduced.

Similar to Haldeman, Kirkaldy-Willis viewed the pathogenesis of LB dysfunction as multifactorial: the rate of progression is not linear and factors that alter the rate are poorly understood. These include sex, body weight, posture, occupation, and activity.

In 1987, the Quebec Workers' Health and Safety Commission empowered a task force to evaluate the current status of scientific evidence for assessment and management of activity-related spinal disorders, due to the rising occurrence and costs of physical therapy interventions for LB disorders.[13] The Quebec Task Force concluded that there was a lack of uniformity in diagnostic terminology, which are based on vague pathologic hypotheses. They proposed an original classification system (Table 5-1) with biologically plausible criteria, exhaustive encompassing classification, mutually exclusive categories, reliability, and simplicity, to facilitate clinical decision-making, evaluation of care, and research. Important to note in this classification system is the relative abandonment of specific diagnosis,

and simplification into 11 categories. Secondary and tertiary classification subsets address time duration and work status. The 11 categories and time stages are correlated to management guidelines, which stress three points for reevaluation: 4 weeks, 7 weeks, and 12 weeks. Other authors have suggested similar time frames: acute (less than 6 weeks), subacute (6–12 weeks), and chronic (more than 12 weeks).[14]

Practitioners increasingly agree on the need to abandon specific tissue diagnosis. Many authors suggest adopting pathomechanic or pathokinesiology classification systems, which identify categories of motion restriction or patterns of symptom provocation. Examples of classification systems based on clinical signs and symptoms are those of McKenzie[15]—derangement, dysfunction, and postural syndromes; Maitland[16]—reproduction of symptoms and reassessment; and Delitto et al.[17]: extension, flexion, and lateral shift syndromes. Delitto et al.[18] have recently gone one step further and suggested a treatment-based classification system.

TABLE 5-1 *Quebec task force on spinal disorders classification system: Classification of activity-related spinal disorders*

CLASSIFICATION	SYMPTOMS	DURATION OF SYMPTOMS FROM ONSET	WORKING STATUS AT TIME OF EVALUATION
1	Pain without radiation	a (<7 days)	Working
2	Pain + radiation to extremity, proximally	b (7 days–7 wks)	Idle
3	Pain + radiation to extremity, distally*	c (>7 wks)	
4	Pain + radiation to upper/lower limb neurologic signs		
5	Presumptive compression of a spinal nerve root on a simple roentgenogram (i.e., spinal instability or fracture)		
6	Compression of a spinal nerve root confirmed by specific imaging techniques (i.e., CT scan, myelography, or MRI) or other diagnostic techniques (EMG, venography)		
7	Spinal stenosis		
8	Postsurgical status, 1–6 mo after intervention		
9	Postsurgical status, >6 mo after intervention		
	9.1 Asymptomatic		
	9.2 Symptomatic		
10	Chronic pain syndrome		Working
11	Other diagnoses		Idle

Abbreviations: CT, computed tomography; MRI, magnetic resonance imaging; EMG, electromyography.
* Not applicable to the thoracic segment
From Spitzer WO,[13] with permission.

In the case of CLBP patients who, in exhibiting inappropriate illness behavior, may not fit into clear-cut pain provocation or motion restriction systems, Mayer et al[19] used suggested a model called "deconditioning syndrome." Baseline measurements of physical status are gathered to make a functional capacity assessment before starting an exercise-based functional restoration program.

In summary, incidence of LBP peaks in adults between the ages of 35 and 55. These adults may attempt to play as hard as when they were 20-year-olds, but are driving bodies that no longer have the same physiologic adaptive capacities or baseline conditioning. Regardless of how LBP is characterized, symptoms from the majority of episodes of LBP will often resolve spontaneously within 6 weeks, although biomechanical and functional deficits may remain undetected. Unfortunately, a few cases will become chronic, and others will suffer reoccurrence. It is these groups that need to be targeted with early intervention, which includes safe, functional movement and exercise.

Functional Anatomy and Biomechanics

The lumbopelvic region has been called the "hub" for both weight-bearing and functional kinetic chain movement.[20,21] In standing, ground reaction forces are transmitted superiorly to the lumbopelvis, and the weight of the head-arms-trunk is transmitted inferiorly. The role of the musculoskeletal tissues of this region is to: (1) transfer forces to surrounding tissues from either ground reaction forces transmitted superiorly at heelstrike or head-UE-trunk compressive forces transmitted inferiorly, (2) absorb forces, and (3) initiate and control movement.

At the simplest level, the spine-pelvis can be functionally viewed as a mechanical joint.[22] The rigid and elastic components of the vertebral column provide intrinsic stability, while the muscles act as tension guy wires to provide extrinsic dynamic stability.[23,24] A model of an optimally balanced and healthy vertebral column-pelvic girdle with muscular guy wires to protect, control, and stabilize it will be used to examine the functional muscular anatomy of the lumbopelvis. Muscles are grouped into those that control the lumbar spine and pelvis and those that control the pelvis and lower extremity (LE). With the pelvis as the hub, 35 bilateral muscles insert into the pelvis, 14 link the pelvis to the spine, and 21 connect the pelvis to the LE.[20,21,25]

TRUNK-PELVIC MUSCLES

The trunk-pelvic muscles are divided into three groups: stabilizers, movers, and monitors. Muscles may serve more than one function.

1. Stabilizers: superficial thoracolumbar fascia and latissimus dorsi, internal and external oblique, transversus abdominis, rectus abdominis, iliopsoas, quadratus lumborum, multifidus, lateral iliocostalis lumborum

2. Movers: erector spinae—(superficial) iliocostalis lumborum and longissimus pars thoracis, (deep) lateral iliocostalis pars lumborum

3. Monitors: multifidus, intertransversarii medialis, interspinalis lateral intertransversarii

Stabilizers

The thoracolumbar fascia consists of three layers of fascia, with both skeletal and muscular attachments.[21,25] The thick posterior layer arises from the lumbar spinous processes, covers the erector spinae, and becomes the lateral raphe when it blends with the other layers at the lateral border of the iliocostalis lumborum. The superficial laminae of the posterior layer is formed by the aponeurosis of the latissimus dorsi. The middle layer attaches to the transverse processes, contributes to the lateral raphe, and becomes the aponeurosis of transversus abdominis and internal oblique. The thin anterior layer is derived from and envelops quadratus lumborum and continues medially to attach to the lumbar transverse processes. Inferiorly, the thoracolumbar fascia has attachments to the sacrum and ilium, and blends with the gluteus maximus fascia.[21] In both the sagittal and transverse planes, the tensile forces of the muscles attached to and contained within the thoracolumbar fascia provide an important passive control of trunk motion. Because of the distance of the contractile portion of latissimus dorsi, it has the largest moment arm on the fascia. Position of the humerus will further affect the length of this moment arm, as will the amount of anterior or posterior pelvic tilt. Increased tensile muscle forces will have a net effect of tightening the thoracolumbar fascia, increasing its rigidity in a stabilizing function.

The abdominal muscles include internal and external oblique, transversus abdominis, and rectus abdominis. Together, the abdominals are commonly described as trunk flexors in the sagittal plane. The investiture of the internal oblique and transversus abdominis into the thoracolumbar fascia, and the fiber orientation of both the external and internal obliques contribute to sagittal control of the pelvis, and transverse and frontal stabilization of the trunk to accommodate UE and LE motion. Porterfield and DeRosa[21] suggest they be viewed as antirotators and antisidebenders; with our functional orientation to the area in our visual field, the abdominals' primary role is to stabilize the trunk on the pelvis in order to accomplish a given task. Although activity of the abdominals is inconclusive in quiet standing and gait, transversus abdominis and obliques become very important in lifting and carrying activities. The abdominals work in synergy with gluteus maximus, quadriceps, and the spinal extensors, which are the primary movers to return from a squat posture while lifting a weight.[21,25–28] This synergy of the abdominals, trunk extensors, gluteals, and quadriceps is a key concept used in neutral spine stabilization postures.

Iliopsoas is traditionally described as a hip flexor. Bogduk[29] feels that the flexion moment on the lumbar spine by the psoas major is negligible and does not justify its description as a lumbar spine muscle. The limited number of psoas EMG studies performed during the 1960s are contradictory. Keagy et al.[30] found electrical si-

lence in resting postures such as sitting and standing, as well as silence during the stance portion of gait. Nachemson,[31] however, recorded psoas activity as a postural stabilizer. More recently, Andersson et al.[32] using fine wire electrodes, measured psoas and iliacus activity in erect sitting but found silence during standing and slumped sitting. They suggest that selective activation of psoas and iliacus occurs in certain tasks. Psoas assists in stabilizing the lumbar spine in the frontal plane when a heavy load is applied on the contralateral side. Iliacus stabilizes the pelvis-hip during contralateral LE extension in standing. The description of iliopsoas as sagittal plane guy wires and intersegmental stabilizers via compression of vertebral segments bears further study.[21,31] It has been suggested that the psoas, when not stabilizing effectively, allows increased lumbar lordosis with relative upper lumbar extension and lower lumbar flexion.[29] Gracovetsky and Farfan[33] present a model that hypothesizes a more significant role for iliopsoas in controlling lordosis, as well as driving the pelvis in gait through its attachments at the lumbar spine and pelvis. It is our belief that iliopsoas is an important postural muscle; it is the only muscle that links the lumbar spine, pelvis, and femur, and it can directly cause lumbar as well as anterior hip pain and dysfunction.

Quadratus lumborum acts to hip "hike" or trunk side-bend. Its most important function is as a lateral guy wire for frontal plane control and stability of the trunk on the pelvis and, indirectly, of the shoulder girdle on the trunk by its attachments to the ribcage. This frontal plane control is coordinated with the pelvic-LE frontal plane stabilizers: the gluteus medius and femoral adductor muscles. Quadratus lumborum also stabilizes in the transverse plane via fiber attachments to the lumbar transverse processes.[21]

Multifidus and the intersegmental muscles (interspinalis and intertransversarii mediales) are considered both spinal stabilizers and proprioceptors. The vertical vector of multifidus makes it a posterior sagittal rotator.[25] Multifidus "bowstring" fascicle attachments also increase lordosis and vertebral compression. Multifidus is considered a stabilizer in the transverse plane, even though EMG studies inconclusively find multifidus silent or active in both ipsi- and contralateral rotation.[25,34] Multifidus forms a force couple with oblique abdominals, the primary trunk rotators in the transverse plane. The obliques simultaneously flex in the sagittal plane as they rotate, while multifidus counteracts their flexion moment.[25] The deep lateral iliocostalis lumborum has both a horizontal and a vertical vector to its fiber orientation, which suggests that it may also work in conjunction with multifidus to stabilize during trunk rotation in the transverse plane. Lateral iliocostalis lumborum decreases anterior shear of L4 on L5 and L5 on S1, and reduces lumbar lordosis.[25]

Researchers have found evidence that the iliolumbar ligament is muscular in neonates and children.[35] Portions are derived from quadratus lumborum[35] and possibly from the L5 fascicle of iliocostalis.[29] The iliolumbar ligament is an important stabilizer of the L5–S1 segment in sagittal, frontal, and transverse planes.[36,37] The relative stability of L5–S1 may explain the greater stresses and injuries sustained at the more mobile L4–L5 segment.

Movers

The superficial erector spinae muscles, iliocostalis lumborum and longissimus pars thoracis, insert into the erector spinae aponeurosis. Together they control eccentric and concentric sagittal spine movements. The deeper division of the erector spinae, lateral iliocostalis lumborum pars lumborum, works with the superficial division during trunk flexion and return to upright. Bogduk and Macintosh[38] calculated the extensor moments of different fibers of the erector spinae and multifidus. The longissimus thoracis contributed 70–86 percent of the total extensor moment at the upper lumbar levels. At the lower lumbar levels, the thoracic fibers contribute 50 percent, multifidus 20 percent, and the lumbar erector spinae contributes the remainder. Each of these muscles also generates compression and shear forces. Iliocostalis lumborum and longissimus pars lumborum and pars thoracis contribute to frontal plane unilateral side-bending due

to their attachments to the vertebral transverse processes and ribs.

Monitors

High spindle density has been found in the slow twitch, type I fibers of the single-segmental intertransversarii medialis and interspinalis[39,40] as well as multifidus.[41] Nitz et al.[42] found the mean spindle density for the small muscles of the back (rotatoris brevis) to be six times that of the multisegmental muscles (semispinalis and multifidus). These short muscles lie so close to their axis of rotation that they are at mechanical disadvantage to contribute much force for movement. Researchers suggest that the short small muscles of the back have primary importance as proprioceptors and might be considered "kinesiologic monitors" and movement modifiers.[29,39–41,43,44] The lateral intertransversarii are not considered true back muscles due to their ventral rami innervation.[29] Due to their single-segment length, they are likely proprioceptive in function.

When working in synchrony, the multiple fascicle insertions of the uni- and polysegmental back muscles, the psoas, and the abdominals are capable of both fine tuning and gross trunk-pelvic control. Fine tuning control is capable of discerning and maintaining the amount of lordosis in any given posture. This is achieved with both sagittal adjustment of the lumbar spine and anterior-posterior rotation (pelvic tilt) of the pelvis. Control and stabilization of this lumbopelvic area allow the larger muscles of the pelvis-LE to perform the workhorse gross movements. Emphasis is changed from shear and torsion at the lumbosacral junction to movement at the femoral-pelvic junction, the hip.

PELVIS-LOWER EXTREMITY MUSCLES

The 21 muscles linking the pelvis with each LE tend to be large powerful muscles and may be divided into four groupings. The anterior and posterior groups may be viewed primarily as movers; the medial and lateral groups primarily as stabilizers. The small monoarticular muscles might also be considered monitors.

1. Anterior thigh muscles: iliopsoas, rectus femoris, sartorius
2. Posterior thigh muscles: gluteus maximus, semitendinosus, semimembranosus, biceps femoris, piriformis, superior and inferior gemelli, obturator internus and externus, quadratus femoris
3. Medial thigh muscles: pectineus, adductor brevis and longus, magnus, gracilis
4. Lateral thigh muscles: gluteus medius and minimus, tensor fascia latae

Movers

Anterior thigh muscles include iliopsoas, rectus femoris, and sartorius. They work primarily in the sagittal plane, causing hip flexion or anterior pelvic rotation, depending on which other muscles are stabilizing. Forward propulsion for locomotion is primarily provided concentrically by the hip flexors, especially as the speed of locomotion increases.[45,46]

The posterior thigh muscles include the powerful gluteus maximus and three hamstrings, as well as the deep hip external rotators, piriformis, superior and inferior gemelli, obturator internus and externus, and quadratus femoris. In the sagittal plane, gluteus maximus and hamstrings control posterior rotation of the pelvis, which results in relative lumbar flexion and femoral extension. The hamstrings, assisted by gluteus maximus, are key in eccentric deceleration of the swing leg before heel strike in locomotion.[45,47] The external rotators act in the transverse plane to stabilize the femoral head in the acetabulum, and decelerate internal rotation of the femur during gait. A neglected concept is their distal effect in controlling closed chain placement of the lower extremity.[47,48] These muscles are critical in ballet, which puts primary emphasis on maintaining closed and open chain LE external rotation.

Stabilizers

Medial thigh muscles include pectineus, adductor brevis, longus and magnus, and gracilis. They are particularly important in frontal plane pelvic control and must work in synchrony with quadratus lumborum and gluteus medius.[21,46,49] Depending on the sagittal position of the femur, they add an internal rotation moment in the transverse plane to counteract the effects of the deep external rotators, iliopsoas, and sartorius. Gluteus medius and minimus, and tensor fascia latae constitute lateral thigh muscles. They impart critical frontal plane pelvic control in stance and locomotion.[45,48,49]

Monitors

There is some evidence that monoarticular muscles are more position sensitive and influenced by central programs, while biarticular muscles are more sensitive to peripheral limb motion.[50] Peck et al.[44] suggest that throughout the body, small short muscles form parallel muscle combinations with larger, longer muscles. In man, small muscles have an average spindle density of 3.76 times as many spindles per gram of tissue as the large ones. Based on these findings, they hypothesize that the small muscles serve as "kinesiologic monitors," giving sensory feedback. Average spindle density of the hip external rotators is 3.5–4.0 times more dense than the hip extensors. Therefore, monoarticular muscles such as the hip external rotators may play the role of pelvic-LE monitors.

In further consideration of the pelvis as the kinetic hub, it is important to consider the sacroiliac (SI) and pubic symphysis joints within the pelvis. The pelvis can be viewed as a boney ring comprised of three joints: two SI joints and the pubic symphysis. Ground forces through the lower extremity and ilium, and trunk forces through the sacrum converge at the SI joint. These are forces that the SI joints generally are well adapted to accommodate. It is accepted that there is movement at the SI joints and that it is small.[21,51,52] Controversy remains concerning the amount of motion and the location of the axis of motion. Problems can occur in hypermobile SI joints of pregnant women, individuals with connective tissue disease, and populations self-selected for flexibility: dancers and gymnasts.

The pubic symphysis allows minimal translatory and rotational movements. The pubic rami provides attachments for multiple large muscles: the adductors, abdominals, and pelvic diaphragm. The symphysis serves as the axis for innominate rotation during gait.[20,53,54] With SI dysfunction, it is easy to see that the symphysis can be affected as part of the same boney ring.

It is important to consider the effect of hip joint dysfunction on the spine. In standing postures, the hip is relatively close-packed. Both the hip and knee display a higher incidence of degenerative joint disease (DJD) than joints less frequently in close-packed position, such as the ankle. As articular tolerance limits are reached in the hip, ground reaction forces are transmitted to the SI joints and lumbosacral junction. A tight hip capsule, commonly seen in conjunction with DJD, results in decreased hip extension ROM. Further effects include anterior rotation moment of the innominate on the sacrum, flexion of the sacrum, and extension of the lumbar spine.

Several authors have examined dysfunction in the hip and lumbar spine to see how they affect each other. In comparing normals to subjects with LBP, Ellison et al.[55] found greater hip internal rotation (IR) in normals and greater ER in subjects with LBP. Mellin[56] found active hip extension ROM had a significant negative correlation with LBP. Cunningham[57] found passive hip extension significantly decreased in his LBP population. Thurston[58] studied kinematics in subjects with significant hip osteoarthrosis (selected for THR). All patients showed increased sagittal and frontal plane pelvic motion compared to controls, and altered spinal movement in the frontal plane.

Biomechanics and Motor Control of the Trunk in Posture and Movement

How do we use the trunk in movement? Walking, lifting, and the more complex movements in sports or dance address important motor control issues. These include maintenance of posture and balance, which requires proprioception, coordination, and stabilization strength.

STATIC POSTURE AND BALANCE

Human *posture* is described as the relationship of the body to the ground and of the body segments to each other. Berg[59] defined *balance* in three ways: the ability to maintain a position, to voluntarily move, and to react to a perturbation. Postural control is the ability to maintain equilibrium and balance in the presence of gravity.[60] Postural adjustments must counterbalance any forces tending to move the center of gravity out of the base of support, and may occur in both static and dynamic contexts.[61] With maximal stability, as in standing with a wide base of support, minimal corrective movements are required to maintain balance. As the body moves toward the limits of stability, more frequent corrective movements are necessary in order to maintain balance and prevent falling. The body attempts to act and react with efficiency to minimize work and energy expenditure.

There is a frequent misconception of some postures, such as relaxed stance, as a static state. Historically, movement therapists such as Mabel Todd (1929, 1937),[62] F. M. Alexander (1932),[63] Lulu Sweigard (1974),[64] and Irene Dowd (1981)[65] have taught that aligning the body parts into a mechanically efficient position yields a balanced posture, which will result in more efficient and effective neuromuscular patterns.[66] The work of Alexander involves manipulating the body's posture—especially the head and neck—to result in smoother movements. He described posture as a dynamic, integral component of voluntary action, and not as a response to stimuli. Patients are trained to adopt this ideal posture in a variety of conditions (sitting, standing) and incorporate it as a component of movement (transfers and locomotion).[67]

Optimal standing posture is efficient, requiring minimal muscular activity to maintain oneself in bone balance. Relaxed standing EMGs of the trunk show minimal to no activity in the abdominals (rectus abdominis and the obliques),[68,69] slight to no activity in the psoas muscle,[31,32,68] and intermittent low activity by lumbar multifidus and erector spinae muscles.[68,70–73] According to Bogduk,[25,29] and Twomey and Taylor,[73] the center of gravity will vary depending on structural relationships such as sacral angle and lumbar lordosis.[25,29,73] If a plumb line is dropped, the line of gravity passes in front of the center of the L4 vertebral body (i.e., in front of the lumbar spine) in 75 percent of individuals. As gravity tends to pull the trunk into flexion, corrective activity of the back muscles is necessary to remain upright. In the 25 percent of individuals with the line of gravity passing behind L4, abdominal activity will be required to correct the tendency of the spine to extend.[25] The dynamic activity of the lumbopelvic musculature will vary depending on whether there is a tendency for gravity to pull the lumbar spine into flexion or extension.

In studying the standing posture on a balance board of the "normal" adult, Woodhull et al.[74] found the ear, shoulder, hip, and knee were forward of the ankle in all subjects. Average center of gravity was positioned 1.4 cm anterior to the knee joint and 1.0 cm posterior to the hip greater trochanter, providing mild gravitational torques tending toward hip and knee joint extension. This has a net effect of tending to decrease pelvic tilt and lumbar lordosis.

Many clinicians have assumed a relationship between abdominal function and degree of lumbar lordosis and pelvic tilt. However, attempts to correlate hip extension ROM, abdominal strength, and pelvic tilt-lumbar lordosis have not been statistically significant.[75,76] Problems exist with the selection of tests of the studies: the validity of the double leg lowering test as an indicator of the abdominals' tension development for postural control is not clear. Assuming that double leg lowering tests iliopsoas and rectus abdominis eccentric strength, there is little relevance with respect to the ability of obliques and transversus abdominis to stabilize in standing posture over time.[77–79]

Functional and structural adaptive changes due to factors such as sedentary life style, poor or imbalanced posture, aging (the average person gains 1 lb and loses one percent of muscle strength per year after age 25[21]), and previous injury may be expressed in more than one alignment strategy. Practitioners frequently describe one type of postural dysfunction: lax abdominals, shortened psoas, increased lumbar lordosis, and anterior pelvic tilt, with increased extension and compression forces on the lumbar spine. Jackson and McManus[80] examined sagittal plane alignment and found decreased total lordosis in patients with LBP (a population also described by McKenzie) compared to a matched control group. There was, however, greater proximal and less distal lumbar lordosis, with a vertical sacrum and greater hip extension in the patient group. Other studies have found little difference in sagittal alignment[81] and diminished hip extension in patients with LBP.[57] Authors agree lumbar lordosis decreases with aging in both sexes.[73]

In the frontal plane, pelvic obliquity is usually associated with either vertebral scoliosis (structural scoliosis) or unequal leg length (functional scoliosis). A statistical association has been found between LBP and leg length inequality, with leg length discrepancy occurring twice as frequently in the LBP population.[73]

The differing responses by the body to stress may depend on body somatotype and structure, amount of joint hyper- or hypomobility, and generalized soft tissue flexibility. Each will react differently to ground and trunk forces. The response of tissues to tensile, compression, torsion, and shear forces during movement, and their ability to transmit or absorb forces, will determine whether there is vulnerability to injury and subsequent structural or functional alteration. Muscle stiffness, or resistance to deformation, is dependent on central nervous system (CNS) "set."[82] An individual's control of muscle stiffness is an important protective and adaptive mechanism in motor control.

DYNAMIC POSTURE AND POSTURAL STRATEGIES

Dynamic posture is defined as the result of the coordinated functioning of proximal and distal neuromuscular strategies to attain a goal or task.[67] Part of dynamic posture is *central set*, the ability of the nervous system to prepare the motor system for upcoming sensory information and to prepare the sensory system for upcoming movements. For example, postural adjustments have been shown to precede self-initiated arm, leg, and trunk movements to minimize postural instability that would have resulted. Central set is used to predict the weight of an object and dynamics of our limbs in complex tasks.[83] One primary function of central set and postural regulation strategies is to maintain axial support during limb movement. There can be no effective movement without the stability offered the limbs by the postural processes. A failure to compensate for imbalance could be indicative of an inability to produce the necessary muscle forces through weakness, lack of preparatory set, improper information processing, impaired motor coordination, or a combination of all.

Frank and Earl[84] summarize Gahery's classification of three postural strategies for regulating posture during movement: *postural reactions* involve feedback crisis management following unexpected perturbations (within 100 ms); *postural preparations* provide a greater margin of safety by increasing the base of support and cocontracting muscles to stiffen the joints in anticipation of an event (e.g., athletes or the elderly); and *postural adjustments* or *accompaniments* precede or coincide, in a feedforward mechanism, the initiation of voluntary movement (30–50 ms). It is hypothesized that postural accompaniments and postural reactions share common motor programs.

Babinski[85] in 1899 was the first to describe postural adjustments. The main purpose of postural adjustments is to maintain equilibrium during movement. This may be accomplished by repositioning the center of mass over a new base of support, resisting displacement of the initial center of mass, or displacing the center of mass in a direction opposite to the movement.[84] Raising a bar by flexing the elbows is accompanied by postural preparations of biceps femoris and erector spinae activity. These precede elbow flexor contraction by 30–50 ms in a distal to proximal sequence.

Nashner and McCollum[86] have extensively studied postural reactions in platform perturbations and found two general strategies. The *ankle strategy* is characterized by a distal to proximal sequence, while the *hip strategy* follows a proximal to distal sequence of muscle contraction to maintain equilibrium. Repetition of some of the work of Cordo and Nashner by Frank and Earl[84] found the erector spinae active in both postural reactions and postural adjustments during voluntary movement. Sequence of muscle contraction was distal to proximal in both types of activities. A third strategy is the *stepping strategy*. If a stable posture cannot be maintained, the subject may step to achieve a new stable posture rather than fall.

GAIT

An understanding of normal lumbopelvic kinematics in gait is crucial to understanding the effects of dysfunction anywhere in the kinetic chain. Historically, analysis of the kinetics and kinematics of gait has focused on the pelvis and lower extremity. A common device to eliminate or simplify any influence of the body above the pelvis is to consider the trunk a rigid column. Researchers refer to the head-arms-trunk as HAT.[87–89] Envisioning HAT as a model of an inverted pendulum, MacKinnon and Winter[87] describe balance as regulated at two primary levels: balance of the total body about the supporting foot, and balance of HAT about the supporting hip. The head-arms-trunk account for 60–70 percent of the total body mass.[89–91] Biomechanical and EMG analysis of standing and gait by Winter et al.[91] suggests that dynamic balance of HAT during gait is the prime responsibility of the hip muscles, with almost no involvement by the ankle muscles. Control of standing balance, however, relies primarily on the ankle muscles. During locomotion, balance of HAT about the hip is dependent upon pelvic control by the hip muscles and the coupling between the pelvis and trunk in both frontal and sagittal planes.[87]

Foot placement is dependent upon hip abduction-adduction moments generated during swing. From heel strike to midstance, frontal plane control initially occurs at the subtalar joint with inversion-eversion corrections, or secondarily at the supporting hip. Activity of the hip external rotators may affect the mechanical advantage of gluteus medius. Analysis of active muscle and joint acceleration moments by MacKinnon and Winter[87] suggests that the hip both generates and absorbs the largest amounts of energy. Increases in subtalar eversion are associated with increased hip abduction forces, and increases in subtalar inversion are associated with decreased hip abduction forces. Hip moments act on the pelvis to regulate motion of the trunk. Coupling between the pelvis and trunk is regulated by the spinal muscles such as lateral flexors.

Kinematics

The weakness of the inverted pendulum model is the assumption that HAT is a rigid segment. Inman[92] describes pelvic motion during gait as listing, rotating, and indulating. The trunk, shoulder girdle, and upper extremities act to counterbalance pelvic motion and maintain consistent visual gaze. Pelvic, trunk, and shoulder girdle kinematics during gait are reviewed and outlined in Table 5-2. The left lower extremity in stance, from heel strike to midstance, is used as an example. As the left leg progresses from heel strike to midstance, the pelvis rotates right or clockwise in the transverse plane, the lumbar and lower thoracic spine also rotate right or clockwise in diminishing amounts. At approximately T7, a transition to counterrotation of the upper thoracic spine and shoulder girdle occurs.[93] From T6 to T1 increasing amounts of counterclockwise or left rotation occur. Gregersen and Lucas[93] suggest that the greater amounts of rotation that occur at the thoracic spine subject thoracic discs to greater torsion, and lumbar discs to greater shearing forces. They also found that in the transverse plane, the pelvis and lumbar spine rotate as a functional unit. Gracovetsky and Farfan[33] suggest that the pelvis-trunk-shoulder girdle represents a "mechanical oscillator": the rotation-derotation resembles a giant spring that stores up energy that can be re-used to help drive the pelvis and shoulder girdle. Total amplitude of trunk rotation in males during self-selected gait has been quantified from 6.8 degrees +/− 2.1 degrees[94] to as high as 12 degrees,[93] and pelvic rotation from 11.5 degrees[94] to 16 degrees.[93] This author found no substantial gait studies that included kinetics or kinematics of the cervical spine and head. Our visual field—used to orient us to our environment—combined with the cervical spine and la-

TABLE 5-2 *Analysis of joint motion during gait occurring from left heelstrike to midstance*

LEFT JOINT	POSITION AT HS	MOTION OCCURRING BY PLANE		
		SAGITTAL	FRONTAL	TRANSVERSE
Foot-STJ	Dorsiflexion	Plantar flexion	Eversion (pron)	Abduction (pronation)
Ankle	Dorsiflexion	Plantarflexion	Eversion	Abduction
Knee	Extension	Flexion	Adduction	Internal rotation
Hip	Flexion	Extension	Adduction	Internal rotation
Innominate	Posterior rotation	Anterior rotation	Superior rotation/Left lateral translation	Right rotation
Sacrum	Extension	Flexion	Right SB (L on L)	Left rotation (L on L)
Lumbar	Flexion	Extension	Left SB	Right rotation
Upper thoracic			Right SB	Left rotation
Shoulder girdle				Left rotation
Cervical				Right rotation

Abbreviations: HS, heelstrike; STJ, subtalar joint; SB, side-bending; L, left.

byrinthine receptors to provide proprioception information, is hierarchically dominant. It is conjectured that a secondary pivot point occurs at the cervicothoracic junction to begin right counterrotation to the shoulder girdle. Counterrotation would progress up the cervical segments to allow the head to remain oriented forward.

As the left heel strikes and moves toward midstance, it is in supination and begins to pronate. In the sagittal plane, the hip is flexed and begins to extend, the pelvic innominate is posteriorly rotated and begins to anteriorly rotate, and the lumbosacral junction begins to extend.[20,95] Maximal peak ground reaction force of 112 percent of body weight appears following heelstrike (25 percent of stance phase).[96] With LE dysfunction, increased forces will be transmitted to the lumbosacral spine. Pronation must occur to unlock a rigid foot, absorb shock, and accommodate the ground.[89,95] Excessive pronation will increase the extensor moment to the lumbar spine. Excessive supination will increase the transmission of ground forces superiorly. Sufficient hip extensor control in the sagittal plane must occur to absorb transmitted forces.[33,96]

In the frontal plane, as the left foot moves from heel strike to midstance, the left innominate moves superiorly as the lumbar spine side bends to the left.[20,89,92,95] Sufficient hip abductor control in the frontal plane must also occur to absorb shock. Total side-bending for the trunk has been measured at 7 degrees.[97]

Further analysis of lumbopelvic arthrokinematics during gait using an osteopathic framework includes the following. The pubic symphysis is the axis of rotation in gait for innominate anterior-posterior rotation.[20,53,54] At left heel strike, the left innominate is in posterior rotation. Through the left stance phase, the left innominate rotates anteriorly, as the right moves posteriorly. Following left heel strike, the left innominate moves superiorly, creating left lumbar side-bending with right rotation. Concurrently, sacral left rotation and right side-bending about the left oblique axis (left on left forward sacral torsion) occurs. Due to coupled motion, the sacrum moves opposite to the lumbar spine. Sacro-

iliac motion is described as occurring about oblique axes in a polyaxial torsional pattern.[20,53,54] From mid-stance to toe-off, the sacrum returns to neutral.

Changes in velocity of locomotion create changes in amplitude of pelvic-spinal movement and pattern. Slow walking shows a pattern of pelvic and shoulder girdle rotation in phase. Opposition occurs as natural walking speeds are approached. The amplitude of pelvic and thoracic rotation increases with walking speed.[94,98]

EMG Patterns

A working knowledge of muscle patterns in normal adult locomotion is also useful in analyzing dysfunction. Winter et al.[49] find in the sagittal plane, hip flexors/extensors dominate control of gait, and in the frontal plane, the hip abductors are dominant. In the frontal plane, there is maximal hip abduction activity (gluteus medius and minimus) from loading at heelstrike through midstance.[48,99] Hip adductor findings are inconclusive, with some authors finding a biphasic pattern during transverse pelvic rotation periods, and others finding activity during loading. In the sagittal plane, hip extensors (gluteus maximus and hamstrings) are consistently active during the swing-stance transition to decelerate, stabilize, and finally extend the hip.[48] There is an inconsistent second and smaller phase during the stance-swing transition. Iliopsoas is consistently found to be active from terminal midstance through midswing. During stance it is probably acting as a lumbar and hip stabilizer.[31,33,48] However, Keagy et al.[30] finds that iliopsoas acts primarily as a hip flexor and less as a postural stabilizer. There may be low level activity in the swing-stance transition.

Abdominal muscle findings are variable. Many authors have found internal and external obliques to be continuously active and rectus abdominis silent; others have found low level biphasic activity of rectus.[48,68,89] Sheffield[69] found no activity in any of the abdominals. Obliques are probably most effective in the transverse and frontal planes. Erector spinae show biphasic activity when pelvic and thoracic rotations are changing direction and as weight support is being shifted, for control in all three planes.[48] Bilateral cocontraction of multifidus and longissimus coincides with the activity of the hip extensors at heel strike.[100] Pauly[101] found greatest activity in multifidus, followed by spinalis, then longissimus. Thorstensson et al.[100] suggest that in walking, the main function of lumbar erector spinae is to dampen excessive trunk movements in the frontal plane. With acceleration to running, these muscles mainly control sagittal plane movements.

Yekutiel[88] suggests that an indirect way to ascertain the role of spinal muscle action is to study intervertebral compression forces. Nachemson found that peak load compression forces of 70 kg at the L3 disc in standing increased to 85 kg in walking.[88] Contraction of muscle around a joint increases the compression force in the joint. Although peak vertical ground reaction forces are approximately 112 percent of body weight at 25 percent of stance phase,[96] muscle contraction forces are probably low, and function primarily to stabilize and align.[88] If a force couple of vertebral rotatory movement is created from the ground upwards, the task of the vertebral muscles may be to control and attenuate forces.

Gait analysis is a frequently used tool in assessment of joint disorders and LE outcome scores, but is often neglected in patients with LBP.[88,102] Diminished walking velocity and stride length, and asymmetric cadence are two gait patterns observed in CLBP patients. Both slow velocity and small steps may occur with elimination of normal pelvic-trunk rotation. Patients with ankylosing spondylitis and surgical fusion display compensatory body movements. The favored adaptation for loss of lumbar hyperextension was hip hyperextension when available, or hip flexion and forward trunk lean when not.[88,102]

Clinical Implications

Carrying loads, particularly asymmetric ones, will also affect gait patterns. Voloshin[103] studied shock attenuation capacity in normals, subjects with painful knees, subjects with menisectomized knees, and subjects with LBP. In finding that the attenuation capacity of the LBP group was about 20 percent less than the other groups, Voloshin suggests the use of viscoelastic inserts to reduce dynamic forces at heel strike. Distal dysfunction can, conversely, affect the lumbopelvic region. Excessive pronation may result in increased hip IR and innominate anterior rotation, causing strain at the SI joint or lumbopelvic junction. Optimally, restoration of normal pelvic-spinal rhythm will provide the most energy efficient gait. When this is not possible, as in certain spinal fusion conditions, optimizing the next best energy efficient pattern should be the goal.

FORWARD BENDING, SQUATTING, AND LIFTING

Researchers have studied muscle activity in forward bending and return to stance with the knees straight (also referred to as stoop lift), squat lifting with kyphotic and lordotic postures, and the effect of loading in all these postures. Current theories of back support mechanisms include intra-abdominal pressure, thoracolumbar fascia, and the posterior ligamentous system.[28,104,105]

Stoop Lifting

During forward bending-knees straight (Fig. 5-3), the moment of forward flexion is caused by gravity, but the rate of descent is controlled eccentrically by the erector spinae and multifidus.[25] Back muscle activity increases proportionally to the angle of flexion and size of the load until about 90 percent of trunk flexion. (At this point, hip flexion is only 60 percent complete.) Back muscle activity ceases at the *critical point* as apposition of the facet joints and tension on the posterior ligaments and fascia supports the trunk. Toussaint et al.[106] found flexion relaxation of lumbar muscles but not at the thoracic level. They suggest that this is due to the mechanical torque advantage of the thoracic fibers of the erector spinae on the aponeurosis. This "flexion-

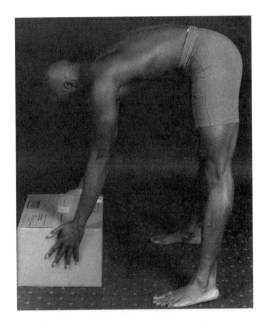

FIGURE 5-3 *Stoop lift.*

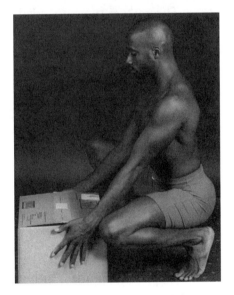

FIGURE 5-4 *Lordotic squat lift.*

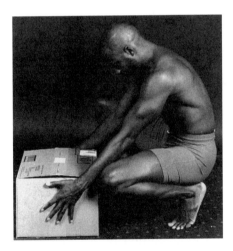

FIGURE 5-5 *Kyphotic squat lift.*

relaxation response" marks a transition from active muscular control to passive ligamentous control.[107] The critical point occurs later in the motion with the addition of weights.

A characteristic lumbopelvic rhythm has been described during forward bending.[108,109]

Paquet et al.[109] found motion of the lumbar spine predominates during the first 75 percent of flexion and the last 75 percent of extension. Hip displacement predominates during the last 25 percent of flexion (after the critical point) and the first 25 percent of extension. Mean values of motion were similar in normal and LBP subjects: 41–49 degrees +/− 10 degrees at the hip and 61–77 degrees +/− 17–23 degrees at the spine.[109] Other authors suggest lumbopelvic motion may be characterized by the direction of movement. Nelson et al.[110] found lumbar and pelvic rotations occurred simultaneously during flexion, and sequentially only during extension. In returning to upright from full flexion, the pelvis must derotate posteriorly, requiring pelvic-hip extensor activity of the gluteals and hamstrings. Peak activity of the pelvic-hip muscles occurs during the early hip predominate portion of extension.[109]

Electromyographic and kinematic investigation of subjects with LBP performing forward bending-knees straight movement have found slower velocities and lack of critical point erector spinae relaxation.[109] In fact, throughout forward bending, LBP subjects showed higher eccentric paraspinal activity, and on return, less concentric EMG activity.[111] Following return to upright, subjects with LBP have displayed prolonged activity of the erector spinae.[112] Nouwen et al.[111] suggest CLBP subjects forward bend differently; they use a hip strategy that emphasizes flexing from the hip while keeping the spine extended. This would also account for the reduced paraspinal EMG activity on return to upright.

Squat Lifting

Analysis of stoop lifting (knees straight) (Fig. 5-3) versus squat lifting (knees bent) (Fig. 5-4) generally agrees that squat lifting requires greater energy expenditure because of the amount of body weight displaced vertically.[104,105,113] Electromyographic comparisons of the two styles found higher quadriceps activity during squat lifting and higher erector spinae activity during stoop lifting.[114] Researchers suggest there is less flexion moment and less compressive forces on the lumbar spine with squat lifting. They have recommended the squat technique as safer for the lumbar spine.[104,105,113,114] Bogduk, in analyzing other research, concludes on the basis of changes in disc pressure and back muscle activity that there are no differences between using a stoop lift or a squat lift.[25] He states that the critical factor is the distance of the load from the body. Squat lifting generally allows the load to be brought closer to the center of mass. It is at this point that the specific motion tolerances of a patient become of primary importance. Individuals with hip DJD have been found to select a stoop lift strategy to minimize stresses on the hip.[58]

Trafimow et al.[113] found the squat lift technique altered to resemble more of a stoop lift style as the quadriceps fatigued or with increased load. A comparison of squat lifting muscle activity and sequencing in weight lifters with asymptomatic controls found early and greater use of gluteus maximus, as well as greater and prolonged use of quadriceps in the weight lifters.[27] This may stabilize the pelvis, permit more efficient use of the erector spinae through improved mechanical advantage, and minimize the forces on the lumbar spine. The authors recommended all lifting muscle groups be strengthened equally through appropriately timed and sequenced lifting tasks.

Researchers have examined muscle activity and forces in lordotic (Fig. 5-4) versus kyphotic (Fig. 5-5) squat lifting.[26,28,104,105,115,116] Electromyographic activity during lifts appears to be related to three factors: the weight of the object lifted, the distance between the center of the body and the object, and the trunk posture during the lift.[68] Paraspinal EMG activity is greater but lumbar flexion moments are lower in the lordotic squat lift. Hip extensors were found to make equal contributions to both types of lifts.[28] Some subjects reported discomfort with kyphotic lifts.[26] Authors concluded that the early portion of the lift is crucial to the success of the lift, and the increased activity of the erector spinae early in the lordotic lift suggests greater contribution to spinal stability with protection of inert structures.[26,28,115]

The argument continues regarding whether lordotic or kyphotic lifting is "better." This may be relevant from a preventive standpoint, but if a modified strategy must be employed for the injured individual, we must work with that person's limitations and stress tolerances.

DIFFERENCES IN MUSCLE ACTIVITY IN INDIVIDUALS WITH CLBP

Neuromuscular control involves the ability to provide the appropriate intensity and timing of muscle contraction to execute movement or stabilize the body while other body parts execute movement. Researchers have sought to develop EMG profiles that differentiate subjects with LBP from controls.[111,112,117–123] Theories as to why profiles of subjects with CLBP might differ include deconditioning, abnormal fiber type composition, protective spasm or inhibition, faulty patterning due to strength and flexibility imbalances, or simply different patterning. Unfortunately, consistent descriptions have not been established. Reports have included excessive recruitment or diminished activity with movement, normal or lack of relaxation at rest, and increased muscle fatigability.

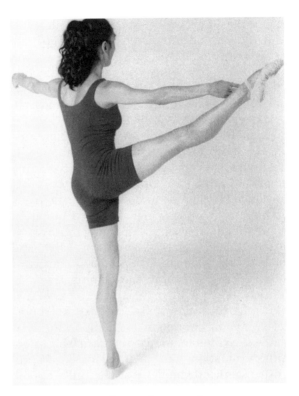

FIGURE 5-6 *Dévelopé a la second.*

Evaluation

Diagnosis of specific tissue injury, even if it were possible, is inadequate, as it does not describe functional repercussions. Normal movement requires normal joint, soft tissue, and muscle motion. Bones, joints, and muscles are maintained in both static and dynamic balance, which enables movement pattern efficiency and effectiveness. Biomechanical efficiency refers to the control of inertia, momentum, and dynamics occurring in a moving object. In examining movement, whether as highly skilled sport-specific as a golfer's swing or a grand ronde jambe in ballet, or as mundane as lifting a box, we need to consider three elements: *shape, timing,* and *dynamics. Shape* refers to postural alignment and balance. *Timing* entails neuromuscular coordination and synchronization. *Dynamics* encompass internal and external force production (which includes momentum accumulated with gravity, etc). The golfer's swing uses the pelvis-torso-shoulder girdle as a pendulum. The ballet dancer moving her leg from arabesque (Fig.

5-1) to à la second (Fig. 5-6) during a grand ronde jambe must synchronize moving her torso and pelvis to the vertical so that the acetabulum can allow her femur to move from the extended position of arabesque to the externally rotated and abducted position of à la second. The act of lifting a box or a weight lifter doing a bent leg dead lift includes synchronization of the hip-knees-ankles as the torso-pelvis moves to the vertical.

Dysfunctional patterns may be acquired through learning or training as easily as a more functional pattern or as a result of compensation for musculoskeletal pathomechanics. Dysfunctional movement patterns may provoke pathomechanics or vice versa. Joint motion restrictions and hypermobilities, muscular restrictions, and muscle insufficiencies have cumulative effects on agonist and antagonist muscles and other joints. The combination of placement and movement discordance might be envisioned an improperly hung door. Every time it swings, most of the door's weight pulls on one hinge instead of even distribution over three. Over time, the stress begins to toggle free the screws that anchor that single hinge to the wall. Someone with lumbosacral dysfunction must cease to move on that one hinge and begin to move in alternate patterns.

Evaluation of the lumbopelvic complex must consider both isolated structural components and functional interrelationships. The guiding principle of evaluation is to introduce forces that reproduce familiar symptoms. This principle is common to many manual therapy evaluation and treatment approaches including those of Cyriax, McKenzie, Maitland, Paris, Porterfield and DeRosa, and Johnson and Saliba. Patterns of weight-bearing, postural, and motion stress tolerances are correlated to structural asymmetries, range of motion, and tissue texture. Abnormal segmental motion is only important as it relates to symptomatic dysfunction. The osteopathic evaluation schema provides a comprehensive segmental analysis of the lumbar spine and pelvis and allows easy correlation to functional analysis.[20,54,124]

STRUCTURAL EVALUATION

A preliminary scan of gait and standing posture provides an overview of areas that may contribute to dysfunction. Postural analysis and gross motion testing in the sagittal and frontal planes begins to focus on specific asymmetries. Vertical compression tests in standing and sitting assess the lumbopelvic system's tolerance for compression and weight-bearing and can identify weak links that are not capable of stabilizing.[125] Assessment of the lumbar protective mechanism evaluates the protective response of the lumbopelvic muscles to manual stress in different planes and diagonals.[125] Repeated gross motion testing, overpressure, and quadrant tests ascertain tolerance for tissue overload in planes and combined planes of movement.

Assessment of pelvic boney landmarks—iliac crest (IC), posterior superior iliac spines (PSIS), anterior superior iliac spines (ASIS)—and tracking PSIS motion in the sagittal plane

during standing forward flexion test (FFT), sitting FFT, and Gillet (or Marcher's) test provides information regarding SI joint symmetry and instability. A positive FFT is one in which the dysfunctional side appears to "jump." A positive standing FFT, with the rotation of the pelvic innominates on the sacrum, is indicative of iliosacral, pubic, or LE dysfunction. A positive Gillet Test, when there is little to no movement on the dysfunctional side (with hip flexion, normal innominate rotation is posterior so the PSIS will drop), confirms the standing FFT. Cummings et al.[126] artificially induced a leg length discrepancy using a heel lift in normal subjects. X-ray and clinical examination consistently found innominate posterior rotation on the side of the lengthened limb. Leg length differences should be corrected with a lift to further assess the SI joint in standing. A positive sitting FFT is indicative of sacroiliac dysfunction as the innominates are locked by body weight. Argument continues regarding the reliability of SI tests. Potter and Rothstein[127] found SI motion tests had low reliability when used separately. (Only two provocative tests were found to be reliable, iliac gapping and compression tests). However, SI tests are seldom used individually; FFT and Gillet tests are compared to supine pubic rami heights, SI gapping and compression, Faber test, and leg length changes from supine to long sit. Cibulka et al.[128] found excellent reliability (K = .88) when using a cluster of SI tests. In general, it is recommended that all active and passive mobility and structural tests be used in clusters.

While in standing, the hip drop test demonstrates the ability of the lumbar spine, and particularly L5–S1, to side-bend. Sagittal plane segmental lumbar motion can be examined and palpated more closely in the seated slump (lumbar flexion) and seated arch (lumbar extension), in quadruped forward bending (camel) and arch (cat), or in heel sit-forward bent and prone prop on elbows, to introduce extremes of forward and backward bending motion. Palpation of the transverse processes ascertains any vertebral rotations occurring in sagittal plane gross motion, indicative of segmental dysfunction. Specifics of sacral torsions and shears may also be assessed in these positions. Provocative sacral and lumbar stress and spring tests in prone provide good confirmatory assessment. Further assessment of positional and postural tolerances that introduce compression, shear, and torsion include supine unilateral and bilateral knees to chest, prone prop and press up, and prone hip extension. Passive motion testing of soft tissue and muscle flexibility, neurologic screening, and neural tension tests are important.

Osteopathic evaluation and discussion of spinal motion build upon the early work of Lovett in 1902, and Fryette in 1954.[53] Spinal side-bending and rotation were found to be coupled motion. This has been confirmed by biomechanists like Panjabi et al,[129,130] who determined that abnormal patterns of coupled motion are associated with patients with LBP. Fryette's Laws of Spinal Motion and Type I and Type II dysfunctions are summarized in Table 5-3. Recent research confirms most of Fryette's work, but suggests that Law II may not be true for lumbar extension. Lumbar extension may in fact revert back to Law I: in normal physiologic motion there is coupled contralateral side-bending and rotation.[20,53] The osteopathic model names a segmental dysfunction by its position. If, while palpating forward bending of L4 on L5, the right L4 transverse process is more prominent or posterior, the positional diagnosis is ERS right L4–L5 (extended, rotated, and side-bent right). The motion restriction is into flexion, rotation, and side-bending left. (For a more complete discussion, the reader is referred to the authors Bourdillon et al.[124] and Mitchell et al.[54]

It is important to remember during the structural evaluation that frontal or sagittal plane asymmetries, even on a segmental level, may be due to any of the following: asymmetric neuromuscular control, spasm, soft tissue restriction, or articular dysfunction.

FUNCTIONAL EVALUATION

Back dysfunction is viewed as the complex interrelationship of the neuromusculo-osteoarticular systems, which manifests in problems in movement. If muscle function can become compro-

TABLE 5-3 *Fryette's laws of spinal motion*

Law I: When the spine is in neutral (facets are idling), side-bending to one side is accompanied by rotation to the other (contralateral coupling).

Comment: There is no "neutral" for the cervical spine. This is for thoracic and lumbar normal physiologic motion.

Law II: When the spine is fully extended or flexed, side-bending to one side is accompanied by rotation to the same side (ipsilateral coupling).

Comment: Because there is no "neutral" for the cervical spine, this is normal physiologic motion for the cervical spine but nonphysiologic motion for the thoracic and lumbar spine.

Law III: When motion is introduced into a segment in one plane, motion in all other planes is reduced.

Types of Spinal Dysfunction

Dysfunctions are named for positional finding not for movement restriction

Type I Dysfunction: Neutral group dysfunction

  Three or more vertebral segments

  Principle restriction is side-bending

  Found above or below a type II dysfunction

  Adaptive or accomodating

  Type I Neutral-Side-bent-rotated dysfunctions are contralateral (abbreviated, NS left or right R right or left)

Type II Dysfunction: Nonneutral Dysfunction

  Single vertebral segment

  Usually traumatic

  Includes a flexion or extension component

  Type II Flexed-Rotated-Side-bent dysfunctions apparent in extension motion (abbreviated, FRS left or right)

  Type II Extended-Rotated-Side-bent dysfunction apparent in flexion motion (abbreviated, ERS left or right)

  Rotation and side-bending are ipsilateral

(Data from Bourdillon JF et al,[53] Ellis JJ,[20] and Mitchell et al.[54])

mised in the presence of an injury to the static structures of a motion segment, the opposite is also true. Altered or abnormal muscle function can place abnormal stresses on a joint. Although therapeutic exercise has been recognized as a key factor to returning the injured LB patient to function, at times exercise is too gross a tool to use on problems of muscle patterning. General exercises may neglect individual muscle contributions to specific movements. If an inhibited muscle is not firing, continued practice of that exercise may never trigger it, thus perpetuating and possibly amplifying impaired muscle function and imbalances. In our clinical approach, two assumptions are made: (1) LBP is a multifactorial problem that lacks specific diagnosis 80 percent of the time, and (2) the neuromuscular-osteoarticular systems are inherently interrelated. The conclusion can then be made that osteoarticular problems will include neuromuscular ones and vice versa. If we examine, for simplicity, peripheral joint pathology, we see certain muscle imbalance patterns emerge. The osteoarthritic hip shows tight iliopsoas and adductors and weak gluteals. The inflamed knee joint presents with hamstring spasm and quadriceps shutdown. The sprained ankle has weak peroneals and altered gluteal function.[131,132] The injured lumbar spine demonstrates paraspinal spasm, gluteal weakness, and iliopsoas tightness.

Sports participation and occupational postures develop characteristic muscle strength and flexibility imbalances. The elderly person who has followed a sedentary lifestyle often displays a characteristic posture including forward head, increased thoracic kyphosis, hip flexion contracture, and tight hamstrings. It is apparent that certain muscles are more easily or frequently accessed (recruited) in our lifespan, lifestyle, and movement habits, as well as with pathology. Janda, Lewit, Kendall, Sahrman[133–140] and others have written extensively about movement dysfunction manifested as imbalance and abnormal movement patterns.

Abnormal Patterns Found in Movement Dysfunction

It is commonly acknowledged that structural lesions produce disturbances of function. Muscular imbalances, ineffective motor patterns, and postural strain cause symptoms by themselves and often precede structural changes.[133–137,139,140] The postural demands of occupation and sedentary modern life, in addition to individual neural biases or predispositions all contribute to abnormal motor patterns, muscle imbalances, and postural strains. The lack of variety of movement in modern life and habitual postures generate muscle adaptations.

TABLE 5-4 *Muscle imbalances*

FACILITATED POSTURAL MUSCLES	INHIBITED DYNAMIC MUSCLES
Lower quadrant	
Thoracic-lumbar erector spinae	Gluteus maximus
Quadratus lumborum	Gluteus medius and minimus
Piriformis	Rectus abdominis
Iliopsoas	External and internal obliques
Rectus femoris	Quadriceps vasti, especially medialis
Short thigh adductors	Peroneals
Tensor fascia latae	Tibialis anterior
Hamstrings	
Gastrocnemius-soleus	
Upper quadrant	
Suboccipitals	Deep neck flexors
Sternocleidomastoid	
Scalenes	Supra- and infraspinatus
Levator scapulae	Serratus anterior
Upper trapezius	Rhomboids
Latissimus dorsi	Middle and lower trapezius
Pectorals	Upper extremity extensors (triceps)
Subscapularis	
Upper extremity flexors (biceps)	

(Data from Bookhout MR,[141] Janda V,[134] Jull GA and Janda V,[137] and Lewit K.[134])

Muscle adaptations are realized in common patterns of imbalance (Table 5-4). Certain muscles react by overactivation and tightness, while others react by inhibition and weakness.[133–137,139] Explanation for these differences has not been correlated to histologic fiber typing or other physiologic characteristics.[131,139,141] These patterns are similar to those found in neurologic disorders such as cerebral palsy and hemiplegia with their characteristic spasticity. Janda[133–137] found that muscles prone to tightness are facilitated, hypertonic, and usually cross more than one joint. Muscles prone to weakness are inhibited, hypotonic, and lengthened. Tight muscles include the iliopsoas, quadratus lumborum, lumbar erector spinae, piriformis, rectus femoris, lower extremity adductors, tensor fasciae latae, hamstrings, triceps surae, upper trapezius, levator scapulae, sternocleidomastoid, scalenes, pectorals, and upper extremity flexors.[137,139,141] Weak muscles include the gluteals, rectus abdominis, internal and external obliques, quadriceps vasti, peroneals, anterior tibialis, lower trapezius, rhomboids, serratus anterior, supra and infraspinatus, deltoids, deep neck flexors, and upper extremity extensors. Inactivity of certain muscle groups and overactivity of other muscle groups result in compensatory patterns to accomplish movement. Habituated compensations perpetuate abnormal sensory input from the locomotor system projected centrally and distribute abnormal stresses to the joints.

Janda[134,137] also described specific postural syndromes of imbalance commonly observed (Tables 5-5 and 5-6).[139] These areas of common muscle imbalance include the pelvic-hip region or Pelvic Crossed Syndrome and the shoulder-neck region or Shoulder Crossed Syndrome. The syndromes are called "crossed" because topographically, the weak-inhibited muscles cross the tight-shortened muscles.[134] Postural repercussions of the Pelvic Crossed Syndrome include increased lumbar lordosis, anterior pelvic tilt, and increased hip flexion. Altered dynamic control is evident in gait and curl up from supine to sitting. These postural changes may also cause increased thoracic kyphosis and forward head, feeding into the Shoulder Crossed Syndrome. In addition to forward head and increased thoracic kyphosis, Shoulder Crossed Syndrome includes elevation, protraction, and abduction of the scapula with altered glenohumeral stability and imbalances. Dynamic control changes are witnessed in movement tests such as the supine head-neck curl up, ability to stabilize the scapula in the push up, and scapula stabilization in standing UE abduction or prone forward elevation. Postural patterns of imbalance were reported by Singer in evaluation of a nonsymptomatic population of 35 students, confirming tendencies of adaptive shortening in the general population.[142]

Lewit found that movement or locomotor dysfunction alone can cause symptoms without structural change.[139] He suggests that movement dysfunction is the most important *cause* of articular dysfunction and precedes degenerative articular changes. Muscles are the primary shock absorbers of the body.[143] Ineffective muscular activity will allow potentially destructive compressive and shear forces to be transmitted to articular cartilage. Degenerative joint changes are the net result of attempts by the body to compensate for movement dysfunction. Asymmetrical compensatory movements produce asymmetries in proprioceptive information, which induce further muscle imbalances, joint injury, and joint changes.

TABLE 5-5 *Pelvic crossed syndrome*

Conditions
    Weak abdominals and tight thoracic-lumbar erector spinae
    Weak gluteus maximus and tight hip flexors
    Weak gluteus medius and minimus and short tensor fascia latae and quadratus lumborum
Results
    Posture includes anterior pelvic tilt, increased lumbar lordosis (upper lumbar), and hip flexion
    Hypermobility in the lower lumbar segments (L4–5 and L4–S1) in sagittal and frontal planes

(Data from Bookhout MR,[141] Janda V,[134] Jull GA and Janda V,[137] and Lewit K.[139])

TABLE 5-6 *Shoulder crossed syndrome*

Conditions
    Weak lower trapezius and serratus anterior and tight upper trapezius, scalenes, and levator scapula
    Weak serratus anterior, rhomboids, supraspinatus, infraspinatus, teres major and minor (external rotators and scapula abductors), and tight pectorals and subscapularis (internal rotators and adductors)
    Weak longus cervicis, longus capitis, longus colli, (deep neck flexors) and tight cervical erector spinae, upper trapezius, suboccipitals, and sternocleidomastoid (neck extensors)
Results
    Posture includes forward head with upper cervical extension, lower cervical flexion, increased thoracic kyphosis, rounded shoulders with scapula elevation, protraction, abduction, and altered glenohumeral stability
    Respiration alters with increased use of accessory inspiratory muscles and diminished diaphragmatic breathing

(Data from Bookhout MR,[141] Janda V,[134] Jull GA and Janda V,[137] and Lewit K.[139])

Movement Assessment

Assessment of movement dysfunction includes evaluation through observation and testing of characteristic postures and movement patterns, as well as muscle strength and flexibility. Standard MMTs are utilized, but palpation and observation of timing and recruitment of muscles participating in a given movement is paramount. Functional and isolated movements will each provide information regarding the contribution or use of any given muscle.

Jull and Janda[137] and Lewit[139] suggest six isolated movements be included in any comprehensive analysis of motor control patterning to ascertain whether traditionally weak muscles are functioning appropriately (Table 5-7). These include hip extension (gluteus maximus), hip abduction (gluteus medius), trunk curl up (rectus abdominis and obliques), prone UE forward elevation (lower trapezius), scapula protraction (serratus anterior), and head-neck curl up (deep neck flexors). The first three are of primary importance in lumbopelvic dysfunction, the latter three in cervicoscapulothoracic dysfunction.

Palpation of the muscle in question through the movement ascertains whether it is firing and when in the sequence it is recruited. MMT may identify weakness if a certain muscle is not recruited, but palpation will confirm what muscle is involved. Janda compared EMG muscle firing patterns during MMTs.[139] In the hip extension MMT, which purportedly tests gluteus maximus strength, Janda found that in normals that the prime movers were hamstrings followed by gluteus maximus, with the lumbar erector spinae assisting. In patients with chronic low back pain, there were instances of a $\frac{5}{5}$ MMT with *no* activity of the gluteus maximus on EMG. The author has found with palpation tests evidence of no gluteal contraction during prone hip extension in dancers with innominate rotation and back pain. Lack of gluteus medius contraction in hip abduction may be manifested in increased use of tensor facia lata and quadratus lumborum. Inability to control curl up will probably be manifested by substitution of hip flexors. Lower trapezius and serratus anterior dysfunction are manifested in poor scapula stabilization. Dancers with poor scapula stability are unable to connect their portebras (arm posture) and shoulder girdle with their torso and pelvis to assist in trunk postural stabilization. Athletes and musicians with poor scapula control display a range of upper extremity problems (see chapter on Upper Extremity).

Several other tests are useful in evaluating the patient's ability to isolate, control, and integrate the lumbopelvic musculature (Table 5-7). Abdominal *bracing* is the maintenance of abdominal isometric contraction without alteration of lumbopelvic alignment. The patient is asked to maintain this in hooklying, and to count out loud to 30 to ascertain ability to brace in an endurance mode with control of breathing and speech. Anterior-posterior pelvic tilts and pelvic clocks (Fig. 5-7) assess general coordination and kinesthetic awareness of this area, ability to isolate movement, as well as tolerance and control of small combined movements. Pain or inability to perform a specific portion of the pelvic clock can often be correlated to segmental vertebral or

TABLE 5-7 *Movement tests for motor control patterning evaluation*

Simple movements for the lumbopelvis
  Gluteus maximus in prone hip extension
  Gluteus medius in sidelying hip abduction
  Rrectus abdominis in curl-up (from hooklying)
  Abdominal bracing in hooklying
Simple movements for the cervicothoracic spine and shoulder girdle
  Lower trapezius in prone forward elevation of the upper extremity
  Serratus anterior in scapula stabilization in quadriped or push-up
  Deep neck flexors in a head-neck curl-up
Combined movements for the lumbopelvis
  Pelvic anterior and posterior tilt in hooklying and standing
  Pelvic clocks
  Gait
  Squatting to lift an object
  Sitting and reaching for an object
Equilibrium
  Stork balance eyes open and closed
  Lunge balance eyes open and closed

(Data from Bookhout MR,[144] Janda V,[134] Jull GA and Janda V,[137] and Lewit K.[139])

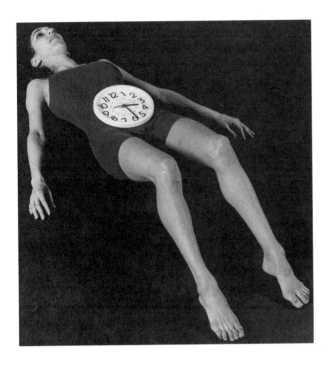

FIGURE 5-7 *Clock orientation for naming pelvic clocks.*

sacral motion restrictions. Bookhout[144] suggests that Type II ERS and FRS dysfunctions can be correlated to pelvic clock quadrant dysfunction (Fig. 5-8). (Reminder: Type II lesions are named for their osteoarticular positional diagnosis. Their movement restriction is in the opposite direction. The actual "dysfunction" may be osteoarticular, neuromuscular, or elements of both). ERS dysfunctions have difficulty moving into the upper clock quadrants from 10:00 through 2:00, which require the ability to move into lumbar flexion. FRS dysfunctions have difficulty moving into the lower clock quadrants 4:00 through 8:00, which require lumbar extension. A patient with an ERS right lesion is unable to move comfortably into 10:00 and 11:00, which requires flexion, rotation, and side-bending left. A patient with an FRS left lesion is unable to move into 4:00 and 5:00, which requires extension, rotation, and side-bending right.

Two extremes of lumbopelvis dysfunction observed by the authors are the rigid ("iron") and hypermobile ("floppy") pelvis. The iron pelvis is so named when a patient is unable to articulate any motion or dissociate the lumbar spine from the pelvis. This is often indicative of a generalized poor kinesthetic awareness and diminished motor control skills such as decreased lumbar rotation and shoulder counterrotation during gait. These people tend to be dominated by sagittal plane movements in the extremities, without some of the compensatory rotations at the proximal joints (pelvis/hips and scapula) that accompany "normal" movement. It can be very difficult for these patients to find and internalize the concepts of neutral spine stabilization. The floppy pelvis is found in individuals with general hypermobility, such as dancers. They respond well to stabilization programs once any structural asymmetries are corrected, but are always at risk when they move into the extremes of their range.

Evaluation of the ability to synchronize all of the neuromuscular-osteoarticular components should include further assessment of walking, squatting, balance, and capability of dissociation, control, and stabilization of the lumbar-pelvis-hip region (Table 5-7). Pelvic tilts and clocks entail fine control and synchronization of trunk and hip extensors, flexors, and rotators. Lack of ability to find these movements is indica-

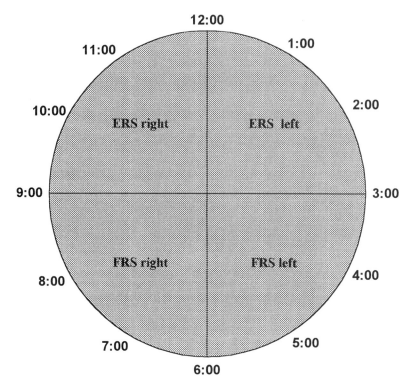

FIGURE 5-8 *Pelvic clock quadrant dysfunction. The positional diagnosis is listed in the quadrant of movement dysfunction. (From Bookout,[144] with permission.)*

tive of poor kinesthetic sense of this region. Parkhurst and Burnett[145] demonstrated a correlation between back proprioception deficits and number of LB injuries. Gait, squatting to lift, and sitting and reaching for an object may further demonstrate areas of stress in the individual's characteristic and habitual movement patterns. Differences have been found between balance responses in normals and subjects with LBP.[146] Subjects with LBP demonstrated increased postural sway, difficulty balancing on one limb with eyes closed, and more posterior center of force. These subjects were more likely to select a hip-back strategy to right themselves compared to the ankle strategy of the normal subjects. The stork (Fig. 5-9) and lunge (Fig. 5-10) balances assess equilibrium on a stable surface.

Evaluation of muscle weaknesses and firing patterns are correlated with evaluation of muscle flexibilities. It is particularly important to assess those facilitated muscles which tend to tighten (Table 5-4). Tests include: Thomas test for iliopsoas, rectus femoris, iliotibial band, and short adductors, quadratus lumborum in sidelying, hamstrings in SLR or straightening the knee with 90 degrees of hip flexion, piriformis in prone with hip in neutral, or supine with hip at 90 degrees.

Modern occupation and leisure activities stress sedentary postures, which emphasize visual and upper extremity fine motor tasks (watching TV, working at computer keyboards, etc). Motor patterns emphasize head-neck-shoulder girdle skills. The lower torso acts to orient the upper torso to the task. Subtleties of control or awareness may be lost regarding integration of lumbopelvic movement. With dysfunction, frequently the majority of lumbar spine motion be-

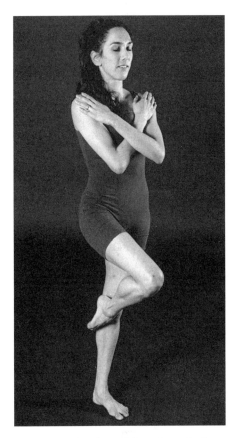

FIGURE 5-9 *Stork or Rhomberg balance.*

mitted in his lumbar spine during his swing. Before injury, he may never have utilized the power and momentum of more distal segments such as his lower extremities and pelvis. Major league baseball pitcher Nolan Ryan's longevity without serious injury to age 47 may be attributed to his emphasis on incorporating the muscle torque of his legs and trunk into his pitch. Life is a process of adaptive adjustment to alterations in both the internal and external environment of an individual through a dynamic homeostasis.[147,148] Often it is a relatively small insult that puts us over the top of our tolerance limits and into overload. Pain and dysfunction is the manifestation of the individual's inability to continue to adapt and adjust. Part of effective treatment may be re-establishment of the patient's inherent homeostasis.

The end goal of treatment is to develop the

gins to occur at only a few segments: particularly L4–5. Frequently, torsion stresses are introduced repeatedly on the L4–5 segment, with rotation in a slumped (flexed) seated posture.

Treatment

The goal of treatment is to maximize the safe return to all combinations of movement and dynamic posture from movement that has become stereotyped, repetitive, and harmful. When injury is more serious, or permanent damage does not permit tolerance of certain planes, combined motions, or forces, rehabilitation still seeks to optimize an individual's movement possibilities within a more controlled safety zone. The golfer may need to reduce the amount of torsion per-

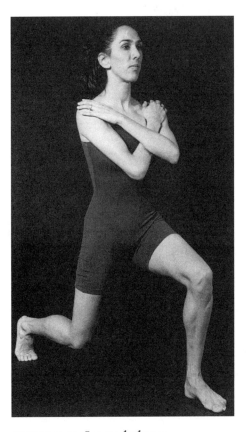

FIGURE 5-10 *Lunge balance.*

individual's kinesthetic awareness and control of the lumbopelvis in order to move safely and effectively to accomplish his or her goals. The orthopedic SAID (specific adaptation of imposed demands) principle is timely and relevant: to prepare the body for the stresses it will encounter according to that patient's lifestyle. Components of treatment include the development of flexibility, coordination, strength, and endurance. The recent guidelines for the treatment of LBP, released by the U.S. Department of Health and Human Services Agency for Health Care Policy and Research, stress early return to activity and exercise.[149] Waddell,[4] in his proposal to approach chronic LBP as an illness rather than purely physical disease, also summarized that management of LBP should emphasize early return to work, minimize bed rest, and promote controlled functional exercise to encourage activity rather than passivity.

It is the author's philosophy that principles of treatment of the lumbopelvis are similar to that of other musculoskeletal areas. Various practitioners have divided treatment into phases, but many phases overlap or occur concurrently. The four phases introduced in Table 5-8 emphasize movement goals. The acute Protected Postures (Phase I) incorporates pain control, biomechanical counseling for protection of the injured area to allow tissue healing, and re-establishment of normal anatomic and biomechanical relationships. Protected Early Motion (Phase II) begins the introduction of controlled forces to initiate early movement of the injured area, maintenance of function, and conditioning of uninjured tissues. Expanding Movement Boundaries (Phase III) increases the individual's general activity and includes exercises to increase flexibility of tight facilitated muscles, cardiovascular exercise, and neuromuscular retraining of inhibited weak muscles. Progressive Movement Challenges (Phase IV) provokes new neuromuscular synergies in complex activities, adds strengthening exercises when warranted, and begins return to complex sport-specific movements.

TABLE 5-8 *Treatment phases*

Protected Postures Phase I
Pain control
  Modalities
  Medication
  Manual therapy (manipulation, mobilization, muscle energy, etc.)
Biomechanical counseling
  Activity modification
  Neutral spine stabilization
  Body mechanics
Re-establishment of normal biomechanical relationships
  Correction of lateral shifts, pelvic assymmetries, leg length discrepancies

Protected Early Motion Phase II
Early mobilization of the injured area
  Passive, active assistive, and active range of movement
  Control of stabilization posture in supported positions
Maintain function of healthy tissues

Expanding Movement Boundaries Phase III
Flexibility
  Stretch facilitated hypertonic muscles
Neuromuscular re-education
  Retrain inhibited hypotonic muscles
  Stimulate automatic righting reactions, proprioceptive training
  Activate postural trunk muscles in differing positions and transfers
Cardiovascular exercise

Progressive Movement Challenges Phase IV
Controlled Activity Progression
  Complex movements, multiplanar, multilevel, increased loading, unstable surfaces
  Manipulation of variables of speed, weight, repetitions, holds
Sport-specific movements
Strengthening and conditioning of target muscle groups

Protected Postures

Protected Postures (Phase I) includes the various manual therapy techniques that may act neuroreflexively in the context of pain, spasm, and circulatory stasis. Manual techniques help to reestablish biomechanical relationships such as lateral shifts, pelvic torsions, and Type II dysfunctions. Analysis of clinical trials of manipulation have found it to be beneficial in the acute stage of LBP for short-term relief.[149–154] Biomechanical counseling teaches the patient about their "safe" nondestructive zones of movement. This includes the concepts of neutral lumbar spine stabilization.[155–157] Saal and Saal[157] were able to demonstrate a 90 percent good or excellent outcome in nonoperative treatment of herniated disc with radiculopathy using an exercise program based on neutral spine stabilization. The patient is educated about postural alignment and balance, assisted in finding their pain-free neutral zone, and instructed in *bracing* (co-contraction of the abdominal wall and trunk extensors aiming toward a corset of muscle protection), which enables them to muscularly control and maintain this posture. Depending on the injury and its acuteness, a patient's "neutral zone" may be only one specific position. In less acute cases, the neutral zone may allow greater motion in the lumbar spine and pelvis.

Biomechanical counseling also includes discussion of activity modification. Just as part of rehabilitation for anterior cruciate ligament deficiency and instability includes counseling about activity modification, low back patients must learn their limitations and manage and modify accordingly. Modified positions of rest such as the constructive rest position in supine with the hips and knees at 90 degrees–90 degrees provide support (allowing muscle relaxation) and pain relief, and assist in re-establishing normal anatomic relations.

Re-establishment of normal biomechanical relationships during Phase I includes both manual therapy techniques and initial patient exercises. These may incorporate side-gliding maneuvers in standing and prone positions, press-up and standing backward bending extension exercises, and supine alternating knees to chest exercises. The centralization of symptoms (resolution of LE radiculopathy) phenomena is a desirable preliminary goal. Donelson et al.[158] found nonoccurrence of centralization was an accurate predictor of poor conservative treatment outcome. Studies reporting favorable findings with extension maneuvers are cited. Extension exercises were judged more effective in the treatment of patients with varying types of instability (spondylolisthesis, normal, or retrodisplacement) than flexion exercises or placebo-control.[159] In another study, patients treated with McKenzie protocol were deemed signifi-

cantly improved compared to Williams protocol.[160] Smith and Mell,[161] studying normals, found the group performing 4 weeks of press-up exercises significantly improved their lumbar extension ROM compared to a control group. Schnebel et al.[162] measured compressive forces and tension in nerve roots of fresh cadavers, and found that flexion of the spine increased and extension decreased nerve root compression forces and tension. They concluded that extension exercise are likely to relieve nerve root tension and decrease compression forces produced at the nerve root. An MRI study of normals found that the lordotic position produced by a lumbar roll in supine caused increased distance from the posterior vertebral body to the nucleus pulposus, compared to the flexion position.[163] There was little change, however, in degenerative disc segments. Interesting to note, prone press-ups have traditionally been considered passive ROM exercises for the lumbar spine. Fiebert and Keller[164] measured greater lumbar paraspinal EMG activity during press-ups than in standing or backward bending in standing.

Protected Early Motion

Protected Early Motion (Phase II) continues to emphasize restoration of normal biomechanic relations with mobilization of the injured area. Mobilization is emphasized with maximal support to minimize the effects of gravity, axial compression, shear, and other forces. Self-mobilization includes activities such as muscle energy-technique isometric contractions for pelvic rotations, foam roll stretching and posterior-anterior mobilization of the thoracic spine, and controlled spinal active range of motion (AROM). Spinal AROM exercises include press-ups, press-ups with rotation or unilateral bridging with rotation for corrected FRS dysfunctions, isolated quadruped trunk flexion, extension, side-bending and rotation, and rotation stretching in upright sitting or standing.

Control of stabilization posture under conditions of maximal support and stability are reinforced. Patients who are unable to perform anterior-posterior pelvic tilts in evaluation, often have a great deal of difficulty learning to estab-

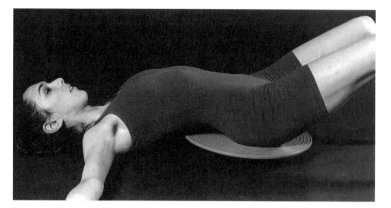

FIGURE 5-11 *Pelvic motion on a sacral rocker.*

lish a neutral posture and then superimpose dynamic abdominal bracing on that posture. Pelvic motion in varying positions such as hooklying using the sacral rocker (Fig. 5-11), sitting on a gym ball, or in quadruped, may assist in establishing a kinesthetic awareness of this region. Other patients are unable to elicit voluntary bracing of the abdominals (especially the obliques). Manually resisted isometric hip flexion in supine, "finger pokes" for manual feedback of the contraction, and functional electrical stimulation can be useful tools. Establishment of dynamic bracing is critical to the patient's management of the stresses encountered in rehabilitation and with resumption of normal activities. Teaching body mechanics includes controlling the new neutral spine posture in varying positions, activities, and movements. Most of the more advanced rehabilitation exercises superimpose increasing challenges while maintaining safe control of the lumbopelvic region. As neutral spine and stabilization concepts are integrated, the patient progresses to postures of diminishing support and stability.

The movement orientation of western culture often emphasizes the periphery or extremities. Athletes in sports like basketball strive to dunk the ball into the basket. The white collar worker manipulates a keyboard or mouse. Eastern disciplines such as Tai Chi (Fig. 5-12) locate the *tan tien* or center of gravity a little below the navel.[165,166] Man's life force or energy, referred to as the *chi* or *hara*, emanates from the *tan tien*. Movement is initiated from this center. A feeling of weightedness of the torso and connection to the ground is taught. The torso is unified with the pelvis and pivoting occurs at the hip joint, which reduces stress to the lumbosacral spine. Many LB patients have lost the connection to their center of gravity. In movement re-education, we attempt to incorporate some of the Eastern *tan tien* pelvic-dominated movement patterns. In teaching transfers from sit to stand or squat to lift, the patient begins to move the trunk-pelvis complex as an integrated unit, with hip, knee, and ankle joints moving synchronously. The gluteals become the powerhouse muscles instead of the smaller lumbar muscles. Trunk muscles are trained to function as stabilizers rather than prime movers.

Cardiovascular exercise is initiated as early as possible to minimize deconditioning syndrome. The initial aerobic exercise selected should be tailored to the patient's positional and loading tolerances. This may include retro or forward walking, biking, arm biking, swimming, or Nordic skiing using legs only.

Expanding Movement Boundaries

Expanding Movement Boundaries (Phase III) stresses flexibility first; the stretching of tight, hypertonic muscles. When Janda[133–137] experimented with remedial exercise to alter pat-

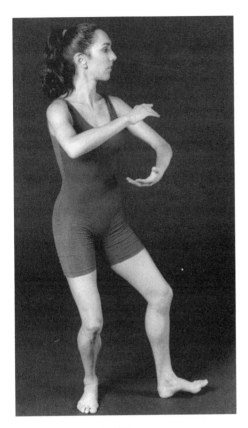

FIGURE 5-12 *Tai Chi.*

such as hip extension standing at a plinth with the torso supported, swimmer (prone alternating arm and leg), and quadruped alternating arm and leg (Fig. 5-13) work the gluteus maximus. Balancing a wand on the back while performing the quadruped alternating arm and leg exercise promotes fine control of lumbopelvic positioning. Wall slides (Fig. 5-14) recruit gluteus medius and minimus as well as maximus as the patient pushes against the wall while abducting the LE. Each exercise emphasizes LE distraction-elongation which assists in appropriate recruitment. Any of the PNF facilitation techniques are helpful. Knott and Voss's[167] concepts of proximal control for distal mobility are emphasized. Appropriate recruitment and sequencing of neuromuscular patterns are considered more important than absolute strength. Khalil et al.[168] examined the effect of stretching versus no stretching on subjects with CLBP undergoing a multimodel physical conditioning program. Both groups showed significant improvement in their functional abilities as measured by pain rating and back extensor strength. The group undergoing aggressive systematic stretching showed a significantly greater decrease in pain level and an increase in static strength and myoelectric output of their back extensors.

Many of the repatterning activities include balance training as a way to increase or normal-

terns of dysfunction, he found that no amount of strengthening of an inhibited muscle was effective until the antagonist facilitated muscle was treated. It is hypothesized that the tight, antagonist, facilitated muscle perpetuates a reciprocal inhibition to the inhibited, hypotonic muscle. Until the inhibited muscle begins to fire, strengthening perpetuates the substitution of synergists. Therefore, Janda stresses the need to stretch the tight muscle and achieve normal muscle length before attempting to strengthen the weak. Passive stretching, contract-relax, and muscle energy are all effective techniques for lengthening muscle.

Often, removal of the inhibitory influence of shortened muscles improves the ability of the patient to recruit "weak" muscles. Specific exercises to facilitate and improve recruitment and timing of these muscles may be given. Exercises

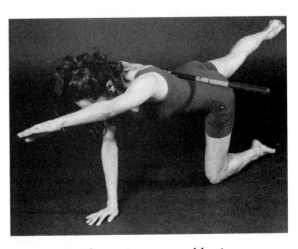

FIGURE 5-13 *Alternating arm and leg in quadriped with balanced wand.*

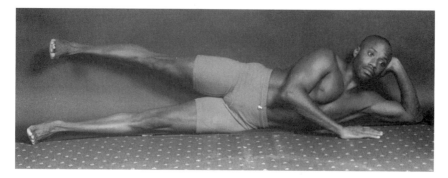

FIGURE 5-14 *Wall slides for gluteals.*

ize joint and muscle afferent input, and trigger better coordinated efferent responses. Balance activities attempt to challenge reorganization of the neuromuscular system to provide new behaviors that may be more efficient and preferable. Although orthopaedic patients are not neurologically impaired in the traditional sense of the word, habitual patterns are often developed that are inefficient and even harmful, and prevent access to movement alternatives. Once a patient is able to elicit voluntary contraction of a "shutdown" muscle, part of our therapeutic goal is to elicit a change in the pattern of coordination. "*Coordination* is defined as the process by which movement components are sequenced and organized temporally, and their relative magnitudes determined, in order to produce a functional movement pattern."[169] The ideas of neural

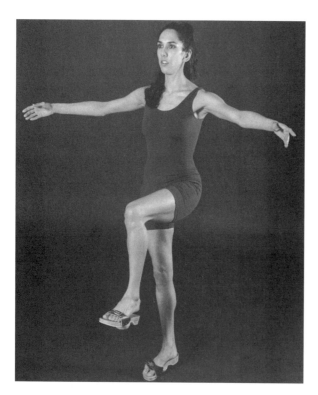

FIGURE 5-15 *Wobble shoes—high marching.*

plasticity are relevant to the orthopedic patient who, in pain, relies on a few stereotyped movement patterns and has lost the richness and relief of movement alternatives. Either more desirable patterns are not within the individual's experience or are no longer available to the individual voluntarily. Novel experiences must be provided in the first instance, or alternative ways to tap into intrinsic patterns must be attempted.

Balance exercises include static and dynamic activities, on stable and unstable surfaces, on two and one legs, with and without visual input. Training in wobble shoes for 1 week was found to facilitate a significant increase in gluteal activity in normals when measured with surface EMG.[170] Patients demonstrate improvements in postural stabilization as they attempt

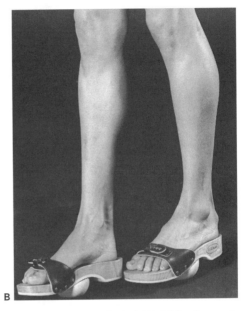

FIGURE 5-16 *Continued.* **(B)** *Wobble shoes close-up.*

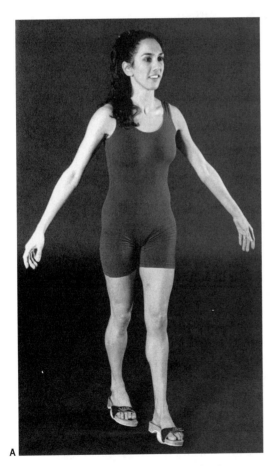

FIGURE 5-16 **(A)** *Wobble shoes—heel-toe.*

progressively more difficult gait patterns in the wobble shoes: walking, high marching (Fig. 5-15), heel-toe walking (Fig. 5-16), and heel-toe balancing. Patients unable to voluntarily stabilize in neutral spine posture have been observed to reflexively accomplish it during wobble shoe activities. Bullock-Saxton, Janda, Lewit, and Gauffin et al.[131,132,139,170,171] have suggested that peripheral or noncentral nervous system injury triggers a central adjustment of (abnormal) motor control in reaction to that injury. Subjects with grades II+ or III ankle sprains demonstrated significant decreases in vibration perception and delayed recruitment of gluteus maximus during hip extension.[131] When training has sufficiently facilitated voluntary control of the gluteals and abdominals, barefoot static stork balance (Fig. 5-9) while maintaining a subtalar neutral posture is attempted, progressing from use of arms for balance to no arms to eyes closed. This is then progressed to a wobble or BAPS board in the same sequence. Other activities such as balance beams, Pilotes equipment (Fig. 5-17), Swiss balls, foam rolls, and mini-trampo-

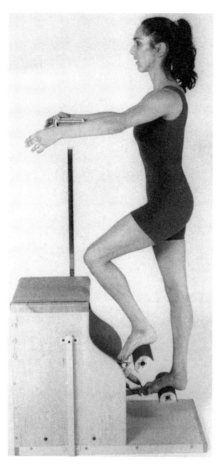

FIGURE 5-17 *Balance exercise on Pilotes equipment.*

lines provide proprioceptive and balance challenges.

Studies of stabilometry performance of athletes and untrained subjects found that athletes tended to experiment more with stances and rely more on proprioceptive cues than did untrained subjects.[66] Nashner and Cordo[172] suggest that attention has an important influence on postural reactions and accompaniments. Postural regulation is generally relegated to subconscious levels, but studies of skilled dancers and other highly trained athletes show a greater degree of conscious control of postural stabilization.[172] Mouchnino et al.[173] studied the differences between naive subjects and dancers performing a

leg movement while standing. In moving from first position to one leg while abducting a straight leg to 45 degrees, dancers were more efficient, minimized center of gravity displacement, and displayed a one-step feed-forward translation strategy that allowed them to maintain the verticality of their trunk. Naive subjects used a two-step inclination strategy that required bending of the trunk. Although certain synergistic patterns may be preprogrammed, there is flexibility in timing and combination of muscles involved.[174] Combinations of the hip and ankle strategies may be selected. The adoption of the term "strategies" is deliberate, to imply the existence of choice. Alterations in environmental conditions, instructions, or following short-term learning may produce varying postural reactions other than the most stereotyped.[175] Anticipatory postural adjustments are primarily acquired by learning through previous experience, or training where voluntary movement causes a postural disturbance.[175] Where disturbance is caused by an external force, postural reactions take place.

During Phase III, the Feldenkrais method provides valuable neuromuscular re-education and reorganization through novel sensory-motor experiences.[176] Feldenkrais teaching occurs in two forms: Functional Integration and Awareness Through Movement. Functional Integration is one-on-one nonverbal tablework in which the practitioner uses passive motions to introduce new sensory information to the client's nervous system in order to establish alternate movement capacities. Self-observation of posture and movement before, during, and following the intervention is emphasized to enhance greater awareness. (Awareness is the term used for conscious knowledge.) Awareness Through Movement is a group teaching method using structured movement sequences in which students develop greater awareness through self-exploration. Recognizing the powerful influence of gravity on neuromuscular organization, many lessons are taught in relatively gravity-eliminated positions. Using developmentally simple motions, the lessons seek to minimize the use of habitual patterns and restore normal joint flexibility and movement ease. Movements are encouraged to be done slowly and effortlessly, with emphasis on the process and not the end result. Visualization is considered more effective for change than action, as improvement in movement only appears after there is a change in the central control of the brain and CNS. Research has demonstrated electrical brain activity in the visual and motor cortex as well as regional cerebral metabolic rate increases, provoked by visual imagery.[177] Studies also demonstrate improved performance with mental rehearsal.[177]

Phase III also emphasizes training the trunk muscles as stabilizers while using the LE or UE muscles as prime movers. Part of stabilizing the spine in differing postures and transfers is learning to make subtle adjustments according to demand. Morgan[156] refers to this as *dynamic stabilization*. As an individual stoops to pick up an object, the trunk must counteract a flexion moment. As the individual lifts an object over his head, a different adjustment is necessary to counteract an extension moment. The effect of task experience on anticipatory postural trunk strategies was examined by Lavender et al.[178] During sudden loading to the torso, subjects demonstrated the development of preparatory response strategies involving increased muscle stiffness by pretensioning of the erector spinae with coactivation of the abdominals (varying ratios of internal and external obliques and rectus abdominus). Although these strategies showed individual differences, each minimized torso displacement, and reduced muscular compression forces with task experience. Lumbar flexion displacement was replaced with hip flexion. Intra-abdominal pressure changes did not appear to function as part of the preparatory strategy. Phase III exercises include the quarterback squat for timed holds, upper body bike, Swiss ball activities (Fig. 5-18), and single or double cable patterns such as chops and lifts, "blue skies" (Fig. 5-19) for the LE, and upper body trunk rotation on a Swiss ball (Fig. 5-20).

The patient is advanced to more difficult cardiovascular exercise as tolerance and control of complex movement increases. This may include stairmaster, fitter, slide board, and Nordic ski machine using arms as well as legs.

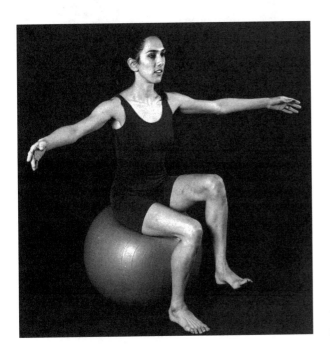

FIGURE 5-18 *Swiss ball marching.*

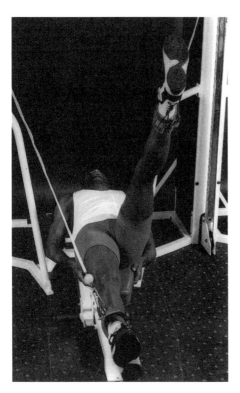

FIGURE 5-19 *Blue skies cable exercise for hamstrings and adductors as well as trunk stabilizers.*

Progressive Movement Challenges

In Progressive Movement Challenges (Phase IV), strengthening and conditioning exercises to specific muscles groups are included if additional endurance or muscle hypertrophy is necessary for the individual's lifestyle. Although practitioners agree on the need for conditioning and strengthening, literature reviewers have reported poor methodologic quality in clinical trials of exercise to determine efficacy.[179] Small sample size and absence of a placebo control group were the most frequently cited study deficiencies. Mayer's[180] functional restoration programs for populations with CLBP have shown improved physical capacity and return to work rates. Return to work rates after 2 years were 87 percent for the treatment group compared to 41 percent for the control group. His program includes a multidisciplinary approach with exer-

cise quotas and operant conditioning. McQuade et al.[181] demonstrated that greater overall fitness was significantly correlated with less physical dysfunction.

There is an association between reduced trunk muscle strength, especially trunk extension, and predisposition or occurrence of low back pain. A Danish general health survey of over 900 30- to 60-year-olds included an extensive low back examination (anthropometric measures and tests of trunk strength and endurance).[9] The 1-year follow-up questionnaire concluded that diminished isometric trunk extension endurance and back hypermobility was a significant predictor of first-time occurrence of LBP among men. There was also a trend that those of either sex with weaker trunk muscles or reduced flexibility of the trunk or hamstrings experienced reoc-

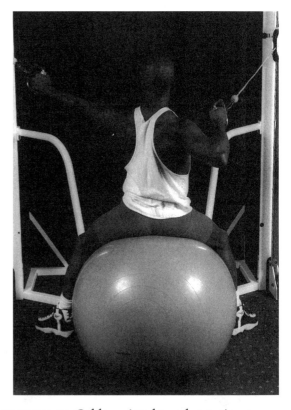

FIGURE 5-20 *Cable resisted trunk rotation on a swiss ball.*

currence more frequently than those with stronger trunk muscles.

CT scan and ultrasound studies have shown ipsilateral atrophy of the lumbar multifidus in subjects with LBP.[182] Paraspinal and multifidus type 2 fiber atrophy has also been demonstrated on biopsy in patients with LBP undergoing discectomy for disc herniation or CLBP.[183,184] Both studies found that training with maximal or submaximal effort may reverse this selective type 2 fiber atrophy. Flicker et al.[185] examined MRI signal intensity changes of the psoas, multifidus, and longissimus/iliocostalis following peak Roman chair exercise. The multifidus was generally most significantly active in normal volunteers, although individual variation was observed. Mayer et al.[19,180] have utilized this exercise as part of their successful restoration program.

Abdominal control is considered a key point in stabilization programs. The goal is to attain abdominal cocontraction with the back extensors. The internal and external obliques are particularly crucial in maximal trunk exertions and

lifting tasks.[186] Richardson et al.[78] examined EMG activity during eight exercises to determine which reflected the most optimal stabilizing pattern. As recruitment of the obliques and back extensors was considered the goal of stabilization (upper rectus abdominis was considered a negative contribution as it adds a flexion moment), exercises that involved trunk stabilization during isometric resisted trunk rotation were judged the most optimal patterns. The most effective bridging with isometric resisted rotation (Fig. 5-21). Crunches and double leg lowering did not provoke coactivation by back extensors, and emphasized upper rectus abdominis recruitment. Jull and Richardson[187] suggest that optimal stabilizing patterns may be absent in currently asymptomatic individuals. They used a model that viewed the function of trunk muscles to be active continuously or repeatedly over long periods of time at relatively low force levels. Assessing automatic stability in hooklying when a leg load was released, Jull and Richardson found two distinct populations: one that displayed a good automatic protective mechanism and one that dis-

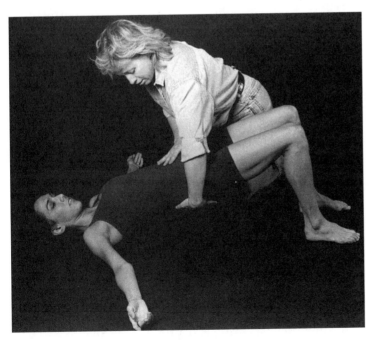

FIGURE 5-21 *Bridging with isometric resisted rotation.*

TABLE 5-9 *Exercise progression*

SIMPLE	COMPLEX
Stable	Unstable
Maximal support	Minimal support (vertical posture, single leg, etc.)
Static	Dynamic (movement)
Single cardinal plane	Multiple planes
No or minimal resistance	Weight progression with decreasing support
Short duration	Time progression for endurance
Minimal repetitions	High repetitions
Simple, isolated, gross movements	Complex patterns, multijoint disassociation
Controlled	Uncontrolled
Slow speed	Fast speeds, or acceleration-deceleration changes
Low force	High force
Isolated, protected	Goal oriented, task-specific

played deficiencies. They suggest that testing under submaximal conditions may be important when assessing motor control.

In Phase IV, exercises are progressed from simple, maximally controlled leg and arm movements superimposed on a stable trunk-pelvis to more complex and challenging activities (Table 5-9). Variables include unsupported postures, unstable surfaces, increased loading, multiple planes, and complex movements. Speed, repetition, weight, and timing can also be manipulated. The synchronization of multiple body parts moving in space to accomplish sport- or task-specific movement embodies the end result of functional exercise. Examples include swinging a golf club and throwing. Pushing and pulling activities challenge the reactiveness of the lumbar protective mechanism; the CNS set of trunk muscle stiffness for stabilization and attenuation of forces. A summary of exercises for lumbar rehabilitation is listed in Table 5-10.

There are two basic concepts in motor learning that should facilitate the achievement of a successful treatment outcome: feedback (visual, auditory, proprioceptive) and adaptation (practicing the desired task under altered contexts, i.e., in as many sensory and environmental conditions as possible).[188,189] Studies show random practice is superior to drill-like blocked practice. Summary or infrequent feedback is superior to immediate feedback. *Skill* occurs with the refinement of practice; successive inhibition of unnecessary motor units allows more efficient or less energy costly movement.[190] An optimal movement pattern entails the appropriate muscle participating at the correct time with the appropriate degree of contraction and having the ability to relax and rest.

Functional Outcomes

Outcome measures are standardized tests that attempt to quantify impairment, disability, or handicap. They may reflect a patient's assessment of function, pain, or satisfaction with treatment received. As pre- and post-tests, these are the only way we have to assess the effectiveness of nonsurgical, surgical, or no intervention. The World Health Organization developed the following definitions pertaining to the assessment of LBP.[191] *Impairment* refers to structural deficits that include deficits in ROM, strength, and radiographic measurements. Impairment is quantified by an observer. *Disability* refers to the functional consequences of impairment, such as the inability to perform ADL tasks such as sitting, walking, and lifting, as well as pain. Disability may be self-reported (pain ratings) or reported by an observer. *Handicap* refers to the disadvantages experienced as a result of impairments and disabilities. Handicap is primarily reported as return to work, since other measures are influenced by an individual's circumstances (such as society, economic and psychosocial background, and injury benefits and compensation).

Although impairment, pain, and disability are logically related, there is no direct relationship.[4] Waddell estimated that physical impairment only accounts for half the disability observed in individuals with CLBP.[4] He suggested that the other half could be attributed to psychological distress resulting in illness behavior rather than physical disease. Waddell observed

TABLE 5-10 *Exercises for lumbar rehabilitation*

Abdominals (increase holding or continuous exercise times)
  Abdominal isometrics in hooklying (counting outloud) with marching
  Half dead bug (1 arm and 1 leg, or legs only)
  Full deadbug (add cuff weights)
  Crunches (diagonal and straight)
  Gym ball crunches
  Graham contractions
  Leg press jumps

Extensors
  Glut squeezes (prone and supine)
  Half prone, half standing hip extension
  Swimmer supine
  Swimmer prone
  Quadriped alternating arm and leg (with cane)
  Bridging with holds
    With marching
    With knee extension
    On Swiss ball
  Half superman
  Full superman

Other Exercises
  Passe
  Wall slides

Balance-proprioception
  Stork (barefoot, maintain subtalar neutral, gluteal contraction)
    Use arms, eyes open
    Cross arms
    Eyes closed
    STAR touchdowns
  Lunges
  Wobble shoes walking
    Marching
    Heel-toe
    Lunge balances
    Heel-toe balances
    Catch
    Partnered push-pull with sticks
  BAPS or KAT wobble board catch
  Minitramp jumps and holds
    2 vs 1 leg
    Catch
  Swiss ball sitting, bridging, supine, prone
    Weight shift
    Upper and lower extremity patterns, cables

Cardiovascular
  Retro-walking on treadmill
    Add incline or hill program
  Arm bike standing in neutral spine posture
  Nordic ski
  Stairmaster trot (with stabilization)
  Bike
  Swimming
  Slide board
  Fitter
  Running

Gym equipment
  Leg press
  Hip machine
  Leg cables bicycle
    Scissors
    Circles
  Kneel sit to stand
  Kneel hip hinging
    Diagonals
    With sport cord
  Trunk flexion (isometrics, short arcs)
  Trunk extension (hinge at hip)
  Roman chair
  Lats
  Cable upper extremity patterns
    Sagittal chops and lifts
    Diagonal chops & lifts
    Rowing/pulling
    Punching/pushing
    On gym ball

Spinal flexibility, mobilization, neuromuscular control
  Press-ups
    Unilateral
    With rotation
  Standing backward bending
  Lateral pelvic shifts (supine and standing)
  Alternating knees to chest
  Sacral rocker in hooklying
  Quadriped cat-camel
    Side-bending
    Rotation
    Rocking
  Swiss ball sitting pelvic motion
  Standing or sitting axial rotation
  Unilateral bridge
    With rotation
  Feldenkrais exercises including:
    Pelvic clocks in hooklying
  Hooklying lower extremity rotation
  Thoracic extension over foam roll
  Segmental roll down from long sit to supine
  Shotgun pelvis

Functional patterns
  Squat quarterback
  Lunges
  Fastex (Biotran)

Stretching
  Piriformis
  Rectus femoris-iliopsoas
  Hamstrings
  ITB
  Quadratus lumborum
  Paraspinals-lats

"nonorganic" behavioral symptoms and signs that cannot be attributed to structural pathology and are not present in normals.[192] Waddell's Nonorganic Physical Signs test (Table 5-11 and 5-12) was developed as a screen to indicate patients who might be poor candidates for surgery or at high risk to develop chronic pain.[192,193] Chan et al.[144] reported a high correlation between high Waddell scores and nonorganic pain drawings, with good interevaluator reliability (73–78 percent). Bradish et al.,[195] however, reported no correlation between the presence of nonorganic signs at initial assessment and subsequent return to work. The authors stressed that the Waddell test should not be used as a predictor of outcome. Werneke et al,[193] on the other hand, found a significant drop in nonorganic signs for patients who successfully returned to work following a functional restoration program. Patients who did not return to work had no reduction in scores. Werneke et al. recommended that the presence of nonorganic signs be used to identify patients who might benefit from additional psychiatric management (Table 5-12).

The most frequently used *impairment* measure is spinal ROM, particularly forward flexion.[191] Most of the American Medical Association Guidelines for evaluation of permanent impairment rely on back motion measurements.[196] Although various techniques for measuring lumbar ROM, such as the inclinometer and the modified Schober technique, are reliable, correlation between ROM, symptoms, and disability are inconsistent.[191,197,198] Menard et al.[199] reported that motor performance in groups with high Waddell scores was lower in all tests, including tests not involving the low back. They conclude that psychological factors may widely affect motor performance. The reader is referred to the work by Clark and Haldeman[197] which describes guidelines for the evaluation of impairment and disability that were developed for the Division of Industrial Accidents (worker's compensation) in California. These guidelines attempt to develop a more comprehensive consideration and correlation of history, subjective complaints, type of work, organic or nonorganic pain patterns, tenderness, ROM, neurologic

TABLE 5-11 *Waddell nonorganic physical signs*

1. Tenderness	Superficial	Widespread sensitivity to light touch of superficial soft tissues (skin, not scar) over lumbar spine is abnormal.
	Nonanatomic	Boney tenderness felt over a wide area is not localized to one structure and often extends to the thoracic spine, sacrum, or pelvis.
2. Simulation	Axial loading	Light pressure (approximately 5 lbs) to skull of standing patient should not significantly increase low-back symptoms.
	Rotation	Back pain is reported when shoulders and pelvis are passively rotated in the same plane, as the patient stands relaxed with the feet together.
3. Distractions	Straight leg raising	Marked difference (approximately 40 to 45 degrees) between leg raising performed in the supine and sitting positions. Record where the back or leg pain is experienced.
4. Regional disturbances	Sensory	Regional sensory alteration or generalized "giving way" indicate possible functional disturbances if they cannot be explained on a neurologic basis, e.g. "stocking effect," cogwheel resistance.
5. Overreaction	Inappropriate overreaction	Guarding/limping, bracing, rubbing (affected area), grimacing, sighing (see definitions).

(From Waddell et al,[192] and Werneke et al,[193] with permission.) The Waddell score is the total number of positive tests of the five rated. Scores are then differentiated into low (0–2) and high (3–5) categories.

TABLE 5-12 *Definitions for inappropriate over-reaction*

CATEGORY	COMPONENTS	DEFINITIONS
Guarding	Assisted movement	Using canes, walkers, objects of furniture during movement (must occur for 3 seconds or more).
	Moderate guarding	Moderately stiff, rigid, or slow movement.
	Extreme guarding	Extremely stiff, rigid, or slow movement.
Bracing	Moderate brace	Using both limbs to support weight or balance while seated. Palms flat on bed or gripping side of bed for 3 seconds or more. Arms are not fully extended and are not supporting weight.
	Extreme brace	Using both limbs to fully support weight during sitting. Palms flat on bed or gripping side of bed for 3 seconds or more. Arms are fully extended and full weight is being supported.
Rubbing	Active rubbing	Hands moving over the affected area; palms down in an up/down or side-to-side motion for 3 seconds or more.
	Grabbing or holding	Clutching, grasping, or squeezing the affected area with hands and fingers for 3 seconds or more.
Grimacing		Obvious facial expression of pain that may include furrowed brow, narrowed eyes, tightened lips and corner of mouth pulled back, and clenched teeth.
Sighing		Obvious exaggerated exhalation of air, usually accompanied by shoulders first rising and then falling, cheeks may be expanded.

(From Werneke MW, et al[193] with permission.)

findings, strength tests, radiologic tests, lifting capacity, and other factors in determining disability. It must be noted that impairment measures are also affected by subjective states, and do not assess function.

Mayer et al[180] used impairment measures of functional capacity (trunk ROM, isometric and isokinetic trunk strength, cardiovascular endurance, static and dynamic lifting, obstacle course, etc.) and handicap measures of return to work rates to compare the effectiveness of a functional restoration program to no treatment.[180] A 2-year follow-up revealed that the treatment group had twice the return to work rate compared to the comparison group, with improvement in functional capacity measures seen in 80 percent of the patients.

The most widely accepted *disability* measures are the Oswestry,[200] Roland-Morris,[201] and Million[202] questionnaires, and the Sickness Impact Profile.[203,204] Deyo,[205] in a literature review, reported high test-retest reliability and good validity for each of the measures. Deyo et al[206] write that outcomes seeking to measure health-related quality of life should include at least one measure each of symptoms, functional status, and role function. The Oswestry, Roland-Morris, and Million questionnaires address disease-specific functional status, while the Sickness Impact Profile addresses generic functional status. Deyo et al. suggest disease-specific functional measures may be more responsive to changes following back intervention.

The most extensively used measure, the Oswestry questionnaire (Table 5-13), was designed to assess failed back surgery patients and is considered better at assessing more severe degrees of disability.[191] A self-report index, there are 10 sections that address ADL, with six levels of disability rating in each section. Fairbank et al.[200] reported a patient test-retest correlation coefficient of r = .99 on consecutive days, and a significant positive change over a 3-week period in patients with a high expectation of spontaneous recovery. Little and MacDonald[207] reported on the use of the percentage change in Oswestry score as an outcome measure in lumbar spinal surgery (all types of procedures combined). They

TABLE 5-13 *Oswestry low back questionnaire*

How long have you had back pain? _____years _____months _____weeks
How long have you had leg pain? _____years _____months _____weeks

This questionnaire has been designed to give information as to how your back pain has affected your ability to manage in everyday life. Please answer every section, and mark in each section only the <u>one</u> statement which applies to you. We realize you may consider that two of the statements in any one section relate to you, but <u>please just mark the one which most closely describes your problem.</u>

PAIN INTENSITY
____ I can tolerate the pain without having to use painkillers.
____ The pain is bad but I can manage without taking pain killers.
____ Pain killers give complete relief from pain.
____ Pain killers give moderate relief from pain.
____ Pain killers give very little relief from pain.
____ Pain killers have no effect on the pain and I do not use them.

PERSONAL CARE (washing, dressing, etc.)
____ I can look after myself normally without causing extra pain.
____ I can look after myself normally but it causes extra pain.
____ It is painful to look after myself and I am slow and careful.
____ I need some help but manage most of my personal care.
____ I need help every day in most aspects of self care.
____ I do not get dressed, wash with difficulty and stay in bed.

LIFTING
____ I can lift heavy weights without extra pain.
____ I can lift heavy weights but it gives extra pain.
____ Pain prevents me from lifting heavy weights off the floor, but I can manage if they are conveniently positioned, eg. on a table.
____ Pain prevents me from lifting heavy weights but I can manage light to medium weights if they are conveniently positioned.
____ I can lift only very light weights.
____ I cannot lift or carry anything at all.

WALKING
____ Pain does not prevent me from walking any distance.
____ Pain prevents me walking more than 1 mile.
____ Pain prevents me walking more than 1/2 mile.
____ Pain prevents me walking more than 1/4 mile.
____ I can only walk using a stick or crutches.
____ **I am in bed most of the time and have to crawl to the toilet.**

SITTING
____ I can sit in any chair as long as I like.
____ I can only sit in my favorite chair as long as I like.
____ Pain prevents me sitting more than 1 hour.
____ Pain prevents me sitting more than 1/2 hour.
____ Pain prevents me sitting more than 10 minutes.
____ Pain prevents me from sitting at all.

STANDING
____ I can stand as long as I want without extra pain.
____ I can stand as long as I want but it gives me extra pain.
____ Pain prevents me from standing for more than 1 hour.
____ Pain prevents me from standing for more than 30 minutes.
____ Pain prevents me from standing for more than 10 minutes.
____ Pain prevents me from standing at all.

(Continues)

TABLE 5-13 *(Continued)*

SLEEPING
___ Pain does not prevent me from sleeping.
___ I can sleep well only by using tablets.
___ Even when I take tablets I have less than six hours sleep.
___ Even when I take tablets I have less than four hours sleep.
___ Even when I take tablets I have less than two hours sleep.
___ Pain prevents me from sleeping at all.

SEX LIFE
___ My sex life is normal and causes no extra pain.
___ My sex life is normal but causes some extra pain.
___ My sex life is nearly normal but is very painful.
___ My sex life is severely restricted by pain.
___ My sex life is nearly absent because of pain.
___ Pain prevents any sex life at all.

SOCIAL LIFE
___ My social life is normal and causes me no extra pain.
___ My social life is normal but increases the degree of pain.
___ Pain has no significant effect on my social life apart from limiting my more energetic interests, eg. dancing, etc.
___ Pain has restricted my social life and I do not go out as often.
___ I have no social life because of pain.

TRAVELLING
___ I can travel anywhere without extra pain.
___ I can travel anywhere but it gives me extra pain.
___ Pain is bad but I manage journeys over two hours.
___ Pain restricts me to journeys of less than one hour.
___ Pain restricts me to short necessary journeys under 30 minutes.
___ Pain prevents me from travelling except to the doctor.

Scoring (not seen by patients): For each section, the total possible score is 5; if the first statement is marked the section score = 0, the last statement = 5.
If all ten sections are completed, the score is calculated as follows:
Example: <u>16</u>   (total scored)   X 100 = 32%
       50   (total possible score)
If one section is missed or not applicable the score is calculated:
Example: <u>16</u>   (total scored)   X 100 = 35.5%
       45   (total possible score)

Interpretation of Disability Scores
0 - 20%   Minimal Disability
20 - 40%   Moderate Disability
40 - 60%   Severe Disability
60 - 80%   Crippled
80 - 100%   These patients are either bed-bound or symptom magnifiers.

(From Fairbank J, et al,[200] with permission.)

found that the level of the patient's subjective improvement, ranked on a scale of 0 to 100, could be correlated with the percentage change in Oswestry score (r = .60). This was then useful to identify which preoperative factors were related to poor outcome. Di Fabio et al.[208] used Oswestry scores, forward bending ROM, maximal isometric lift, and work status as outcome measures of a physical therapy program involving multiple interventions (including exercise and manual therapy). Overall, there was improvement in each dependent measure at discharge, with the high compliance group showing greatest improvement in Oswestry score (12 percent) (average score 25) and the low compliance group showing the least (5 percent) (average score 38). There was an 18 percent improvement in Oswestry score (average score 12) and 80 percent return to work in patients with acute symptoms compared with only 7 percent improvement in Oswestry score (average score 35) and 44 percent return to work in patients with chronic symptoms. Timm[209] reported on the change in status of CLBP as measured by Oswestry score, trunk ROM, and lift test in a randomized controlled study. All patients were screened for and did not demonstrate Waddell nonorganic signs. Comparing 8-week treatment efficacy of five groups—control, physical agents, manipulation, low-tech exercise, and high-tech exercise— Timm concluded that only the low-tech and high-tech exercise were effective treatments for CLBP. Low-tech and high-tech exercise groups demonstrated 20.5 and 18.0 percent improvement in Oswestry scores (averages 14.46 and 15.06) respectively. Low-tech also produced the longest period of relief and was most cost-effective, depending on patient compliance. Return to work status was not reported.

Saal and Saal[157] reported outcomes in a retrospective cohort study of the nonoperative treatment of patients with herniated lumbar disc with radiculopathy. The authors used the Oswestry scale, pain self-rating, work status, and self-rating of outcome. There was a 92 percent return to work rate and 90 percent good or excellent self-rating of outcome. Good and excellent self-ratings averaged 20 and 16.6, respectively, in

TABLE 5-14 *The Quebec back pain disability scale*

This questionnaire is about the way your back pain is affecting your daily life. People with back problems may find it difficult to perform some of their daily activities. We would like to know if you find it difficult to perform any of the activities listed below, because of your back. For each activity there is a scale of 0 to 5. Please choose one response option for each activity (do not skip any activities) and circle the corresponding number.

Today, do you find it difficult to perform the following activities because of your back?

1. Get out of bed.
2. Sleep for at least 6 hours.
3. Turn over in bed.
4. Travel one hour in a car.
5. Stand up for 20–30 minutes.
6. Sit for 4 hours.
7. Climb one flight of stairs.
8. Walk a few blocks (300–400 m).
9. Walk several miles.
10. Reach up to high shelves.
11. Throw a ball.
12. Run two blocks.
13. Take food out of the refrigerator.
14. Make your bed.
15. Put on socks (panty hose).
16. Bend over a sink for 10 minutes.
17. Move a table.
18. Pull or push heavy doors.
19. Carry two bags of groceries.
20. Lift 40 lb.

(From Kopec JA, Esdaile JM, Abrahamowicz M, et al,[204] with permission.)

Oswestry scores, which is the lowest disability category.

Seeking a more sensitive measure for the less impaired back patient, Kopec et al.[204] compared a new scale, the Quebec Back Pain Disability Scale (Table 5-14), to the Oswestry and Roland measures. The test includes six areas of activity: (1) bed rest, (2) sitting/standing, (3) ambulation, (4) movement, (5) bending/stooping, and (6) handling large/heavy objects. The Quebec scale displayed high test-retest reliability, and correlated strongly with the Oswestry and Roland scales for validity measures. Frequency distributions of scores were symmetrical like the Roland, with the Oswestry skewed to the right. The scale was also found to detect relatively small changes in level of disability over time, both for short and long intervals.

Conclusion

LBP is a multifactorial problem that lacks specific diagnosis much of the time. In this chapter, back dysfunction is presented as the complex interrelation of the neuromuscular-osteoarticular systems, which is manifest in problems in movement. This chapter has attempted to provide a link between structural injury, movement dysfunction, exercise, and return to function. Rehabilitation emphasizes maximizing movement options within the individual's tolerance. Part of our task as movement educators is teaching the patient how to control the lumbopelvic area to optimize function.

The field of motor control, using kinetic and kinematic analysis with tools such as force plates, EMG telemetry, videotape, and electrogoniometry, has greatly enhanced our understanding of normal movement. Further research should enlarge our understanding of abnormal movement following injury and the effectiveness of treatment intervention. Some of the most fulfilling, creative, and fun challenges of physical therapy rehabilitation can be in assisting the patient to bridge the gap from functioning at a basic ADL level to resume or initiate for the first time sports participation, dance, and other riches of human movement.

References

1. Frymoyer JW: Back pain and sciatica. N Engl J Med 318:291–300, 1988
2. Cassidy JD, Wedge JH: The epidemiology and natural history of low back pain and spinal degeneration. p. 3. In Kirkaldy-Willis WH (ed): Managing Low Back Pain. 2nd Ed. Churchill Livingstone, New York, 1988
3. Kelsey JL, White AA: Epidemiology of low back pain. Spine 6:133–142, 1980
4. Waddell G: A new clinical model for the treatment of low-back pain. Spine 12:632–644, 1987
5. Bigos S, Spengler D, Martin N et al: Back injuries in industry: a retrospective study. Spine 11:246–256, 1986
6. Cherkin DC, Deyo RA, Loeser JD et al: An international comparison of back surgery rates. Spine 19:1201–1206, 1994
7. Mooney V: Where is the pain coming from? Presidential Address, International Society for the Study of the Lumbar Spine. Spine 12:754–759, 1987
8. Taylor VM, Deyo RA, Cherkin DC et al: Low back pain hospitalization: recent United States trends and regional variations. Spine 19:1207–1213, 1994
9. Biering-Sorenson F: Physical measurements as risk indicators to low-back trouble over a one-year period. Spine 9:106–109, 1984
10. Nachemson AL: Advances in low back pain. Clin Orthop 200:266–278, 1985
11. Haldeman S: Failure of the pathology model to predict back pain. Presidential Address, North American Spine Society. Spine 15:718–724, 1990
12. Kirkaldy-Willis WH: The pathology and pathogenesis of low back pain. p. 49. In Kirkaldy-Willis WH (ed): Managing Low Back Pain. Churchill Livingstone, New York, 1988
13. Spitzer WO: Quebec task force on spinal disorders: scientific approach to the assessment and management of activity-related spinal disorders. Spine 12:S1–S58, 1987
14. Wheeler AH, Hanley EN: Spine update: nonoperative treatment for low back pain. Spine 20:375–378, 1995
15. McKenzie RA: The Lumbar Spine: Mechanical Diagnosis and Therapy. Spinal Publications, Waikanae, 1981
16. Maitland GD: Vertebral Manipulation. 4th Ed. Butterworths, London, 1981
17. Delitto A, Shulman AD, Rose SJ: On developing expert-based decision-support systems in physical therapy: the NIOSH low back atlas. Phys Ther 69:554–558, 1989
18. Delittlo A, Erhard RE, Bowling RW: A treatment-based classification approach to low back syndrome: identifying and staging patients for conservative treatment. Phys Ther 75:470–489, 1995
19. Mayer TG, Gatchel RJ, Kishino N et al: Objective assessment of spine function following industrial injury. Spine 10:482–493, 1985

20. Ellis JJ: Lumbo-Pelvic Integration, Course Notes. Institute of Physical Arts, San Anselmo, CA, 1993

21. Porterfield JA, DeRosa C: Mechanical Low Back Pain: Perspectives in Functional Anatomy. W. B. Saunders, Philadelphia, 1991

22. Andersson GBJ, Ortengren R, Schultz AB: Analysis and measurement of the loads on the lumbar spine during work at a table. J Biomech 13: 513–520, 1980

23. Ladin Z, Murthy KR, DeLuca CJ: Mechanical recruitment of low-back muscles. Spine 14: 927–938, 1989

24. Seroussi RE, Pope MH: The relationship between trunk muscle electromyography and lifting moments in the sagittal and frontal planes. J Biomech 20:135–146, 1987

25. Bogduk N: The lumbar back muscles and their fascia. p. 83. In Bogduk N, Twomey LT (ed): Clinical Anatomy of the Lumbar Spine. 2nd Ed. Churchill Livingstone, Melbourne, 1991

26. Hart DL, Stobbe TJ, Jaraiedi M: Effect of lumbar posture on lifting. Spine 12:138–145, 1987

27. Noe DA, Mostardi RA, Jackson ME et al: Myoelectric activity and sequencing of selected trunk muscles during isokinetic lifting. Spine 17: 225–229, 1992

28. Vakos JP, Nitz AJ, Threlkeld AJ et al: Electromyographic activity of selected trunk and hip muscles during a squat lift. Spine 19:687–695, 1994

29. Bogduk N: Anatomy and function of the lumbar back muscles and their fascia. p. 111. In Twomey LT, Taylor JR (ed). Physical Therapy of the Low Back. 2nd Ed. Churchill Livingstone, New York, 1994

30. Keagy RD, Brumlik J, Bergan JJ: Direct electromyography of the psoas major in man. J Bone Joint Surg 48-A:1377–1382, 1966

31. Nachemson A: Electromyographic studies on the vertebral portion of the psoas muscle. Acta Orthop Scand 37:177–190, 1966

32. Andersson E, Oddsson L, Grundstrom H et al: The role of the psoas and iliacus muscles for stability and movement of the lumbar spine, pelvis and hip. Scand J Med Sci Sports 5:10–16, 1995

33. Gracovetsky S, Farfan H: The optimum spine. Spine 11:543–573, 1986

34. Donish EW, Basmajian JV: Electromyography of deep back muscles in man. Am J Anat 133:25–36, 1972

35. Luk KDK, Ho HC, Leong JCY: The iliolumbar ligament. A study of its anatomy, development, and clinical significance. J Bone Joint Surg 68B: 197–201, 1986

36. Chow DHK, Luk KDK, Leong JCY et al: Torsional stability of the lumbosacral junction: significance of the iliolumbar ligament. Spine 14: 611–615, 1989

37. Yamamoto I, Panjabi MM, Oxland TR et al: The role of the iliolumbar ligament in the lumbosacral junction. Spine 15:1138–1141, 1990

38. Bogduk N, Macintosh JE, Pearcy MJ: A universal model of the lumbar back muscles in the upright position. Spine 17:897–913, 1992

39. Amonoo-Kuofi HS: The density of muscle spindles in the medial, intermediate and lateral columns of human intrinsic postvertebral muscles. J Anat 136:509–519, 1983

40. Barker D, Milburn A: Development and regeneration of mammalian muscle spindles. Sci Prog Oxf 69:45–64, 1984

41. Sirca A, Kostevc V: The fiber type composition of thoracic and lumbar paravertebral muscles in man. J Anat 141:131–137, 1985

42. Nitz AJ, Peck D: Comparison of muscle spindle concentrations in large and small human epaxial muscles acting in parallel combinations. American Surgeon 52:273–277, 1986

43. Bastide G, Zadeh J, Lefebvre D: Are the little muscles what we think they are? Surg Radiol Anat 11:255–256, 1989

44. Peck D, Buxton DF, Nitz A: A comparison of spindle concentrations in large and small muscles acting in parallel combinations. J Morphology 180:243–252, 1984

45. Montgomery WH, Pink M, Perry J: Electromyographic analysis of hip and knee musculature during running. Am J Sports Med 22:272–278, 1994

46. Mann RA, Moran GT, Dougherty SE: Comparative electromyography of the lower extremity in jogging, running, and sprinting. Am J Sports Med 14:501–510, 1986

47. Winter D: Foot trajectory in human gait: a precise and multifactorial motor control task. Phys Ther 72:45–53, 1992

48. Shiavi R: Electromyographic paterns in normal adult locomotion. p. 97. In Smidt GL (ed): Gait in Rehabilitation. Churchill Livingstone, New York, 1990

49. Winter DA, MacKinnon CD, Ruder GK et al: An integrated EMG/biomechanical model of upper

body balance and posture during human gait. Progress in Brain Research 97:359–367, 1993

50. Van Ingen Schenau GJ, Pratt CA et al: Differential use and control of mono- and biarticular muscles. Human Movement Sciences 13: 495–517, 1994

51. Alderink GL: The sacroiliac joint: review of anatomy, mechanics, and function. J Orthop Sports Phys Ther 13:71–84, 1991

52. Walker JM: The sacroiliac joint: a critical review. Phys Ther 72:903–916, 1992

53. Bourdillon JF, Day EA, Bookhout MR: Anatomy and biomechanics. p. 13. In Bourdillon JF, Day EA, Bookhout MR (eds): Spinal Manipulation. 5th Ed. Butterworth-Heinemann Ltd, Oxford, 1992

54. Mitchell FL, Moran SP, Pruzzo NA: An Evaluation and Treatment Manual of Osteopathic Muscle Energy Procedures. Mitchell, Moran, and Pruzzo, Valley Park, MO, 1979

55. Ellison JB, Rose SJ, Sahrman SA: Patterns of hip rotation range of motion: a comparison between healthy subjects and patients with low back pain. Phys Ther 70:537–541, 1990

56. Mellin G: Correlations of hip mobility with degree of low back pain and lumbar spinal mobility in chronic low back pain patients. Spine 13: 668–670, 1988

57. Cunningham K: Comparison of hip extension range of motion in normals to people with low back pain. Masters Thesis, Long Island University, 1992

58. Thurston AJ: Spinal and pelvic kinematics in osteoarthrosis of the hip joint. Spine 10:467–471, 1985

59. Berg K: Balance and its measure in the elderly: a review. Physiother Can 41:240–246, 1989

60. Horak FB: Clinical measurement of postural control in adults. Phys Ther 67:1881–1885, 1989

61. Friedli WG, Cohen L, Hallet M et al: Postural adjustments associated with rapid voluntary arm movements. II: Biomechanical analysis. J Neurol Neurosurg Psychiatr 51:232–243, 1988

62. Todd ME: The Thinking Body. Dance Horizons, Brooklyn, 1975

63. Alexander FM: The Use of the Self. Centerline Press, Long Beach, CA, 1989

64. Sweigard LE: Human Movement Potential: Its Ideokinetic Facilitation. Harper & Row, New York, 1974

65. Dowd I: Taking Root to Fly. Contact Collaborations, New York, 1981

66. Debu B, Werner L, Woollacott MH: Influence of athletic training on postural stability. p. 281. In Woollacott MH, Shumway-Cook A (eds): Development of Posture and Gait Across the Life Span. University of South Carolina Press, Columbia, SC, 1989

67. Reed ES: Changing theories of postural development. p. 3. In Woollacott MH, Shumway-Cook A (eds): Development of Posture and Gait Across the Life Span. University of South Carolina Press, Columbia, SC, 1989

68. Ortengren R, Andersson GBJ: Electromyographic studies of trunk muscles, with special reference to the functional anatomy of the lumbar spine. Spine 2:44–52, 1977

69. Sheffield FJ: Electromyographic study of the abdominal muscles in walking and other movements. Am J Phys Med Rehab 41:142–147, 1962

70. Jonsson B: The functions of individual muscles in the lumbar part of the spinae muscle. Electromyography 10:5–21, 1970

71. Portnoy H, Morin F: Electromyographic study of postural muscles in various positions and movements. Am J Physiol 186:122–126, 1956

72. Valencia FP, Munro RR: An electromyographic study of the multifidus in man. Electromyogr Clin Neurophysiol 25:205–221, 1985

73. Twomey LT, Taylor JR: Lumbar posture, movement, and mechanics. p. 57. In Twomey LT, Taylor JR (eds): Physical Therapy of the Low Back. 2nd Ed. Churchill Livingstone, New York, 1994

74. Woodhull AM, Maltrud K, Mello BL: Alignment of the human body in standing. Eur J Appl Physiol 54:109–115, 1985

75. Heino JG, Godges JJ, Carter CL: Relationship between hip extension range of motion and postural alignment. J Orthop Sports Phys Ther 12: 243–247, 1990

76. Walker ML, Rothstein JM, Finucane SD et al: Relationships between lumbar lordosis, pelvic tilt, and abdominal muscle performance. Phys Ther 67:512–516, 1987

77. Miller MI, Medeiros JM: Recruitment of internal oblique and transversus abdominis muscles during the eccentric phase of the curl-up exercise. Phys Ther 67:1213–1217, 1987

78. Richardson C, Toppenberg R, Jull G: An initial evaluation of eight abdominal exercises for their ability to provide stabilisation for the lumbar spine. Aust J Physiother 36:6–11, 1990

79. Wohlfahrt D, Jull G, Richardson C: The relationship between the dynamic and static function of

abdominal muscles. Aust J Physiother 39:9–13, 1993

80. Jackson RP, McManus AC: Radiographic analysis of sagittal plane alignment and balance in standing volunteers and patients with low back pain matched for age, sex, and size. Spine 19:1611–1618, 1994

81. Hansson T, Sandstrom J, Roos B et al: The bone mineral content of the lumbar spine in patients with chronic low back pain. Spine 10:158, 1985

82. Prochazka A: Sensorimotor gain control: a basic strategy of motor systems? Progr Neurobiol 33:281–307, 1989

83. Horak FB: Assumptions underlying motor control for neurologic rehabilitation. p. 11. In Lister MJ (ed): Contemporary Management of Motor Control Problems: Proceedings of the II STEP Conference. Foundation for Physical Therapy and APTA's Neurology Section and Section on Pediatrics, Fredericksberg, 1991

84. Frank JS, Earl M: Coordination of posture and movement. Phys Ther 70:855–863, 1990

85. Babinski J: De l'aynergie cerebelleuse. Rev Neurol 7:806–816, 1899

86. Nashner LM, McCollum G: The organization of human postural movements: a formal basis and experimental synthesis. Behav Brain Sci 8:135–172, 1985

87. MacKinnon CD, Winter DA: Control of whole body balance in the frontal plane during human walking. J Biomech 26:633–644, 1993

88. Yekutiel MP: The role of vertebral movement in gait: implications for manual therapy. J Manual & Manip Ther 2:22–27, 1994

89. Perry J: Gait Analysis: Normal and Pathological Function. Slack, Thorofare, NJ, 1992

90. Thelen E, Ulrich BD, Jensen JL: The developmental origins of locomotion. p. 25. In Woollacott MH, Shumway-Cook A (eds): Development of Posture and Gait Across the Life Span. University of South Carolina Press, Columbia, 1989

91. Winter DA, Patla AE, Frank JS: Assessment of balance control in humans. Medical Progress Through Technology 16:31–51, 1990

92. Inman VT, Ralston HJ, Todd F: Human Walking. Williams & Wilkins, Baltimore, 1981

93. Gregersen GG, Lucas DB: An in vivo study of the axial rotation of the human thoracolumbar spine. J Bone Joint Surg 49-A:247–262, 1967

94. Murray MP: Gait as a total pattern of movement. Am J Phys Med 46:290, 1967

95. Gray G: The relationship of low back pain to the foot. Biomechanics 2:61–64, 1995

96. Chao EYS, Cahalan TD: Kinematics and kinetics of normal gait. p. 45. In Smidt GL (ed): Gait in Rehabilitation. Churchill Livingstone, New York, 1990

97. Thurston AJ, Harris JD: Normal kinematics of the lumbar spine and pelvis. Spine 8:199–205, 1983

98. Stokes VP, Anderson C, Forssberg H: Rotational and translational movement features of the pelvis and thorax during adult human locomotion. J Biomech 22:43–50, 1989

99. Michaud TC: Foot Orthoses. Williams & Wilkins, Baltimore, MD 1993

100. Thorstensson A, Carlson H, Zomlefer MR et al: Lumbar back muscle activity in relation to trunk movements during locomotion in man. Acta Physiol Scand 116:13–20, 1982

101. Pauly JE: An electromyographic analysis of certain movements and exercises. I: Some deep muscles of the back. Anat Rec 155:223–234, 1966

102. Smidt GL: Gait in musculoskeletal abnormalities, p. 199. In Smidt GL (ed): Gait in Rehabilitation. Churchill Livingstone, New York, 1990

103. Voloshin A: An in vivo study of low back pain and shock absorption in the human locomotor system. J Biomech 15:21–27, 1982

104. Sullivan MS: Back support mechanisms during manual lifting. Phys Ther 69:38–45, 1989

105. Sullivan MS: Lifting and back pain. p. 329. In Twomey LT, Taylor JR (eds): Physical Therapy of the Low Back. 2nd Ed. Churchill Livingstone, New York, 1994

106. Toussaint HM, de Winter AF, de Haas Y et al: Flexion relaxation during lifting: implications for torque production by muscle activity and tissue strain at the lumbo-sacral joint. J Biomech 28:199–210, 1995

107. Wolf LB, Segal RL, Wolf SL et al: Quantitative analysis of surface and percutaneous electromyographic activity in lumbar erector spinae of normal women. Spine 16:155–161, 1991

108. Cailliet R: Low Back Pain Syndrome. FA Davis, Philadelphia, 1991

109. Paquet N, Malouin F, Richards CL: Hip-spine movement interaction and muscle activation patterns during sagittal trunk movements in low back pain patients. Spine 19:596–603, 1994

110. Nelson JM, Walmsley RP, Stevenson JM: Relative lumbar and pelvic motion during loaded spinal flexion/extension. Spine 20:199–204, 1995

111. Nouwen A, Van Akkerveeken PF, Versloot JM: Patterns of muscular activity in patients with chronic low back pain. Spine 12:777–782, 1987

112. Soderberg GL, Barr JO: Muscular function in chronic low-back dysfunction. Spine 8:79–85, 1983

113. Trafimow JH, Schipplein OD, Novak GJ et al: The effect of quadriceps fatigue on the technique of lifting. Spine 18:364–367, 1993

114. Higgins M, Fisher T, Elbaum L: Rectus femoris and erector spinae activity during simulated "knees-bent" and "knees-straight" lifting, abstracted. J Orthop Sports Phys Ther 13:257, 1991

115. Delitto RS, Rose SJ: An electromyographic analysis of two techniques for squat lifting and lowering. Phys Ther 72:438–448, 1992

116. Holmes JA, Damaser MS, Lehman SL: Erector spinae activation and movement dynamics about the lumbar spine in lordotic and kyphotic squat-lifting. Spine 17:327–334, 1992

117. Cassisi JE, Robinson ME, O'Conner P et al: Trunk strength and lumbar paraspinal muscle activity during isometric exercise in chronic low-back pain patients and controls. Spine 18: 245–251, 1993

118. Dolce JJ, Raczynski JM: Neuromuscular activity and electromyography in painful backs: psychological and biomechanical models in assessment and treatment. Psychol Bull 97:502–520, 1985

119. Grabiner MD, Koh TJ, El Ghazawi A: Decoupling of bilateral paraspinal excitation in subjects with low back pain. Spine 17:1219–1223, 1992

120. Kravitz E, Moore ME, Glaros A: Paralumbar muscle activity in chronic low back pain. Arch Phys Med Rehab 62:172–176, 1981

121. Robinson ME, Cassisi JE, O'Connor PD et al: Lumbar iEMG during isotonic exercise: Chronic low back pain patients versus controls. J Spinal Dis 5:8–15, 1992

122. Roy SH, De Luca CJ, Emley M et al: Spectral electromyographic assessment of back muscles in patients with low back pain undergoing rehabilitation. Spine 20:38–48, 1995

123. Wolf SL, Nacht M, Kelly JL: EMG feedback training during dynamic movement for low back pain patients. Behav Ther 13:395–406, 1982

124. Bourdillon JF, Day EA, Bookhout MR: Detailed examination of the spine. p. 103. In Bourdillon JF, Day EA, Bookhout MR (eds.): Spinal Manipulation. 5th Ed. Butterworth-Heinemann, Oxford, 1992

125. Johnson G, Saliba V: Functional Orthopaedics I, Course Notes. The Institute of Physical Art, San Anselmo, CA, 1988

126. Cummings G, Scholz JP, Barnes K: The effect of imposed leg length difference on pelvic bone symmetry. Spine 18:368–373, 1993

127. Potter NA, Rothstein JM: Intertester reliability for selected clinical tests of the sacroiliac joint. Phys Ther 65:1671–1675, 1985

128. Cibulka MT, Delitto A, Koldehoff RM: Changes in innominate tilt after manipulation of the sacroiliac joint in patients with low back pain: an experimental study. Phys Ther 68:1359–1363, 1988

129. Oxland TR, Crisco JJ, Panjabi MM et al: The effect of injury on rotational coupling at the lumbosacral junction: a biomechanical investigation. Spine 17:74–80, 1992

130. Panjabi M, Yamamoto I, Oxland T et al: How does posture affect coupling in the lumbar spine? Spine 14:1002–1011, 1989

131. Bullock-Saxton JE: Local sensation changes and altered hip muscle function following severe ankle sprain. Phys Ther 74:17–31, 1994

132. Bullock-Saxton JE, Bullock MI: Changes in hip and knee muscle strength associated with ankle injury. N Zealand J Physiother 21:10–14, 1993

133. Janda V: Muscles, central motor regulation, and back problems. p. 27. In Korr IM (ed.): The Neurologic Mechanisms in Manipulative Therapy. Plenum Press, New York, 1978

134. Janda V: Muscles and cervicogenic pain syndromes. p. 153. In Grant R (ed): Physical Therapy of the Cervical and Thoracic Spine. Churchill Livingstone, New York, 1988

135. Janda V: Muscle weakness and inhibition (pseudoparesis) in back pain syndromes. p. 197. In Grieve GP (ed.): Modern Manual Therapy of the Vertebral Column. Churchill Livingstone, London, 1986

136. Janda V: Pain in the locomotor system—a broad approach. p. 148. In Glasgow EF, Twomey LT, Scull ER et al. (eds.): Aspects of Manipulative Therapy. Churchill Livingstone, Melbourne, 1985

137. Jull GA, Janda V: Muscles and motor control in low back pain: assessment and management. p. 253. In Twomey LT, Taylor JR: Physical Therapy of the Low Back. Churchill Livingstone, New York, 1987

138. Kendall FP, McCreary EK: Muscles: Testing and Function. 3rd Ed. Williams & Wilkins, Baltimore, MD, 1983

139. Lewit K: Manipulative Therapy in Rehabilitation of the Motor System. Butterworths, London, 1985

140. Sahrman S: Postural applications in the child and adult: adult posturing. p. 295. In Kraus SL (ed.): TMJ Disorders: Management of the Craniomandibular Complex. Churchill Livingstone, New York, 1988

141. Bookhout MR: Examination and treatment of muscle imbalances. p. 314. In Bourdillon JF, Day EA, Bookhout MR (eds.): Spinal Manipulation. 5th Ed. Butterworth-Heinemann, Oxford, 1992

142. Singer KP: A new musculoskeletal assessment in a student population. J Orthop Sports Phys Ther 8:34–41, 1986

143. Radin EL: Role of muscles in protecting athletes from injury. Acta Med Scand, suppl 711: 143–147, 1986

144. Bookhout MR: Exercise as an adjunct to manual medicine, Course notes. Minneapolis, 1994

145. Parkhurst TM, Burnett CN: Injury and proprioception in the lower back. J Orthop Sports Phys Ther 19:282–295, 1994

146. Byl NN, Sinnott PL: Variations in balance and body sway in middle-aged adults: subjects with healthy backs compared to subjects with low-back dysfunction. Spine 16:325–330, 1991

147. Hoag JM: The musculoskeletal system: a major factor in homeostasis. Thomas L. Northrup Lecture, J Am Osteopathic Assoc, 1976

148. Little KC: Toward a more effective manipulative management of chronic myofascial strain and stress syndromes. J Am Osteopathic Assoc 68: 675–685, 1965

149. Bigos S, Bowyer O, Braen G et al: Acute Low Back Problems in Adults. Clinical Practice Guideline, Quick Reference Guide Number 14. U.S. Dept of Health and Human Services, Public Health Service, Agency for Health Care Policy and Research, AHCPR Pub No 95–0643, Rockville, MD, 1994

150. Di Fabio RP: Clinical assessment of manipulation and mobilization of the lumbar spine: a critical review of the literature. Phys Ther 66:51, 1986

151. Jayson MIV, Sims-Williams H, Young S et al: Mobilization and manipulation for low-back pain. Spine 6:409, 1981

152. Shekelle PG, Adams AH, Chassin MR et al: Spinal manipulation for low back pain. Ann Intern Med 117:590–598, 1992

153. Twomey L, Taylor J: Spine update: exercise and spinal manipulation in the treatment of low back pain. Spine 20:615–619, 1995

154. Zhu Y, Haldeman S, Starr A et al: Paraspinal muscle evoked cerebral potentials in patients with unilateral low back pain. Spine 18: 1096–1102, 1993

155. Porterfield JA: Dynamic stabilization of the trunk. J Orthop Phys Ther 6:271–276, 1985

156. Morgan D: Concepts in functional training and postural stabilization for the low back injured. Topics in Acute Care Trauma Rehab 2:8–17, 1988

157. Saal JA, Saal JS: Nonoperative treatment of herniated lumbar intervertebral disc with radiculopathy: an outcome study. Spine 14:431–437, 1989

158. Donelson R, Silva G, Murphy K: Centralization phenomena: its usefulness in evaluating and treating referred pain. Spine 15:211–213, 1990

159. Spratt KF, Weinstein JN, Lehmann TR et al: Efficacy of flexion and extension treatments incorporating braces for low-back pain patients with retrodisplacement, spondylolisthesis, or normal sagittal translation. Spine 18:1839–1849, 1993

160. Ponte DJ, Jensen GJ, Kent BE: A preliminary report on the use of the McKenzie protocol versus Williams protocol in the treatment of low back pain. J Orthop Sports Phys Ther 6:130–139, 1984

161. Smith RL, Mell DB: Effects of prone spinal extension exercise on passive lumbar extension range of motion. Phys Ther 67:1517–1520, 1987

162. Schnebel BE, Watkins RG, Dillin W: The role of spinal flexion and extension in changing nerve root compression in disc herniations. Spine 14: 835–837, 1989

163. Beattie PF, Brooks WM, Rothstein JM et al: Effect of lordosis on the position of the nucleus pulposus in supine subjects. Spine 19: 2096–2102, 1994

164. Fiebert I, Keller CD: Are "passive" extension exercises really passive? J Orthop Sports Phys Ther 19:111–116, 1994

165. Da Liu: Tai Chi Chuan and I Ching: A Choreography of Body and Mind. Harper & Row, New York, 1972

166. Durckheim KG: Hara: The Vital Centre of Man. Mandala-Harper Collins, London, 1962

167. Knott M, Voss DE: Proprioceptive Neuromuscular Facilitation, 2nd Ed. Harper & Row, Philadelphia, 1968

168. Khalil TM, Asfour SS, Martinez LM et al:

Stretching in the rehabilitation of low-back pain patients. Spine 17:311–317, 1992

169. Scholz JP: Dynamic pattern theory—some implications for therapeutics. Phys Ther 70: 827–843, 1990

170. Bullock-Saxton JE, Janda V, Bullock MI: Reflex activation of gluteal muscles in walking. Spine 18:704–708, 1993

171. Gauffin H, Tropp H, Odenrick P: Effect of ankle disk training on postural control in patients with functional instability of the ankle joint. Int J Sports Med 9:141–144, 1988

172. Nashner LM, Cordo PJ: Relation of automatic postural responses and reaction-time voluntary movements of human leg muscles. Exp Brain Res 43:395–405, 1981

173. Mouchnino L, Aurenty R, Massion J et al: Coordination between equilibrium and head-trunk orientation during leg movement: a new strategy built up by training. J Neurophysiol 67: 1587–1598, 1992

174. Pedotti A, Crenna P, Deat A et al: Postural synergies in axial movements: short and long term adaptation. Exp Brain Res 74:3–10, 1989

175. Massion J: Movement, posture and equilibrium: interaction and coordination. Progr Neurobiol 38:35–56, 1992

176. Feldenkrais M: Awareness Through Movement. Harper & Row, New York, 1977

177. Warner L, McNeill ME: Mental imagery and its potential for physical therapy. Phys Ther 68: 516–521, 1988

178. Lavender SA, Marras WS, Miller RA: The development of response strategies in preparation for sudden loading to the torso. Spine 18: 2097–2105, 1993

179. Koes BW, Bouter LM, van der Heijden G: Methodological quality of randomized clinical trials on treatment efficacy in low back pain. Spine 20: 228–235, 1995

180. Mayer TG, Gatchel RJ, Mayer H et al: A prospective two-year study of functional restoration in industrial low back injury. J Am Med Assoc 258: 1763–1767, 1987

181. McQuade KJ, Turner JA, Buchner DM: Physical fitness and chronic low back pain. Clin Orthop Rel Res 233:198–204, 1988

182. Hides JA, Stokes MJ, Saide M et al: Evidence of lumbar multifidus muscle wasting ipsilateral to symptoms in patients with acute/subacute low back pain. Spine 19:165–172, 1994

183. Rantanen J, Hurme M, Falck B et al: The lumbar multifidus muscle five years after surgery for a lumbar intervertebral disc herniation. Spine 18: 568–574, 1993

184. Rissanen A, Kalimo H, Alaranta H: Effect of intensive training on the isokinetic strength and structure of lumbar muscles in patients with chronic low back pain. Spine 20:333–340, 1995

185. Flicker PL, Fleckenstein JL, Ferry K et al: Lumbar muscle usage in chronic low back pain: magnetic resonance image evaluation. Spine 18: 582–586, 1993

186. Zetterberg C, Andersson GBJ, Schultz AB: The activity of individual trunk muscles during heavy physical loading. Spine 12:1035–1040, 1987

187. Jull GA, Richardson CA: Rehabilitation of active stabilization of the lumbar spine. p. 251. In Twomey LT, Taylor JR (eds.): Physical Therapy of the Low Back. 2nd Ed. Churchill Livingstone, New York, 1994

188. Keshner EA: How theoretical framework biases evaluation and treatment. p. 37. In Lister MJ (ed.): Contemporary Management of Motor Control Problems: Proceedings of the II Step Conference. Foundation for Physical Therapy, APTA, Alexandria, VA, 1991

189. Schmidt RA: Motor learning principles for physical therapy. p. 49. In Lister MJ (ed.): Contemporary Management of Motor Control Problems: Proceedings of the II Step Conference. Foundation for Physical Therapy, APTA, Alexandria, VA, 1991

190. Basmajian JV: Motor learning and control: a working hypothesis. Arch Phys Med Rehab 58: 38–41, 1977

191. Thomas AMC: The spine. p. 94. In Pynsent PB, Fairbank JCT, Carr A (eds.): Outcome Measures in Orthopaedics. Butterworth-Heinemann, Oxford, 1994

192. Waddell G, McColloch JA, Kummel E et al: Nonorganic physical signs in low-back pain. Spine 5:117–125, 1980

193. Werneke MW, Harris DE, Lichter RL: Clinical effectiveness of behavioral signs for screening chronic low-back pain patients in a work-oriented physical rehabilitation program. Spine 18: 2412–2418, 1993

194. Chan CW, Goldman S, Ilstrup DM et al: The pain drawing and Waddell's nonorganic physical signs in chronic low-back pain. Spine 18: 1717–1722, 1993

195. Bradish CF, Lloyd GJ, Aldam CH et al: Do nonorganic signs help to predict the return to activity

of patients with low-back pain? Spine 13: 557–560, 1988

196. Clark WL, Haldeman S, Johnson P et al: Back impairment and disability determination: another attempt at objective, reliable ratings. Spine 13:332–341, 1988

197. Clark W, Haldeman S: The development of guideline factors for the evaluation of disability in neck and back injuries. Spine 18:1736–1745, 1993

198. Shirley FR, O'Connor P, Robinson ME et al: Comparison of lumbar range of motion using three measurement devices in patients with chronic low back pain. Spine 19:770–783, 1994

199. Menard MR, Cooke C, Locke SR et al: Pattern of performance in workers with low back pain during a comprehensive motor performance evaluation. Spine 19:1359–1366, 1994

200. Fairbank JCT, Couper J, Davies JB et al: The Oswestry low back pain disability questionnaire. Physiotherapy 66:271–273, 1980

201. Roland M, Morris R: A study of the natural history of low-back pain. Part I: development of a reliable and sensitive measure of disability in low-back pain. Spine 8:141–144, 1983

202. Million R, Hall W, Nilson KH et al: Assessment of the progress of the back-pain patient. Spine 7:204–212, 1982

203. Bergner M, Bobbitt RA, Carter WB et al: The sickness impact profile: development and final revision of a health status measure. Med Care 19:787–805, 1981

204. Kopec JA, Esdaile JM, Abrahamowicz M et al: The Quebec back pain disability scale. Spine 20: 341–352, 1995

205. Deyo RA: Measuring the functional status of patients with low back pain. Arch Phys Med Rehab 69:1044–1053, 1988

206. Deyo RA, Andersson G, Bombardier C et al: Outcome measures for studying patients with low back pain. Spine 19:2032S–2036S, 1994

207. Little DG, MacDonald D: The use of the percentage change in Oswestry disability index score as an outcome measure in lumbar spinal surgery. Spine 19:2139–2134, 1994

208. Di Fabio RP, Mackey G, Holte JB: Disability and functional status in patients with low back pain receiving workers' compensation. Phys Ther 75: 180–193, 1995

209. Timm KE: A randomized-control study of active and passive treatments for chronic low back pain following L5 laminectomy. J Orthop Phys Ther 20:276–286, 1994

6

Functional Evaluation and Treatment of the Lower Extremity

WALT JENKINS

SHAW BRONNER

ROBERT MANGINE

A recent trend in the rehabilitation of lower extremity (LE) injuries has been toward functional closed kinetic chain (CKC) exercise.[1,2] Advances in bio- and pathomechanics research has had a significant influence on our practice. Instead of treating isolated joint complexes, emphasis is on the entire lower quadrant. Due to these changes in perspective, the clinician must gain a better understanding of the intricate relations and interactions between all of the structures that make up the lower kinetic chain complex in order to safely and completely treat the specific lesion. Thorough evaluation must include specific joint and muscle assessment as well as functional analysis of extremity and body movement control and skills.

Over the past two and a half decades significant effort has gone into researching the sequela following anterior cruciate ligament (ACL) tears, which has transformed how we treat most LE injuries. Researchers studied the tensile stiffness and strength of various tissues to ascertain which tissue might function as an ACL replacement.[3] Artificial grafts quickly fell out of favor, as

did externally augmented[4,5] and acute repairs.[6,7] Researchers examined the effects of immobilization and early motion on cartilage[8] and surgical tissue healing and strength.[3,9] The deleterious effect of immobilization on cartilage and the ability of the new ACL graft to tolerate full extension, immediate motion, and immediate weight bearing was learned. Over the years, surgical instrumentation (arthroscopically assisted) and techniques including graft placement, isometric tension, and fixation have been analyzed and refined.[10,11] These advances have diminished tissue morbidity and enhanced early rehabilitation. Authors documenting outcomes of ACL reconstruction in the early days reported graft integrity using Lachman's and KT testing, range of motion (ROM), and assessed strength with isokinetic tests.[4,5] As researchers learned more, they realized that these tests did not explain the ability of some athletes to return to former levels of competition while others could not. This was particularly obvious in the ACL-deficient population.[12]

During this period clinicians also began to

report their observations of patients with structurally stable ankles who repeatedly reinjured themselves.[13–15] As it became apparent that isolated joint and muscle testing could not accurately predict readiness for return to play, functional tests were included in assessment. Functional outcome scoring systems were developed as a result to better ascertain treatment effectiveness. Some systems focused subjectively on patient self-report of ability to perform activities of daily life (ADL) and sport activities. Other systems developed objective functional skills tests, seeking to more accurately predict readiness to return to play.

Preceding and paralleling the development of functional tests was the biomechanical analysis of forces on the joints, and electromyographic (EMG) activity of the muscles of the lower quadrant. Researchers learned there were differences between open kinetic chain (OKC) and CKC movements, due to the "concurrent shift" contraction of biarticular muscles and axial compression forces of weight bearing in CKC.[1,16] Subsequent rehabilitation encorporating CKC activities has led to aggressive accelerated programs that result in earlier return to full activities.[17] Improved outcomes have been reported with these accelerated programs, including improved and earlier achievement of ROM, strength, stability on KT testing, decreased incidence of arthrofibrosis, less patellofemoral pain, less joint stiffness, and greater patient compliance and satisfaction.[17,18] When used appropriately, these aggressive accelerated programs appear to have no deleterious effects on tissue healing and ultimate strength on short-term follow-up.[2] Although much of the basic research was conducted in relation to knee injury, our understanding of tissue mechanics has enhanced treatment of all LE injuries. A good example is the case of achilles tendon repairs, where the same advances that have made ACL reconstruction a less morbid, more predictable result are being applied. New methods of fixation, early mobilization, early weight bearing, and function oriented rehabilitation have resulted in as good or better outcomes following achilles tendon repair.[19,20]

Imperative in using accelerated rehabilitation programs is understanding normal and pathomechanics, biologic tissue healing parameters, and putting the pieces together in neuromuscular evaluation in functional weight-bearing contexts.[21] In this chapter, functional rehabilitation refers to evaluation, treatment, and testing in which forces exert the same effect on loading and moving muscles and joints as occurs in life. Movement frequently involves more than one joint, with complex interactions between muscles working as prime movers, assisters, stabilizers, or antagonists, with isometric, concentric, or eccentric contractions. This chapter discusses lower kinetic chain evaluation, treatment, and testing using functional movement.

Stance and Locomotion

A thorough analysis of standing posture and locomotion forms the foundation for the treatment of LE dysfunction. One approach is to break down motion into the cardinal planes and assess the control and tolerance of joint and muscle function within each plane. Donatelli refers to predominance of joint motion in one cardinal plane as *planar dominance*.[22] This may restrict motion in another plane and provoke dysfunction. Sagittal plane motion, the primary motion in walking, running, and biking, involves the largest and strongest muscles of the LE. Frontal and transverse plane muscles may play their most important role in stabilizing weight shift and weight acceptance onto one limb, and fine tuning the placement of the limbs for skilled movement. The practitioner must bear in mind, however, that muscles are working and limbs are moving in multiple planes simultaneously. Gray[23] expanded this idea in dividing gait into the "pronation response" and the "supination response." In describing the gait cycle using foot terminology, it is important to stress that control and initiation of movement may occur proximally as well as distally.

For simplicity, initial analysis of standing and gait uses the model "Six Criteria of Nor-

TABLE 6-1 *Six criteria of normalcy*

1. Bisection of the calcaneus is parallel to the long axis of the lower leg
2. Plantar surface of the metatarsal heads is perpendicular to a bisection of the calcaneus
3. Ankle joint must allow 10 degrees of dorsiflexion with the knee extended and subtalar joint in neutral
4. No force is exerted on the talus from the lower extremity due to abnormal anterior or posterior attitude
5. No force is exerted on the talus from the lower extremity due to abnormal valgus or varus attitude
6. No force is exerted on the talus from the lower extremity due to abnormal rotation or torsion

(From McPoil T[25] and Root ML et al,[24] with permission.)

malcy" (Table 6-1).[24,25] These criteria represent a static ideal relation of osseous structures in stances necessary for efficient locomotion.

Criteria number 1 states that when the subtalar joint is neutral, the calcaneus and lower leg are vertical and therefore in parallel alignment. Deviation from this is within the frontal plane and may occur at any joint within the kinetic chain. The most common compensation is at the subtalar joint during the weight acceptance phase of gait. Normal subtalar motion includes 4 degrees pronation and 12 degrees supination from neutral.[26]

Criteria number 2 refers to the relation of the midtarsal and forefoot. Compensation is seen during midstance and push-off phase of gait. The term *metatarsal break* refers to the composite axis of motion of the five metatarsophalangeal joints during push-off in stance.[27] This axis should occur 50–70 degrees to the long axis of the foot. Great toe dorsiflexion ranges of 55–90 degrees are necessary at push-off.[27,28]

Criteria number 3, which refers to the talocrural joint, and number 4, which refers to the knee or hip, reflect deviations within the sagittal plane. This frequently means loss of motion. The talocrural joint requires 10 degrees of dorsiflexion for walking and 25 degrees for running.[26,28] The knee must extend 0 degrees and flex a minimum of 50 degrees[26] to 60 degrees.[28] The hip must extend a minimum of 10 degrees, and flex 30–40 degrees.[26,28] A significant improvement in

gait economy as measured by maximum oxygen consumption was demonstrated following a hip extension stretching program in asymptomatic males with tight hip flexors.[29] Waters et al.[30] compared walking speed and oxygen consumption in subjects with unilateral arthrodesis of the hip and ankle to normals. They found average walking speed for each group was 84 percent of normal gait velocity. The ankle arthrodesis group's mean rate of oxygen consumption was 3 percent more than normal walkers, with a gait efficiency of 90 percent. The hip arthrodesis group had a 32 percent greater mean rate of oxygen consumption than normal walkers, with a gait efficiency rate of 53 percent.

Criteria number 5 refers to frontal plane deviation at the knee or hip. An increase in the valgus or varus alignment of the knee or hip will affect the loading of these joints as well as the foot. Criteria number 6 involves transverse plane deviations observed in the femur or tibia. Both Michaud[26] and Perry[28] suggest that the hip must rotate a minimum of 15–20 degrees. Total tibial rotation is approximately 18 degrees during gait.[31]

The static Six Criteria of Normalcy correlate well with the six determinants of gait defined by Saunders et al.[32] These include (1) pelvic rotation, (2) pelvic tilt, (3) knee flexion, (4) hip flexion, (5) knee and ankle interaction, and (6) lateral pelvic displacement. The authors described locomotion as "the translation of the center of gravity through space along a path requiring the least expenditure of energy." The interrelation of each of the six determinants of gait summate to minimize vertical and horizontal displacements in order to conserve energy. Pathologic gait might be viewed as a compensatory attempt to minimize energy expenditure by exaggerating motion at unaffected areas, relieving the area of dysfunction, and diminishing pelvic displacement.

The Criteria of Normalcy model, as established by Root et al.,[26] has been challenged by research findings regarding the reliability of measurement of subtalar neutral, the observed normal foot alignment, and the position of the subtalar joint during the stance phase of walking. Measurement of subtalar neutral is, at best, moderately reliable.[33–35] The assumption that a majority of the population would meet the criteria for a normal foot has been shown to be false, challenging the validity of the criteria of normalcy model.[36] Finally, McPoil and Cornwall[37] showed that the subtalar joint usualy does not reach the neutral position during the stance phase of walking.[35] The position obtained during walking corresponds closely to the relaxed calcaneal position described by McPoil.[25] Presently, the criteria of normalcy model is effective in identifying relations between the joints of the foot, ankle, and leg. A combination of this evaluation with identification of the tissues being stressed can determine the most effective treatment.[38] Static evaluation must always be accompanied by dynamic evaluation and close attention to the mechanical status of the injured tissues. Treatment must be guided by relief of patient complaints and return to function, not merely accomodation to a model.[38]

The mechanical axes of the foot are not perpendicular to the cardinal planes.[22,24,39] Motion actually occurs across all three planes and is described as triplanar motion. The terms pronation and supination were developed to describe this combined motion occurring at the subtalar and midtarsal joints. Pronation in the CKC refers to combined calcaneal eversion and talus plantar

flexion and adduction.[22,40] OKC pronation involves eversion, dorsiflexion, and abduction. Supination in the CKC refers to calcaneal inversion and talus dorsiflexion and abduction, while OKC supination entails inversion, plantar flexion, and adduction. Because the motion of the foot is triplanar, resulting motion up the LE kinetic chain is also triplanar in the weight-bearing, closed chain context (Table 6-2). In the CKC, pronation results in LE flexion and internal rotation, while supination results in extension and external rotation.

It is well known that pronation "unlocks" the joints to provide a flexible foot for shock absorption and accommodation to the ground surface.[22,25] Pronation occurs following heel strike, maximizes at foot flat, and occurs again following toe-off during the swing phase. Supination provides a rigid lever and muscle pulley system for push-off from midstance through toe-off. Gray describes pronation as giving into gravity to accommodate and absorb.[23] Muscle activity is primarily eccentric to decelerate. Supination overcomes gravity to propel. Its muscle action is primarily concentric to accelerate. In analyzing different postures and gait, it is important to observe of the amount of collapsing that occurs through the kinetic chain during pronation response, and whether there is planar or specific joint dominance in movement. An individual

TABLE 6-2 *Triplanar joint motion during CKC pronation and supination*

JOINT	SAGITTAL	FRONTAL	TRANSVERSE
		Pronation Response	
Subtalar	Plantarflexion (talus)	Eversion (calcaneus)	Adduction (talus)
Ankle	Dorsiflexion/Plantarflexion	Eversion	Abduction
Knee	Flexion	Abduction	Internal rotation
Hip	Flexion	Adduction	Internal rotation
L5–S1	Extension	Side-bending (tow)	Rotation (away)
		Supination Response	
Subtalar	Dorsiflexion (talus)	Inversion (calcaneus)	Abduction (talus)
Ankle	Plantarflexion	Inversion	Adduction
Knee	Extension	Adduction	External rotation
Hip	Extension	Abduction	External rotation
L5–S1	Flexion	Side-bending (away)	Rotation (tow)

(From Tiberio D,[122] with permission.)

asked to balance on one leg may respond with poor gluteus medius stabilization and allow his pelvis to drop and his trunk to shift. This may carry over into walking and running. This is an excessive pronation response. A patient complaining of chronic Achilles tendinitis who walks and runs on his toes demonstrates an excessive supination response. A patient with extreme forefoot abduction and limited dorsiflexion ROM (less than 5 degrees) displays transverse planar dominance.

When observing the motor control dynamics of walking and running, it is useful to pay attention to key muscle groups. In the OKC with the foot free, proximal segments take precedence in determining limb progression and foot placement for subsequent heel strike and weight acceptance.[41] Winter et al.[41] find that in gait the ankle muscles are not as important as in stance, because the balance requirements are altered. The ankle muscles are capable of fine tuning movement and placement. They are too small and too distant from the head-arms-trunk (HAT), which comprises two-thirds of the body's mass, to effectively control acceleration and deceleration. The gluteals and hamstrings primarily provide eccentric deceleration of the momentum of hip flexion and knee extension in late swing.[28,42] In stance, they act to restrain forward momentum of the pelvis and trunk. Gluteus medius is the primary frontal plane stabilizer of the pelvis and is active from late swing through heel-off. As the largest muscles of the body, the gluteals are key shock absorbers.

In walking, jogging, running, and sprinting, the hip flexors are primarily responsible for increasing the speed of movement.[43,44] Researchers disagree on the function of the gastrocnemius-soleus muscles. Peak activity of all calf muscles occurs during midstance in walking[22] and running,[45] while eccentrically controlling ankle dorsiflexion. Several authors report that there is little or no gastrocnemius-soleus activity past heel-off, suggesting that forward propulsion is primarily a factor of rapid hip flexion rather than calf muscle push-off.[43–45] Winter[42] and Rodgers,[46] on the other hand, report that plantar flexors are primarily responsible for propulsion

at push-off, with activity increasing exponentially with increasing speed. Michaud[26] writes gastrocnemius-soleus are active at heel-off to assist with heel lift, but more importantly, supinate the subtalar joint and thus externally rotate the tibia and femur. A secondary consequence of controlling tibial motion into dorsiflexion is a contribution to stabilizing the knee.

Comparison of EMG activity profiles during running shows that the quadriceps and posterior ankle muscles (gastrocnemius, soleus, posterior tibialis) have almost identical activity profiles, indicating that they work in concert to stabilize the foot, ankle, tibiofemoral, and patellofemoral joints during the stance phase.[44,45] The phasic activity of the hamstring muscles may be indicative of their role in transferring power up and down the lower extremity.

Tibialis anterior is active in late swing through foot flat to control the deceleration of plantar flexion and stabilize against eversion.[46,47] It is concentrically active following toe-off to dorsiflex the foot. Reber et al.[45] report that during running tibialis anterior shows the highest rate of sustained activity of any of the leg muscles. It contracts during more than 85 percent of the gait cycle, at a level greater than 20 percent of maximal voluntary contraction (MVC). Monad[48] suggests that muscles sustaining contraction at levels above 20 percent of MVC are susceptible to fatigue overload. This may manifest in overuse injuries such as shin splints. Tibialis posterior is considered another important stabilizer by decelerating pronation forces in early stance, and supinating at midstance.[49] When the pace is increased in running, the peroneals work harder to stabilize during midstance. This is probably because with little or no heel strike, ground reaction forces are rapidly transmitted to the mid- and forefoot and the stabilizing effect of the supinated subtalar joint is eliminated.[45]

In a motor control analysis of the energetics of gait, Winter finds four mechanical power phases in gait that affect step length and cadence: ankle push-off, hip pull-off, knee extensors at push-off, and knee flexors at end of swing.[42] Step length and velocity is increased by increasing concentric plantar flexor activity at push-off, and increased concentric hip flexor activity at pull-off. Concomittant with increased push-off impulse is increased absorption of energy at the knee by eccentric quadriceps contraction. The hamstrings must increase their eccentric work to decelerate the limb during swing for foot placement. Step length can be decreased by increasing eccentric quadriceps activity in late stance and hamstring activity in late swing.

Peak vertical ground reaction force values increase from 1.1 to 1.3 times body weight in walking to 2.5 to 3.5 times body weight in running, depending on speed.[46,50] In running, there are two periods of "float," when neither foot is in contact with the ground. Stance phase is divided into absorption and propulsion components. With increasing velocity, there is decreased stance time and increased float time. At any given velocity of running, vertical rise per stride is an average of 4 cm greater in the poor runner, and better runners have a greater length of stride and lower stride frequency.[51] The location of initial foot contact plays an important role on the pattern of force development, most significantly in running. Runners may be forefoot, midfoot, or rearfoot strikers. Mean peak to peak ampli-

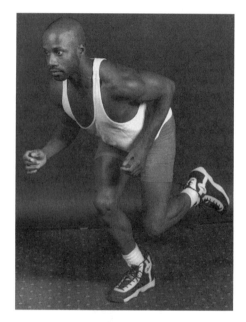

FIGURE 6-2 *One-legged squat.*

tude for mediolateral ground reaction force (the smallest of the three components of ground reaction force) has been measured at three times greater in midfoot strikers compared to rearfoot strikers.[52] Other researchers have reported midfoot strikers have greater impact forces at slower speeds but the reverse at higher speeds compared to rearfoot strikers.[50] At sprint paces, forefoot strikers displayed the highest impact forces. The center of pressure path may also vary depending on initial foot contact.[46]

Other movements useful in LE assessment include two- (Fig. 6-1) and one-legged squatting (Fig. 6-2). Shift in weight-bearing pattern, compensatory movements, or avoidance altogether will provide useful information. In initial evaluation of acute problems, total ROM as measured at the knee or at hip and knee, or ROM until compensation takes place are one method of quantifying two- and one-legged squatting. Qualitative changes such as compensatory proximal or distal joint motion, and shift in weight-bearing away from the involved side should also be noted. A grid Polaroid photo allows measurement at a later time.

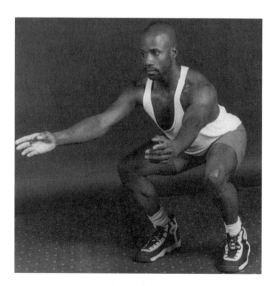

FIGURE 6-1 *Two-legged squat.*

Balance

Balance was defined earlier in this text (see ch. 5) as the ability of an individual to maintain a position, to voluntarily move, and to react to a perturbation.[53] This may occur in both static and dynamic contexts as in standing on one leg to put one's trousers on, landing on one leg from a jump, or pivoting to change direction. Problems in balance may occur in individuals with *mechanical instability* such as ACL deficiency or multiple ankle sprains due to ligamentous laxity. The term *functional instability* was first introduced by Freeman et al.[13] to describe individuals who reported frequent "giving way" of their limbs, some of which had no apparent anatomic instability. Functional instability is defined as joint motion beyond voluntary control but not necessarily exceeding physiologic ranges, while mechanical instability is joint motion that exceeds normal physiologic limits.[15,53] It is hypothesized that both mechanical and functional instabilities have contributing proprioception deficiencies. Authors report using a modified Rhomberg test (eyes open and closed) to screen for functional instability.[13,55,56] Freeman et al.[13] proposed that functional instability of the ankle follows in 40 percent of all ankle injuries. Ryan reported only 24 percent of the ankles with functional instability demonstrated mechanical instability in a sample of 45 subjects.[57]

The Rhomberg test is a useful clinic screen but is imprecise and unquantifiable (Fig. 5-9, Ch. 5). Tropp et al.[53,58] found stabilometry to be an objective quantification of a modified Rhomberg test. Stabilometry using forceplate measures has demonstrated increased postural sway in the frontal plane on the injured limb of individuals with unilateral inversion ankle sprains and a positive anterior drawer, 1 week postinjury.[15] Fridén et al.[59] found that compared to a control reference group, even the uninjured limb showed impaired equilibrium, suggesting centrally impaired postural control may predispose for injuries. This was supported by Löfvenberg et al.[60] who found increased peroneal reaction times in both injured and contralateral ankles in subjects with unilateral ankle sprain. They suggested that functional stability is affected by changes in the gamma motor system, which regulates stiffness and sensitivity to stretch. Ligamentous injury can alter muscular response by reducing postural tone.[60–62] Increased frontal plane postural sway has also been demonstrated in the injured leg of individuals with ACL deficiency and in both legs compared to referenced controls.[63]

The stabilometry results of Tropp et al.[53,58] did not support those of Freeman et al.,[13] Fridén et al.,[15] or Garn and Newton.[55] No increased postural sway was recorded on the involved limb of individuals with previous ankle injury. They concluded that ankle injury alone did not result in persistent functional instability. Selection by Tropp et al.[58] of a combined sagittal and frontal plane measurement to give a total body sway ellipse may not have provided a sufficiently sensitive test. Friden et al.[15] believed that the frontal plane was the plane of greatest potential instability. Cornwall and Murrell[64] examined postural sway in both sagittal and frontal planes in subjects with a history of unilateral inversion sprain compared to controls. Increased sway amplitude was demonstrated in each plane on the involved limb (the uninvolved limb was not tested). The dependent variables used by these authors were possibly more sensitive to alterations in sway than those of Tropp et al.

Muscle weakness has also been proposed as a contributing factor to instability. Ryan[57] has noted lower inversion peak torque isokinetic values on the involved side of individuals with unilateral functional instability. Frontal plane balance was impaired on the involved limb, with greater time spent in the adducted position, despite normal eversion strength values. Ryan concluded that his results supported proprioception impairment as the cause of functional instability. Other authors have reported peroneal weakness in athletes with functional instability compared to those with normal ankles.[14] Lentell et al.[56] found no significant bilateral differences in isokinetic or isometric measurements of inversion-eversion torque in individuals with unilateral chronic ankle instability. The modified

Rhomberg test did determine gross differences in stability in these subjects.

Delayed peroneal response perhaps due to denervation has been suggested as a causative factor in ankle functional instability. Sudden inversion stress using a trapdoor measured a trend toward increased peroneal response time in unilateral instability.[65,66] There was also a high correlation between postural sway and peroneal reaction time.[65]

Denervation may be caused by a traction lesion of the peroneal nerve resulting in mild axonotmesis.[67] Kleinrensink et al.[68] found reduced nerve conduction velocity at 4–8 days postinjury in 22 patients with grades I–III inversion ankle sprains; in the superficial peroneal nerve compared to the contralateral leg and control group, and in the deep peroneal nerve of both legs compared to the control group. There were no findings of denervation. By 5 weeks postinjury, values were normal. No correlation was found between nerve conduction velocity and degree of sprain. Although these subjects were not a population with a chronic history of sprains, the authors suggest that the lack of correlation between degree of sprain and nerve conduction velocity may explain the presence of functional instability without apparent mechanical instability.

Nitz et al.[67] reported the incidence of both peroneal and posterior tibial nerve injury in 66 consecutive patients with grade II or III ankle sprains. (Grade I sprains were not included, as a pilot study revealed no denervation changes.) Nerve conduction velocities were unaltered, but mild to moderate denervation potentials were found in the peroneal nerve distribution of 17 percent (5) and in the posterior tibial nerve distribution of 10 percent (3) of the 30 patients with grade II ankle sprains. Moderate to severe denervation potentials were found in the peroneal nerve distribution of 86 percent (31) and in the posterior tibial nerve distribution of 83 percent (30 in 36) patients with grade III sprains. Time to return to full activity averaged 1.6 weeks for the grade II group and 5.3 weeks for the grade III group. In follow-up EMG studies at 3 months postinjury, continuing abnormalities were present in only two of the 14 examined.

Differences between the Nitz et al.[67] and Kleinrensink et al.[68] studies include the definition of grade and type of ankle sprain, the time of initial EMG measurement (2 weeks versus 4–8 days), and the type of EMG analysis (needle versus surface). It is not clear why one group found changes in motor action potential and no changes in nerve conduction velocity while the other group found opposite results. Further studies are needed to examine both motor denervation (due to traction injury) and articular deafferentation (due to direct mechanoreceptor trauma) and the interaction of both in arthokinetic reflexes. A third explanation is neurogenic inflammation.[60,69] There is evidence that chemosensitive and other receptors in the joint and muscle lead to alterations in both direct muscle function and the CNS control of the muscle.[69,70,71]

It is recommended that all LE dysfunction be screened with a modified Rhomberg test: eyes open and closed. The literature suggests a test of 30 seconds duration with eyes open and closed. Touch-down by the opposite foot, hopping, or wobbling at any joint stops the clock. In the absence of age- and activity-specific norms, a percentage of the uninvolved limb time is one way to compare limb data. Dancers may be screened at a higher level, in a pressure releve balance. At the appropriate time, athletes, dancers, and active individuals should also be evaluated in their ability to stabilize in landing from vertical and distance hops, or other sport-specific postures and movements.

Lower Extremity Function

Pathomechanics in LE movement are quite common. It is extremely rare for individuals to completely comply with the Six Criteria of Normalcy. As noted earlier, the incidence of normal foot alignment is relatively small. Smith-Oricchio and Harris[35] found that only 15 percent (3 of 20 subjects) and McPoil et al.[36] found that 17 percent (20 of 116) of subjects stood in a subtalar neutral position. The degree of compliance with the criteria is not in and of itself an indicator of pathology; it is an ideal model on which to base an evaluation. Individuals who have significant structural deformity may be completely asymptomatic while others with relatively minor variance have profound dysfunction. Many of us have also observed people who run seemingly incorrectly, but win races and remain uninjured. Tamper with their mechanics and they fall apart. Other factors that make up a patient's adaptive potential include activity level, body weight and distribution, and neuromuscular integration. In the instance of structural abnormality, the neuromuscular system is the unknown variable. It is difficult to predict the implications of structural abnormality because the neuromuscular system can adapt significantly to limit dysfunction. It is also in this system where treatment can have a major influence.

ANKLE-FOOT

Abnormal pronation is the most common problem associated with the foot. Congenital rearfoot varus (the most frequent), midtarsal varus, forefoot varus, and ankle equinus can each result in compensatory overpronation.[49] In a survey of 58 normal females between the ages of 18 and 30, McPoil found subtalar varus present in 83.6 percent (97 feet) of the samples.[36] Rearfoot varus was defined as the sum of subtalar varus and tibial varum. In another study, McPoil et al.[72] found that all subjects had 4.6 to 8.7 degrees of tibiofibular varum. Forefoot valgus was present in 44.8 percent (52 feet), forefoot varus in 8.6 percent (10 feet), and plantar flexed first ray in 14.7 percent (17 feet). Garbalosa et al., on the other hand, found forefoot valgus in 8.7 percent and forefoot varus in 86.7 percent of a sample of 240 feet.[73] Perhaps the extreme differences reported in the two studies is due to the poor interrater reliability of measuring subtalar neutral.

Maximum pronation is usually reached at completion of 25 percent of stance phase (foot flat).[31] Compensatory pronation often continues past 50 percent of stance phase (heel-off), and thus the foot may never reach supination. The velocity of overpronation as well as where it oc-

curs in the stance phase will determine what structures become symptomatic. Rearfoot varus results in increased and rapid pronation early in stance.[22,26] Midtarsal and forefoot varus result in prolonged pronation into the propulsion phase. Forefoot varus may be the most destructive, as the foot never locks to become a rigid lever in supination. Ankle equinus, a sagittal plane deformity, results in decreased dorsiflexion of the talocrural joint. Compensatory pronation to allow dorsiflexion of the midfoot on the rearfoot, results in a prolonged pronation period.[24] Excessive subtalar joint pronation has been causally related to more proximal problems including shin splints, iliotibial band syndrome, patellofemoral dysfunction, medial knee problems, trochanteric bursitis, and pelvosacroiliac dysfunction.

Excessive, prolonged subtalar pronation will cause increased frontal plane valgus stress to the knee, resulting in increased tibial internal rotation, knee flexion, and femoral internal rotation.[49,74,75] Coplan, in the OKC, measured significantly greater total tibial rotation at 5 degrees knee flexion in pronating subjects (mean, 18.5 degrees) compared to normals (mean, 11.4 degrees).[76] She suggested that the torsional forces of excessive pronation produced pathologic laxity at the knee.

While many authors refer to the increased Q angle present on static evaluation,[77] Tiberio[74] points out that the effect of increased tibial internal rotation would be to dynamically decrease the Q angle. In the CKC, the tibia must internally rotate during the first 15–20 degrees of knee flexion and externally rotate with knee extension; there is an obligatory action of automatic rotation. Because tibial rotation automatically occurs with subtalar pronation-supination, the actions of the knee and subtalar joint are interdependent synchronous actions. With excessive pronation, supination and tibial external rotation are delayed, creating a biomechanical dilemma at the tibiofemoral joint. The knee is extending as the limb approaches push-off, but is unable to acquire tibial external rotation. Compensatory femoral internal rotation allows the necessary rotation but creates relative lateral tracking and compression of the patella. Orthotic inserts have been found to be effective in diminishing the degree of pronation, total period of pronation, and reported symptoms in walking and running.[75,78,79] Nawoczenski et al.[80] found a significant orthotic effect on reduction of transverse plane tibial internal rotation in the first 50 percent of stance phase of running in subjects with LE pain.

Excessive prolonged pronation diminishes the ability of peroneus longus to stabilize the first ray, important for propulsion.[26] Over time, this may create a hypermobile first ray, leading to destructive forces on the first metatarsophalangeal joint. Further changes can lead to hallux valgus, or hallux limitus, and finally hallux rigidus. Extrinsic deformities contributing to compensatory pronation include femoral ante- or retroversion, increased valgus knee angle, tibial torsion, and structural or functional leg length discrepancy.

While abnormal pronation frequently results from a hypermobile foot, abnormal supination results from a relatively rigid foot. The foot is unable to effectively absorb shock or adapt to uneven terrain, which can result in tissue inflammation and joint destruction locally or transmitted elsewhere in the kinetic chain.[49] Forefoot valgus is often seen together with a pes cavus foot.[26] Common muscular imbalances seen with abnormal supination include weakness of the dorsiflexors, peroneals, and gastrocnemius-soleus group, and overactivity of abductor hallicis and foot intrinsics.[49] Michaud suggests that rigid forefoot valgus symptoms will be primarily provoked during impact.[26]

KNEE

Ligaments appear to have a neurophysiologic as well as mechanical function.[61,62,81–84] Morphologic verification of mechanoreceptors within the cruciates,[81,83] and the dynamic reflex effects on fusiform neurons in hamstrings and gastrocnemius with stretch of the ACL and PCL (posterior CL)[61,62] point to the active as well as the passive role that inert structures have on joint function through their primary afferent discharge. Their reflex pathways to the gamma motor system may contribute to preparatory muscle stiffness for joint protection. This arthrokinetic reflex may also be true for other joint ligaments and capsule.[85,86]

When injury disrupts the mechanical and neurosensory effectiveness of passive restraints, new demands are made on dynamic restraints. EMG analysis of movements in individuals with ACL deficiency suggests alteration in firing patterns as a compensatory device for changes in reflex-mediated stiffness control.[84,87,88] Cocontraction of agonist-antagonist is thought to commonly occur around most limb joints in order to achieve skilled, accurate movement. Baratta et al.[86] compared the hamstring-quadriceps coactivation patterns in the OKC of normal knees of nonathletic and athletic subjects. Athletes with hypertrophied quadriceps (no hamstring exercise) demonstrated depressed hamstring coactivation compared to athletes who exercised their hamstrings (as well as their quadriceps) and nonathletic subjects. Antagonist coactivation in the final 40 degrees of OKC extension and flexion increased for both the quadriceps and hamstrings of normal knees as limb velocity increased.[89] Hamstring cocontraction has been effective in reducing anterior displacement and internal rotation of the tibia in the 15–80 degree but not the 0–15 degree knee flexion ROM in cadaver knees.[90] Lutz et al.[91] found that muscular cocontraction of either hamstrings or quadriceps in the CKC occurs at those points in ranges where higher potential anterior shear forces exist in the OKC environment.

Walla et al.[92] reported that CKC "reflex" hamstring activity causing reduction of the pivot shift test was associated the closest with high functional outcome scores (compared to isokinetic strength and power tests) in ACL-deficient knees. Beard et al.[93] studied the mean reflex latency of the hamstrings and found that the latency of the injured limb was almost twice that of the uninjured limb in subjects with ACL deficiency. They reported a significant correlation between hamstring reflex latency and functional Lysholm score. Individuals were able to normalize their hamstring contraction latency values with proprioception training, with concurrent significant improvement in their Lysholm scores.

Wojtys and Huston[87] found voluntary muscle timing and recruitment order in response to anterior tibial translation (CKC with weightbearing of 20–30 lb) altered with time from ACL injury. These changes correlated with activity level, subjective functional evaluation, and degree of dynamic anterior tibial laxity, and provided a descriptive difference between best and worst outcome ranked ACL-deficient groups. Acute ACL-deficient individuals recruited muscles (quadriceps first) in an order different from normals, best semiacute ACL-deficient subjects, and best chronic ACL-deficient individuals (hamstrings-quadriceps-gastrocnemius). Muscle reaction time remained slower than normal, regardless of time from injury. There was no difference in the quadriceps strength, and in equal or increased hamstrings strength in the best ACL-deficiency groups compared to normal. The evidence suggests that central nervous system reprogramming occurs to implement joint protection.

A "quadriceps avoidance" or hamstring substitution pattern has been suggested as a way to minimize anterior tibial translation.[94] Their findings indicate that patients use a gait pattern with reduced knee flexion moment that requires decreased quadriceps activity. In comparing the level walking gait of ACL-deficient varus knees with those of controls, Noyes et al.[95] reported 40 percent lower knee flexion movements (related to quadriceps activity) and 50 percent higher extension movement (as relates to hamstrings). Tibone et al.[96] found little difference between ACL-deficient and uninjured knees during level walking. Longer duration of medial hamstrings in stance phase of running, earlier cessation of quadriceps activity with knee extension in stair-climbing, and decreased angle of cut in the cross-cut maneuver (no difference in straight cut) was recorded in ACL-deficient subjects.

Branch et al.[97] compared ACL-deficient and normal subjects in a more challenging activity: sidestep cutting. The ACL-deficient subjects used increased medial hamstring and decreased quadriceps and gastrocnemius activity in stance to accomplish the movement.

Ciccotti et al.[98] reported increased muscle activity and altered patterns in rehabilitated ACL-deficient subjects compared to similar profiles in ACL-reconstructed and normal knees. Their ACL-deficient subjects used increased vastus lateralis and anterior tibialis activity during six of the seven functional movements tested (walking, ascending and descending ramps and stairs, running, but not cross-cutting). This was attributed to a protective mechanism of diminished tibial internal rotation to avoid a pivot-shift. The activity and subjective outcome levels of the ACL-deficient subjects were not reported. The authors concluded that surgical reconstruction should be supported, as rehabilitation was not successful in restoring EMG patterns of the normal and bone-patella, tendon-bone reconstructed knees.

It has been suggested that movement and muscle activity will differ in the ACL-deficient patient who is compensating well (with high Lysholm or other functional outcome [FO] scores), compared to the patient who is doing poorly (low Lysholm scores, activity modification, or reports of frequent instability). Many of the EMG studies testing ACL-deficient subjects are conducted before reconstruction, implying that the patient has failed conservative measures. One reason the patient may fail is lack of achievement of successful adaptive patterns.[96] Andriacchi[99] urges the use of testing activities that stress the knee in different ranges of motion to assess functional adaptive capabilities. In walking, jogging, stair climbing, running to stop, and running to lateral sidestep, Andriacchi found greater knee extension moments at heel strike and avoidance of peak flexion moments.[99,100] Avoidance of quadriceps contraction as ACL-deficient subjects neared full knee extension at mid-stance was most significant in level walking. The greatest adaptations tend to occur as the knee nears extension; they tend to disappear when knee flexion is greater than 45 degrees.[100] Alteration was also observed in the unaffected limbs of patients who developed adaptations. One conclusion is that patients who are successful in the conservative management of ACL deficiency have undergone a central reprogramming of locomotor patterns.[100]

Gauffin and Tropp found both compensatory movement and muscular patterns in a one-legged jump for distance in patients with old ACL ruptures and good knee function (Lysholm knee score greater than 90).[101] Mean hop quotient (injured/uninjured) was 93 percent. With the involved leg, there were higher hip flexion angles at touch-down and when forces peaked. There were higher knee flexion angles at touch-down. Quadriceps EMG activity was significantly lower on the involved leg at take-off and touch-down, but no differences were found in hamstring activity. The findings suggest that use of increased hip and knee flexion allow improved hamstring ability to prevent both anterior tibial translation and internal and external rotation. Decreased quadriceps activity indicates quadriceps avoidance compensation.

Lass et al.[102] reported on level and increasing gradient treadmill walking in ACL-deficient subjects with mean Lysholm scores of 74. Compared to controls, they found earlier onset and longer duration of EMG activity in all muscles studied (vastus medialis and lateralis, medial and lateral hamstrings, medial gastrocnemius). This was most significant in lateral hamstrings and medial gastrocnemius. Several of the same authors compared a high Lysholm score (more than 84) with good/excellent stability group to a low Lysholm score (less than 64) with poor stability group using the same study parameters.[103] Only medial gastrocnemius displayed significant differences between the two groups. Earlier onset, earlier peak, prolonged burst duration, and on inclines greater root mean square (RMS) amplitudes were measured in the good/excellent group. Two subjects from the poor group were trained with visual feedback to change the recruitment of gastrocnemius to a pattern similar to that of the good/excellent group. After a 15-week training program, recruitment patterns altered, and knee stability improved as measured by a significant improvement in Lysholm score. The authors concluded that increased coactivation of muscles at the knee can partly compensate for the impaired reflex-mediated stiffness

control. They emphasize the importance of muscle coordination in successful rehabilitation of ACL-deficient patients.

Patellofemoral pain has been attributed to static patella malalignment and/or dynamic extensor mechanism dysfunction. Static malalignment causes include increased femoral anteversion, external tibial torsion, and lateral displacement of the tibial tubercle,[104] which can cause an increased Q angle and lateral tracking of the patella.[105] Other authors have found no difference in the Q angle[106] or femoral anteversion-patellofemoral characteristics[107] of symptomatic and asymptomatic subjects. Tight rectus femoris, iliotibial band,[108] hamstrings, and lateral retinaculum, increased pronation, and patella alta are other causes. Malalignment may also be manifested in abnormal patella tilt, lateralization, congruence angles,[109] and patella shape.[110] The interaction of malalignment measures and quadriceps contraction reminds us of the importance of muscle dynamics. Guzzanti et al.[109] compared static and dynamic patellofemoral malalignment measures in subjects with anterior knee pain. Quadriceps contraction altered the malalignment in both type and severity in 52 percent of the cases.

Malalignment may be associated with increased patellofemoral contact force, reduced patellofemoral contact area, or both.[111] In vitro studies demonstrate that induced changes in biomechanics of the patellofemoral joint can lead to changes in the magnitude and distribution of contact pressures. Studies on normal subjects found that knee movement, patellofemoral joint reaction force, and patellofemoral joint stress were significantly greater at 0-degree and 30-degree knee flexion in the OKC compared to CKC leg press.[112] At 60-degree and 90-degree knee flexion, the three parameters were greater on the leg press. Patellofemoral joint stress intersected at 48 degrees of knee flexion.

Dynamic extensor dysfunction may be either morphologic—hypotrophy of vastus medialis oblique (VMO), or functional (due to altered meural mechanisms)—or may have elements of both.[113] With hypotrophy of VMO, force production may be insufficient to maintain patella alignment. Alternatively, neural activation of

VMO may be of insufficient magnitude or inappropriately timed. This has been measured in altered EMG timing patterns and ratios, and kinematic measurements.

Dillon et al.[114] compared the level and downhill gait of women with symptoms of chondromalacia patellae with matched controls. During swing phase, symptomatic women displayed decreased knee flexion and increased femoral external rotation, followed by radical internal rotation immediately preceding heelstrike on both surfaces. During single support stance on the level surface, they had significantly less knee flexion. Dillon et al.[114] question whether this gait pattern may be a contributing cause rather than result of the chondomalacia patella. Hébert et al.[115] compared normal and patellofemoral pain syndrome subjects performing three squat tests. They hypothesized that subjects with painful knees would decrease their use of knee extensors and compensate with increased use of hip extensors and ankle plantar flexors. Results were exactly opposite. Subjects with painful knees increased their use of knee extensors and used less hip extensors. This does not answer the question of whether these patterns are a cause of or compensation for painful knees. It is this author's observation that patients with anterior knee pain often appear to walk from their knees (a knee dominant gait), exhibiting a snapping into extension as they reach midstance. On manual muscle test (MMT), proximal hip muscles are found to be weak.

Information on the EMG patterns during gait of subjects with patellofemoral pain would be useful to assess firing patterns and ratios of the VMO: vastus lateralis (VL). None were found in a recent literature search. Reynolds et al.[116] found a normalized VMO:VL ratio of 1 : 1 in normal females moving from a 30 degree kneesstraight squat to standing. Mariani and Caruso[117] reported VM:VL ratios of less than 1 : 1 in subjects with patella subluxation preoperatively, and approximately equal ratios following realignment. It is unfortunate that they did not measure VMO. The majority of the literature reporting VMO:VL ratios is in OKC. Subjects report that their functional pain is in CKC: walking, ascending and descending stairs, and prolonged sitting. More functionally appropriate research is needed.

Voight and Weider[118] reported altered reflex response times to patella tendon tap in subjects with patellofemoral knee pain compared to normals. In normal subjects, VMO fired significantly faster than VL. In subjects with patellofemoral pain, this was reversed. Although VMO onset firing time was consistent in the two populations, it was the increase in VL firing onset that constituted the altered firing order. Their findings suggest a neurophysiologic motor control imbalance, with the reversal in firing order contributing to problems in patella tracking.

Absolute reflex latency values reported by Voight and Weider[118] are strongly correlated with subject height. Karst and Willet[113] challenged their findings by examining relative reflex latencies that eliminated the effect of height. No differences were found between VMO and VL relative reflex latencies in symptomatic and normal subjects. There was also no difference between groups in voluntary VMO/VL onset timing in CKC lateral step-ups or OKC knee extension.

Bennet and Stauber[119] found OKC eccentric torque deficiencies in subjects with anterior knee pain. Instead of eccentric torque exceeding concentric torque, symptomatic subjects produced significantly diminished eccentric torque between 30 degrees and 60 degrees of knee flexion. The majority of subjects reported resolved symptoms within 4 weeks of concentric-eccentric training. Those subjects available for retesting showed normalization of eccentric-concentric torque curve relations. The short period required for rehabilitation suggests that neural adaptation was involved.

It may be that current tools lack the sensitivity necessary to resolve neuromotor control questions concerning patellofemoral dysfunction. Magnetic resonance imaging (MRI) evaluation of the VMO/VL following various exercises may provide additional information regarding differences in usage patterns.[111]

HIP

EMG analysis of walking, running, and jumping activities underscores the primacy of the hip musculature in driving movement. It is unfortunate that EMG investigations of pathology frequently neglect comprehensive analysis of the entire lower quadrant. The authors hypothesize that hip muscle weakness is present in many LE pathologies. Whether this precedes the injury or reflects a subsequent motor control adjustment to injury remains unknown. Beginning with the investigation of ankle joint mechanoreceptors by Wyke,[120] authors have observed that joint injury to sensory receptors not only influences muscle function at that joint,[85] but also can lead to altered muscle function in more proximal joints.[121–123]

Early OKC isokinetic peak torque strength testing by Nicholas et al.[124] revealed significant correlation between patterns of thigh muscle weakness and joint pathology in nonsymptomatic individuals. Significant relations between ipsilateral ankle-foot problems and abductor and adductor weakness, knee ligamentous instability and quadriceps weakness, and patella lesions and quadriceps, hamstrings, and hip flexor weakness were demonstrated. The most distal injury had the greatest total limb weakness. Subjects' uninvolved limbs served as controls and were not compared to uninjured age- and activity-matched normals. This 1976 study pointed to the importance of addressing the entire lower quadrant in rehabilitation.

Bullock-Saxton and Bullock[122] performed isometric strength tests at different muscle lengths of hip and knee flexors and extensors in army subjects with severe ankle sprains compared to matched controls. Strength was significantly lower in all muscles in the left ankle injury group, and in all muscle except hip flexors in the right injury group. Specific range of motion differences were also found. It is unfortunate the authors only investigated sagittal plane muscle groups. With findings of greater balance deficiencies in the frontal plane in subjects with ankle sprains,[15] altered frontal (and possibly transverse) plane hip function might be anticipated.

Further investigation on the same population by Bullock-Saxton[123] revealed significant decreased ankle vibration perception and delays in gluteus maximus recruitment in the injured group. Muscle recruitment of gluteus maximus lagged behind that of bilateral erector spinae and biceps femoris in prone hip extension in the injured group. The control group activated all muscles almost simultaneously. Information regarding correlation with walking patterns, and the length of time this pattern alteration remains would be of interest.

Hip joint pathology is manifested recognizably in a Trendelenberg gait pattern due to decreased hip abduction strength in the involved limb during stance. Loss of hip extension ROM is also common, which can result in a shortened stance phase on the involved side. However, other compensations include increased anterior pelvic tilt and/or increased lumbar lordosis.[28]

LUMBOPELVIS

The interrelation of the lumbopelvis and hip musculature has been previously addressed in the preceding chapter on the spine. The lack of stabilization or coordination of these structures has potential repercussions in any of the more distal segments.

Treatment Strategies

Kegerreis wrote about functional progression of sports injuries in the early 1980s.[125,126] Based on the SAID (Specific Adaptation to Imposed Demands), principle, functional progression directs rehabilitation to prepare the individual for the stresses encountered in daily life. Those stresses will differ for the secretary, plumber, ballet dancer, and hockey player. Goals of rehabilitation include varying degrees of movement components such as strength, power, coordination, agility, and balance. Functional exercises should emphasize biomechanically safe movement and loading patterns at levels the injured segment can tolerate.

Exercise progression includes manipulation of the variables of force, direction, speed, support, and complexity (Table 6-3).[127] In closed chain exercise, force is manipulated by varying

TABLE 6-3 *Treatment progression variables*

Force reduced body weight > full body weight > increased body weight

Direction secondary links and planes > primary links and planes

Support double support > single support > double nonsupport > single nonsupport stable level surface > unstable or irregular

Speed slow > fast, consistent > acceleration—deceleration static > dynamic

Complexity changing combinations of all variables

the amount of body weight and impact loading. Reduced body weight exercises can be accomplished on equipment such as the leg press, shuttle, or total gym, seated, in a pool, or upright supported by external devices such as Zuni-unloading or handrails. Greater impact loading is introduced with running and pliometric activities. Direction involves the planes of motion in which an exercise occurs. Speed may vary from static to dynamic: slow to rapid, or combinations of each with acceleration and deceleration. Support includes bilateral weight bearing, progresses to unilateral, and then to nonsupport drills. Support also includes stable or unstable surfaces such as wobble boards, trampolines, or irregular playing fields. Nonsupport refers to one or both legs off the ground as in jumping, hopping, and running.[128] Complexity may entail combinations or changes of planes and levels, and speed and direction.

In understanding the degree of stress an exercise may produce on an injured joint, Tiberio[129] recommends analyzing the joints and planes involved in the movement. Planes are considered primary (the plane of injury and most stressful) or secondary, and joints are classified as primary (the injured joint) or secondary links. A progression from least to most stressful would begin with emphasis to a secondary link and secondary plane, progress to a secondary link in the primary plane, followed by the primary link in a secondary plane, and end with the primary link in the primary plane (Fig. 6-3). Using the example of an inversion ankle sprain, the talocrural joint is the primary link and the frontal plane is the primary plane (although elements of the transverse and sagittal plane may be involved depending on the severity of injury). Initial exercises might emphasize secondary links and planes such as the hip or knee in the sagittal plane. The stage of recovery and level of stress tolerance might initially dictate greater support, as in a double leg squat exercise, or be progressed to a single leg squat or step-up. Heel raises constitute a primary link in a secondary plane. Activities such as cross over cuts or side to side one-legged jumps would be the highest level of exercise, stressing the primary link in the primary plane with unilateral nonsupport.

A patient should be able to tolerate full, symmetrical weight bearing to initiate double support activities. Symmetrical gait pattern should be achieved before beginning single support activities. Certain equipment allows us to introduce movements in a reduced weight-bearing context before full weight bearing has been achieved: squats and heel raises can be performed on a leg press, shuttle, or total gym; walking and running can be performed in a pool or Zuni-unloading apparatus. Wobble boards and shoes can be used while sitting, or on a leg press (Fig. 6-4), shuttle, or total gym. The amount of

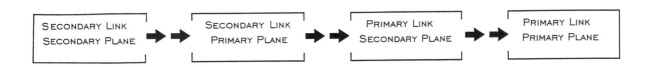

FIGURE 6-3 *Links and planes: progression of rehabilitation exercises in the closed chain. (From Tiberio D,[129] with permission.)*

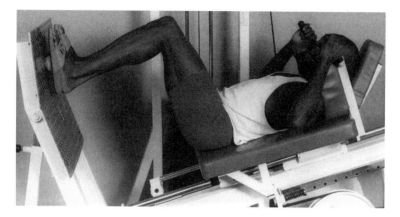

FIGURE 6-4 *Wobble shoes on the leg press.*

motion tolerated within a given plane should also be considered. No motion (isometric), or short arcs are introduced before full motion.

An exercise may be altered to relieve stress to a particular joint or joint compartment, or to add additional planes. The squat is primarily a sagittal plane activity, with the majority of the motion occurring at the hips and knees. Patients with hip and knee pathology have been shown to reduce hip and knee movement and substitute with trunk flexion, which results in more of a stoop-lift pattern.[130,131] (Refer to Ch. 5 for further discussion of types of lifts.) In the frontal plane, a varus knee with medial compartment degeneration may need to be brought into more valgus alignment to tolerate the squat. This might entail intrinsic adjustment by the patient or extrinsic assistance by placing a towel under the lateral aspect of his foot. In the transverse plane, control of the hip rotators and subtalar joint will also enhance control of hip-knee-ankle alignment in the sagittal squat. As control of the squat is mastered, the addition of motion in the sagittal, secondary plane or frontal, primary plane with sport cord, slide board, or fitter adds new challenges and complexity.

One of the postoperative problems following ACL reconstruction is patellofemoral pain and catching. It is often assumed that this is primarily due to the compromised patella tendon following bone-patella-bone graft harvesting. Concurrent with this is decreased patella mobility

and lateral tracking due to quadriceps weakness and imbalance. It is frequently observed by the authors that increased femoral internal rotation is occuring throughout the stance phase of gait and during exercises such as the squat. Focus on transverse plane hip control by engaging hip external rotators (Fig. 6-5) (which are often weak) is often a key to correcting the observed pathomechanics. Knutzen and Price[132] identified the hip as the most important contributor to rearfoot movement in the prediction of degree of pronation. The principle of proximal stability for distal mobility is important to remember: are the large proximal pelvic-hip muscles performing appropriately? Conditioning variables are also manipulated according to tissue stress tolerances. These include intensity, volume (amount of work), frequency, and recovery.

NEUROPHYSIOLOGIC FACILITATION

Proprioception is defined as the combined afferent neural input to the central nervous system (CNS) from mechanoreceptors in joint capsule, skin, muscles (muscle spindles), tendon (Golgi tendon organs), and ligaments.[133] The cumulative result on a reflexive spinal cord level is excitation or inhibition of motor neurons. *Kinesthesia* is the conscious awareness of position and movement, the sense of which is developed from proprioceptive input.[55] *Balance* must integrate proprioception, with the visual, vestibular, kin-

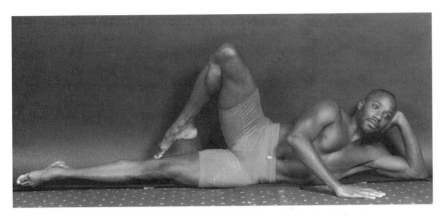

FIGURE 6-5 *Passé exercise for hip external rotation strengthening.*

esthesia, and motor systems using feedback and feedforward mechanisms. Neurophysiologic facilitation activities, more commonly called proprioceptive training, seek to enhance balance and coordinated motor control on both reflexive and voluntary levels. It is hypothesized that CNS adaptation occurs with the acquisition of skilled movement patterns in response to appropriate movement tasks and challenges.[134] Efferent neural responses, manifested in coordinated movement, become more efficient with cumulative motor learning. Studies on the effect of muscular training on joint position sense in ballet dancers and Navy SEAL trainees show enhanced kinesthetic function despite induced fatigue.[135]

Emphasis on the quality of an activity—postural alignment of body segments; kinesthetic sense of which muscles are used to correctly control alignment with motion, speed, or timing, coordinated sequencing; and movement dynamics—are important in facilitating recovery. Selection of the appropriate level of proprioceptive training must consider articular deafferation and motor deefferation. Decreased motor unit recruitment and muscle fiber atrophy and impaired sensory input may result in early fatigue with deterioration of performance quality.

STATIC BALANCE

Progression of proprioceptive training follows the treatment progression variables (Table 6-3). Static balance activities include progression from eyes open to closed, bilateral to unilateral, arms outstretched for balance assistance to no arms, and stable surface to unstable surface. Maintaining a one-legged stork balance with sneakers on, arms outstretched, and eyes open for 30 seconds becomes quite difficult when barefoot, maintaining subtalar neutral, crossing the arms, and closing the eyes (see Fig. 5-9, ch. 5). Performing the same task on a trampoline or a wobble board adds an unstable surface. Holding a deep lunge, eyes closed, with the front foot in subtalar neutral and the rear limb with knee bent and foot in a push-off posture requires hip-knee-ankle stabilization and static balance (see Fig. 5-10, ch. 5). Exercises with additional complexity include the distraction of attention from balancing toward throwing and catching tasks. Examples are plio-ball toss on one leg, or a game of catch on two legs on a large wobble board or kinesthetic activity trainer (K.A.T.).

The ability to perform static balance is particularly important to gymnasts, figure skaters, and dancers. This includes balance on a unilaterally plantar flexed foot (relevé) in demi or full pointe (see Fig. 8-1, 8-2, ch. 8). A relevé balance on a wobble board in a dance-specific posture (Fig. 6-6) provides such a challenge.

The integration of static and dynamic control is also important to these athletes. A simple exercise like the "karate kid" involves static balance on the standing limb combined with movement of the unweighted or gesture limb. This ex-

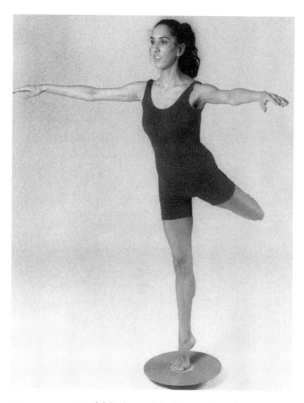

FIGURE 6-6 *Wobble board balance in relevé.*

around the calf, thigh, or pelvis to encourage increased use of specific muscles for stabilization can be added in many of the exercises.

DYNAMIC BALANCE

Most functional activities require dynamic postural balance and control. Dynamic proprioceptive training includes gait drills, wobble boards and shoes, pliometrics (from squats to jumping on a minitrampoline or box drills), and running agility drills. A simple static exercise like balancing on one leg is progressed to a dynamic balance and strengthening exercise by imposing controlled movement. This includes motion in a single plane or circles on a wobble board, or moving from foot flat to plantar flexion with knee straight or bent on the unstable surface of a trampoline. Studies on normals[136] and subjects with ankle functional instability have shown im-

ercise can be performed with the gesture leg sliding on a power board or slide board (Fig. 6-7). Movement of the gesture limb in the sagittal plane progresses to movement in the frontal plane. The addition of pivoting the trunk and gesture leg around the stance limb develops transverse plane control. The same karate kid movement on a balance beam (Fig. 6-8) with only part of the support limb on the beam adds further difficulty. Patients who could benefit from this functional progression are dancers and gymnasts, who must balance on one limb in flat foot or relevé while moving the gesture limb to complete an arabesque or developpé (Fig. 5-1, 5-6, ch. 5), or a construction worker, who may need to walk and balance on beams and girders.

Changing the level while maintaining balance in an exercise such as the star (Fig. 6-9), is performed in different planes and moving at one joint (the hip) or all three (hip-knee-ankle) concurrently. Placing theraband or sport cord

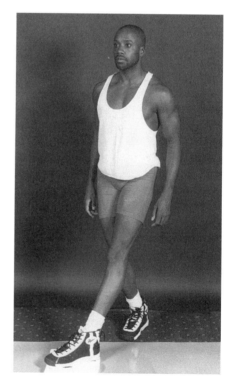

FIGURE 6-7 *Single limb movement in frontal plane on slide board.*

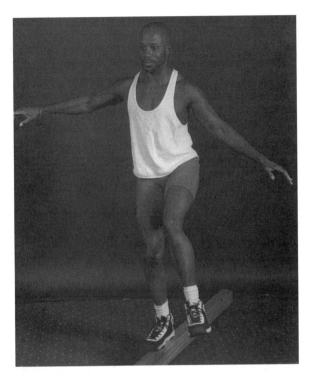

FIGURE 6-8 *"Karate kid" exercise on balance beam.*

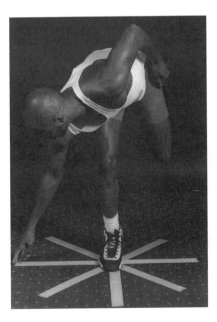

FIGURE 6-9 *Star exercise.*

proved stabilometry measures and diminished subjective feelings of giving way following wobble board training.[13,14,101,137] Gauffin et al.[101] reported uninvolved as well as involved limb improvements following training on the involved limb only. Tropp and Askling[137] also reported improvements in isokinetic eversion and dorsiflexion torque measurements following 10 weeks of wobble board training. Balogun et al.[138] found isometric force improvements in knee extensors and flexors, and ankle plantar and dorsiflexors (invertor and evertors were not tested) in normal patients following weeks of wobble board training.

Forward and retro walking, marching, and heel-toe drills in wobble shoes (see Fig. 5-15, 5-16, Ch. 5) are an alternate way to provoke ankle, hip, and pelvic stabilization and integration. A study on normals by Bullock-Saxton et al.[139] showed significant facilitation of gluteal activity after one week of practice walking on wobble shoes.

RETROMOVEMENT

Early well-tolerated gait activities include retromovement. Although movement trajectories of the limb in forward and backward walking mirror each other, most of the limb muscles change their pattern of activity in relation to gait phases.[140] In backward walking, patterns of angular displacement are almost completely reversed; the hip flexes and knee extends during the support phase and the hip extends and the knee flexes during swing. Rectus femoris (as both hip flexor and knee extensor) and other quadriceps muscle activity is greatly increased and for a longer duration—for most of support phase.[140,141] Instead of the eccentric action during forward stance, they primarily work concentrically during retrostance.

Current locomotion theory suggests that muscle patterns are generated by a central program. Similar neural mechanisms may be at work in backward walking, but Thorstensson[140] suggests that retro capabilities imply inherent neural modifiability. It is easy to observe in the clinic how a patient with a newly formed habit of decreased stance time and decreased stride length on a recently reconstructed ACL limb, is instantaneously capable of symmetrical gait when walking, marching, or tiptoeing backward. Brunnstrom[142] and Bobath[143] also recommended retromovement many years ago to affect motor control of neurologically involved (hemiplegic) patients.

Studies of normal patients show that average cadence increases and stride length decreases in backward walking.[140,141] Subjects are able to modify cadence and stride length to one similar to forward walking with a metronome-set stride frequency.[140] Cardiopulmonary demands and metabolic costs of backward walking are higher than forward walking at the same speed.[141,144] These findings are also true in retrorunning.

Comparisons of forward and backward running suggest that backward running can increase quadriceps muscle strength while decreasing the loads of the knee. Threlkeld et al.[145] found that the peak vertical component of ground reaction force is significantly less (30 percent) in backward running. Peak patellofemoral joint compressive forces occur later in retrostance and are significantly reduced.[146] Flynn and Soutas-Little[141] reported that during early to midstance,

eccentric quadriceps work is significant in forward running. As there is minimal change in knee joint ROM during this period in retrorunning, quadriceps activity is primarily isometric, and from midstance on becomes concentric. Threlkeld et al.[145] compared the effects of an 8-week forward and mixed 70:30 forward-backward running and training regime in normal patients. The mixed regime group produced concentric quadriceps isokinetic torque increases after 8 weeks. As individuals with patellofemoral dysfunction often have pain with eccentric activity, retrotraining is often tolerated and used as a strengthening tool.

Retrorunning may not be appropriate for mid- and forefoot problems. There is no heel strike in backward running, which diminishes impulse loading of the limb. This also puts greater stress on the mid- and forefoot.

AGILITY AND PLIOMETRICS

Mastery of static balance, stabilization, and control in tests like the stork balance (30 seconds) (see Fig. 5-9, ch. 5) and single-leg half-squat (Fig. 6-2) indicates readiness for basic jumping exer-

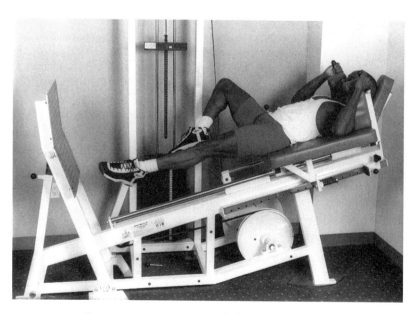

FIGURE 6-10 *Leg press jumps on single leg.*

cises.[147] Initially, timing and recruitment can be practiced on a leg press or shuttle before working against gravity and full body weight. A key component in jumping technique is landing. Integration of the full foot, ankle, knee, and hip in sharing shock absorption as well as storing energy for take-off is critical. Sets of one-legged jumps on the leg press provide an excellent eccentric lower extremity power drill (Fig. 6-10).

Although trampoline jumping (see Fig. 8-22, ch. 8) differs in impact and timing from jumping on firmer surfaces, postural alignment and synchronization of upper extremity motion for additional momentum can be learned. Plio-lunge patterns incorporate push-off from the forward or rear limb in varying planes. Equipment such as the fitter and slide board require balance and co-ordination in frontal plane movement (They may also be used for sagittal plane activity as well).

When forward and backward running are tolerated, running drills in large circles, figures of eight, full sprints, and cuts are added. Drills that require acceleration and deceleration, change of direction, and pivoting can incorporate sport cord, or cones. The Fastex is an excellent tool for practicing quick reaction to a visual stimulus with changes of direction (Fig. 6-11). It can be programmed for length of drill or sport-specific patterns.

Landings from complex jumps or the final position of intricate movements must often be maintained statically. An example is a gymnast's dismount. Jumping sequences that finish in a static posture may be performed on a mini-tram-

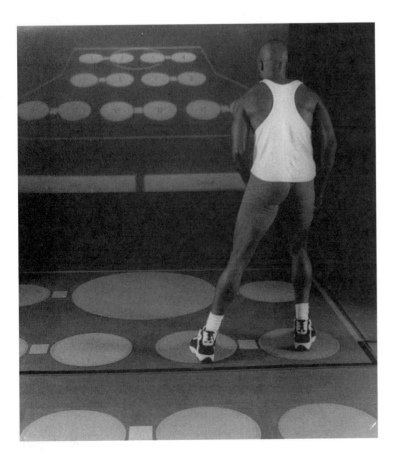

FIGURE 6-11 *Fastex.*

poline, back and forth from the trampoline to the floor, on the Fastex.

The ultimate objective of these drills is the attainment of coordination and agility. Kottke et al.[148] defines *coordination* as the development of a central nervous system engram that directs the skilled sequencing of motor activity on an unconscious level.[148] *Agility* has been defined by Yamamoto[149] as the ability one possesses for rapid directional changes without loss of joint stability or body balance.

Lower Extremity Functional Tests and Outcome Rating Scores

Evaluation and outcome determination must follow a systematic and standardized approach. The goal in evaluation is to develop a differential diagnosis initially, and with repeat assessments, determine the individual's progress toward resumption of full activity. At the time of initial assessment, the patient attempts to describe the injury through a subjective analysis. This information is integrated into the objective physical examination, leading to diagnosis, goals, and treatment planning.

Functional testing is conducted on a periodic basis as part of the evaluative process. It is used to assess readiness to progress to another level of rehabilitation, to return to athletic practice, play, or discharge. Selection of the appropriate battery of tests is important to maximize information about the patient's functional capacities.

Outcomes are changes in status that are attributed to treatment intervention. Outcome rating systems have been divided into subjective (patient-rated) and objective (clinical examination with or without functional tests), or combinations of both. Miller and Carr[150] suggest that outcome systems consider the following areas: functional level (preinjury, presurgery, and at follow-up), symptoms and impairments, clinical examination, and ancillary tests. Functional level should delineate activity level, intensity, and frequency of participation. Confounding factors important to identify are whether a reduction in activity is injury-related or patient-related.[150,151] Patients may alter their activities due to persisting symptoms (injury-related) or, as they grow older, due to change in interest, lifestyle, and type of sports participation (patient-related).

Perception of outcome may differ between medical personnel and patient. Separation of scores for each of the components of assessment is considered most appropriate. Combined assessment of multiple factors may involve more than one scorer (patient and medical personnel) and be misleading. Because different pathology (even different ligament injuries) affect function in different ways, clinical findings should be separated from functional rating scores.[152] A functional performance test measures performance at that moment in time. A rating score is seeking information about average function 7 days a week. Subjective patient-rated outcomes are used by many clinicians as another tool in assessment. Used periodically (every 4–6 weeks) and combined with frequent functional testing, they provide additional insight into the patient's progress and their perception of it.

OBJECTIVE FUNCTIONAL TESTING

Commonly used athletic field tests include one- and two-leg vertical jump test, one-leg timed hop, one-leg hop for distance, shuttle run, M-K staircase test, figure of eight run, T-test, Barrow zig-zag run, and Illinois agility run. Single-leg tests such as the vertical jump, hop-for-distance, timed 6-m hop, triple hop, crossover hop, and 30-meter agility hop, have been found to have high reliablity (.77—.99),[153–155] limb symmetry (less than one percent dominant to nondominant difference),[155] and positive correlation to athletic performance for normal subjects. However, the sensitivity for prediction of successful return to full activity following injury (ACL-deficient and reconstructed populations) has been mixed.[156,157]

The goal in rehabilitation is to return the patient to their preinjury activity status, or barring that, to maximize their potential activity level. Functional rehabilitation entails the clinician's attempt to re-educate the patient to regain systematic control of their movement through movement analysis and integration. This requires a program that involves both perceptual and intellectual abilities in order for the patient to regain the neuromuscular patterns necessary to compensate for injury and surgery. Sensitivity of functional testing is improved with the use of a scaled or analog system, to ensure achievement of the highest possible function. This is not always feasible in many simple-to-administer clinical tests. Quantification by time or distance in comparison to the uninvolved limb does not account for the quality of movement control.

The primary goal of functional tests is to assess the lower extremity's ability to perform dynamic activities. Variables such as joint pain and effusion, patellofemoral and tibiofemoral pathology, neuromuscular control, strength, coordination, and passive restraints, are components of functional tests. Functional tests can be used to determine readiness to progress to more difficult exercise challenges. As mentioned earlier, ability to balance and control movement in the 30-second stork balance and single-leg 1/2-squat are used as criteria for readiness for simple jumps. Lunsford and Perry recently reported standing plantar flexion (heel raises) norms for 203 subjects.[158] The average number of heel-raises performed was 27.9 for all age groups and genders, suggesting that MMT standards may need revision. A patient who is status post Achilles tendon repair might be tested in this revised context for readiness to jog.

A hierarchy of hop tests is illustrated in Figure 6-12. Qualitative and quantitative ability to perform a single-leg hop-for-distance tests ability to land with control of the body. Following mastery of one hop, the single-leg triple hop-for-distance requires multiple landing and push-off combinations of eccentric and concentric control patterns. A single-leg timed 6-m hop requires the performance of work. The most difficult hop pattern is a single-leg crossover triple hop for distance. This pattern requires control in multiple planes.

The results of functional tests are based on contralateral limb scores. An 85 percent symme-try index score was found in more than 90 percent of the normal population for the single-leg hop-for-distance and single-leg timed hop tests.[156] The literature generally recommends achievement of 85 percent of the contralateral score as an acceptable measure.[155,156] The clinician also needs to take into account the quality of execution of the test task. Successful completion of a test on the basis of time or distance alone may give a false impression of the individual's ability to control movement dynamics with the resumption of higher level activities.

The gold standard for discharge for many years was isokinetic test symmetry (within 85 percent of the uninvolved limb). A review of literature attempting to correlate isokinetic testing with functional tests proves mixed. In general, it is felt that there is not a strong correlation between isokinetic torque and functional tasks.[12,159] Positive correlation may require selection of appropriate low isokinetic test speeds.[156,157] Lephart et al.[12] studied the relation between selected functional tests and clinical examinations in ACL-deficient athletes. They found that ligamentous laxity and isokinetic peak torque correlated poorly with the three functional tests: carioca, shuttle run, and semicircular cocontraction test. Fridén et al. found reduced quadriceps low velocity (0 and 30 deg/sec) isokinetic torque was associated with reduced hop for distance and Lysholm functional knee score in ACL-deficient patients.[59] However, patients with less than ten percent quadriceps isokinetic deficit still displayed significant functional disability. The authors suggest that these patients have little to gain from conventional strengthening but might benefit from programs that emphasize coordination. Barber et al.[156] found a positive correlation between low velocity (60 degrees/sec) isokinetic quadriceps deficit and the single-hop test.

A variety of functional tests have been reported in the knee literature. Single-leg tests allow a comparison between involved and uninvolved sides. Tegner et al.[160] reported turn (figure of eight) running, spiral stair running, and slope running detected differences within a rehabilitated ACL-deficient group compared to nor-

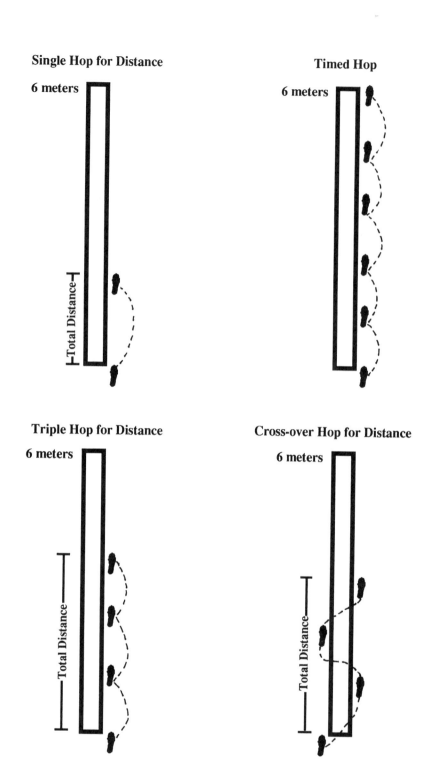

The courses for the four fuction tests.

FIGURE 6-12 *Illustration of the legs tests for function testing of the knee. (From Noyes FR et al.,*[157] *with permission.)*

mals. The degree of sensitivity was not determined. Lephart et al.[12] compared functional results of two groups of ACL-deficient athletes. Combining the results of three performance tests: shuttle run, carioca, and cocontraction semicircular test, the authors found that subjects who returned successfully to competition scored significantly higher on the performance tests than those who were unable to return to pre-injury levels of competition. Extensive examination by Barber et al[156] of hopping, jumping, and cutting (shuttle run) tests in normal and ACL-deficient populations found that cutting and vertical jump tests did not detect functional limitations reliably. Analysis of four different single-leg hop tests (single-hop, triple-hop, timed hop, crossover hop) by Noyes et al.[157] found low sensitivity in using any one test. Combining any two of the four tests was more sensitive than only one, but was still not highly sensitive. They concluded that these functional tests should be used to confirm abnormal limb symmetry but not as a sole screen.

Our goal with function testing is to provide an environment for the individual to perform under control certain patterns of movement that demonstrate successful completion of a comprehensive rehabilitation program. The clinician must be aware that the patient who scores normally on objective testing may still be at risk while performing actual ADL or athletic activities. The next step is to take the individual into the actual environment and progress them through that environment.

Future research needs to select reliable, valid, and sensitive outcome tests, and standardize them for implementation in multiple facilities. In this way we can better compare methods of rehabilitation and assure equivalency of outcome findings.

SUBJECTIVE OUTCOME RATING SCORES

Patient-rated or subjective rating systems were for many years considered soft science. O'Doherty states "it is surprising that we can accept a patient's description of their symptoms for clinical decision-making but find the same descrip-

tions suspect when describing the outcome of treatment".[161] This attitude is changing as we re-examine our health care policies and fiscal responsibilities.

Patient-rated scoring systems exist in both binary (yes/no or able/not able) and linear scoring systems. Linear scoring systems allow greater detail of information.[152] In the lower extremity scoring systems, there are clear diagnostic biases. Outcome expectations for total hip and knee replacement are greatly different from expectations for ligament recontruction. The populations are widely disparate in age, pathology, and activity requirements. Orthopaedics is unlike other medical pathologies such as cancer and heart disease, which may base outcomes on morbidity or survival rates. Orthopaedics rating systems must delineate functional levels and symptoms to qualify surgical and treatment success. (The majority of hip outcome systems are used to assess outcome for total hip replacement. Outcome measures for total hip and knee replacement will be discussed in Chapter 9.)

The most widely used knee outcomes were developed for knee ligament injuries. These include the modified Lysholm function score (Table 6-5),[152,162] the Tegner activity score (Table 6-6),[152] the Cincinnati Knee Rating System (Table 6-7),[151] and the modified Noyes questionnaire (Table 6-8).[17,151,163] The Visual Analog Pain Scale has also been used as a knee scale. There is currently no accepted system for assessing patients with patellofemoral dysfunction.[150] Visual Analog, Lysholm, Tegner, and modified Noyes scores have been reported in the literature for this population.[164–166] The modified Noyes is currently used in the clinic by several of the authors for monitoring outcomes of patellofemoral patients. McMullen et al.[166] reports outcomes on static versus isokinetic treatment of chodromalacia patella using the modified Noyes system.

The modified Lysholm[152] and modified Noyes questionnaires[17,151,163] are "subjective" patient rated systems that assess function, symptoms, and impairments. The Tegner activity score quantifies different activity levels by participation in competive or recreational sports

TABLE 6-4 *Modified Lysholm knee score*

LIMP

5 _____ None
3 _____ Slight or periodical
0 _____ Severe and constant

SUPPORT

5 _____ None
2 _____ Stick or crutch
0 _____ Weight-bearing impossible

LOCKING

15 _____ No locking or catching sensations
10 _____ Catching sensation but no locking
6 _____ Locking occasionally
2 _____ Locking frequently
0 _____ Locked joint on examination

INSTABILITY

25 _____ Never gives way
20 _____ Rarely during athletics or other severe exertion
15 _____ Frequently during athletics or other severe exertion (or incapable of participation)
10 _____ Occasionally in daily activities
5 _____ Often in daily activities
0 _____ Every step

PAIN

25 _____ None
20 _____ Inconsistent and slight during severe exertion
15 _____ Marked during severe exertion
10 _____ Marked on or after walking more than 2 km
5 _____ Marked after walking less than 2 km
0 _____ Constant

SWELLING

10 _____ None
6 _____ On severe exertion
2 _____ On ordinary exertion
0 _____ Constant

STAIR-CLIMBING

10 _____ No problems
6 _____ Slightly impaired
2 _____ One step at a time
0 _____ Impossible

SQUATTING

5 _____ No problems
4 _____ Slightly impaired
2 _____ Not beyond 90 degrees
0 _____ Impossible

(From Tegner Y and Lysholm J,[152] with permission.)

TABLE 6-5 *Tegner activity score*

LEVEL 10: COMPETITIVE SPORTS
Soccer: national and international elite

LEVEL 9: COMPETITIVE SPORTS
Soccer, lower divisions, ice hockey, wrestling, gymnastics

LEVEL 8: COMPETITIVE SPORTS
Bandy, squash or badminton, athletics (jumping, etc), downhill skiing

LEVEL 7: COMPETITIVE SPORTS
Tennis, athletics (running), motorcross, speedway, handball basketball
RECREATIONAL SPORTS
Soccer, bandy, and ice hockey, squash, athletics (jumping), cross-country track—recreational and competitive

LEVEL 6: RECREATIONAL SPORTS
Tennis and badminton, handball, basketball, downhill skiing, jogging at least five times/week

LEVEL 5: WORK
Heavy labor (building, forestry)
COMPETITIVE SPORTS
Cycling, cross-country skiing
RECREATIONAL SPORTS
Jogging on uneven ground at least twice weekly

LEVEL 4: WORK
Moderately heavy work (truck driving, heavy domestic work)
RECREATIONAL SPORTS
Cycling, cross-country skiing, jogging on even ground at least twice weekly

LEVEL 3: WORK
Light labor (nursing)
COMPETITIVE AND RECREATIONAL SPORTS
Swimming
Walking in forest possible

LEVEL 2: WORK
Light labor, walking on uneven ground possible but impossible to walk in forest

LEVEL 1: WORK
Sedentary work, walking on even ground possible

LEVEL 0: SICK LEAVE or DISABILITY due to knee

(From Tegner Y and Lysholm J,[153] with permission.)

TABLE 6-6 *The Noyes knee rating system*

Patient name		Date of visit	Involved knee ☐right ☐left	Date of original injury

DIRECTIONS:

Using the KEY (at right), check the appropriate boxes on the four scales below which indicate the highest level you can reach WITHOUT having symptoms.

KEY:

Scale	Description
10	Normal knee, able to do strenuous work/sports with jumping, hard pivoting
8	Able to do moderate work/sports with running, turning and twisting; symptoms with strenuous work/sports
6	Able to do light work/sports with no running, twisting or jumping; symptoms with moderate work/sports
4	Able to do activities of daily living alone; symptoms with light work/sports
2	Moderate symptoms (frequent, limiting) with activities of daily living
0	Severe symptoms (constant, not relieved) with activities of daily living

1. PAIN _____ / 10

10 —— 8 —— 6 —— 4 —— 2 —— 0

2. SWELLING (actual fluid in the knee; obvious puffiness) _____ / 10

10 —— 8 —— 6 —— 4 —— 2 —— 0

3. PARTIAL GIVING-WAY (partial knee collapse, no fall to the ground) _____ / 10

10 —— 8 —— 6 —— 4 —— 2 —— 0

4. FULL GIVING-WAY (knee collapse occurs with actual falling to the ground) _____ / 10

10 —— 8 —— 6 —— 4 —— 2 —— 0

Pain	Location of pain	☐ inner side	☐ outer side	☐ front / kneecap	☐ back of knee	☐ all over
	Type of pain	☐ sharp	☐ aching	☐ throbbing	☐ burning	
	Pain occurs on	☐ sitting	☐ standing	☐ stairs	☐ squatting	☐ running / jumping
	Pain relieved	☐ by not doing sports	☐ by limiting daily activities		☐ by rest / medications	☐ pain not relieved
	Kneecap grinding? ☐ yes ☐ no		Knee stiffness? ☐ yes ☐ no			

| **Catching/ Locking** | 1. Check one box: ☐ yes ☐ no My knee **catches** -- it does not move for a few seconds but works out. |
| | 2. Check one box: ☐ yes ☐ no My knee **locks** -- it does not move for five or more minutes at a time. |

| **Work Activity** | My job title is: | Work status: ☐ full time ☐ part time | ☐ full duty ☐ light duty ☐ not working |
| | When I work, I experience: ☐ no limitations ☐ mild limitations ☐ moderate limitations ☐ severe limitations | | |

| **Exercise Program** | In my exercise program, I am: ☐ making good progress ☐ slow progress, but better ☐ some problems with exercise ☐ exercise causes pain, problems ☐ doesn't apply |

| **Follow-up Progress** | Following my last visit, I am: ☐ making good progress ☐ slow progress, but better ☐ staying the same ☐ symptoms worse ☐ doesn't apply |

Patient Grade

Rate the overall condition of your knee at the present time. Circle one number below.

1 — 2 poor — 3 — 4 fair — 5 — 6 good — 7 — 8 — 9 — 10 normal

poor -- I have significant limitations that affect activities of daily living.
fair -- I have moderate limitations that affect activities of daily living, no sports possible.
good -- I have some limitations with sports but I can participate; I compensate.
normal/excellent -- I am able to do whatever I wish (any sport) with no problems.

| **Average** | Pain (x2) _____ + swelling _____ + partial giving way _____ + full giving way _____ | Subtotal = _____ = _____ / 5 |

SYMPTOM RATING FORM — CINTI KNEE RATING SYSTEM

(Continues)

TABLE 6-6 *(Continued)*

Patient Name		Involved Knee	Date of Visit
		Right_____ Left_____	mo_____ day_____ yr_____

Sports Activity Scale

Check the box which describes your level of sports activity before your original knee injury. Then, check the box which describes your level of sports activity at this time.

BEFORE INJURY		CURRENT LEVEL	

Level I (participates 4-7 days/week)
☐ 100 ☐ Jumping, hard pivoting, cutting (basketball, volleyball, football, gymnastics, soccer)
☐ 95 ☐ Running, twisting, turning (tennis, racquetball, handball, ice hockey, field hockey, skiing, wrestling)
☐ 90 ☐ No running, twisting, jumping (cycling, swimming)

Level II (participates 1-3 days/week)
☐ 85 ☐ Jumping, hard pivoting, cutting (basketball, volleyball, football, gymnastics, soccer)
☐ 80 ☐ Running, twisting, turning (tennis, racquetball, handball, ice hockey, field hockey, skiing, wrestling)
☐ 75 ☐ No running, twisting, jumping (cycling, swimming)

Level III (participates 1-3 times/month)
☐ 65 ☐ Jumping, hard pivoting, cutting (basketball, volleyball, football, gymnastics, soccer)
☐ 60 ☐ Running, twisting, turning (tennis, racquetball, handball, ice hockey, field hockey, skiing, wrestling)
☐ 55 ☐ No running, twisting, jumping (cycling, swimming)

Level IV (no sports)
☐ 40 ☐ I perform activities of daily living without problems
☐ 20 ☐ I have moderate problems with activities of daily living
☐ 0 ☐ I have severe problems with activities of daily living; on crutches, full disability

Highest Level (before injury) _____ / 100
Highest Level (current) _____ / 100

Change in Sports Activities

Check the box which best describes any change you have had in sports activities since your injury / surgery.
My sports activities have:

Not Changed
If yes, check one box below:
☐ I have no / slight problems (c)
☐ I have moderate / significant problems (d)

Decreased
If yes, check one box below:
☐ I now have no / slight problems (e)
☐ I now have moderate / significant problems (d)
☐ For reasons not related to my knee (g)

Stopped -- given up all sports
If yes, check one box below:
☐ I have moderate / significant problems when I play sports (f)
☐ For reasons not related to my knee (g)

Level_____

Function ADL

Check the problems you have during:

1. Walking
check one box:
40 ☐ normal, unlimited
30 ☐ some limitations
20 ☐ only 3-4 blocks possible
0 ☐ less than 1 block; cane, crutch

2. Stairs
check one box:
40 ☐ normal, unlimited
30 ☐ some limitations
20 ☐ only 11-30 steps possible
0 ☐ only 1-10 steps possible

3. Squatting / kneeling
check one box:
40 ☐ normal, unlimited
30 ☐ some limitations
20 ☐ only 6-10 possible
0 ☐ only 0-5 possible

Level_____ / 3=_____

Function Sports

Check the problems you have during:

1. Straight running
check one box:
100 ☐ fully competitive
80 ☐ some limitations, guarding
60 ☐ definite limitations, half speed
40 ☐ not able to do

2. Jumping / landing on affected leg
check one box:
100 ☐ fully competitive
80 ☐ some limitations, guarding
60 ☐ definite limitations, half speed
40 ☐ not able to do

3. Hard twists / cuts / pivots
check one box:
100 ☐ fully competitive
80 ☐ some limitations, guarding
60 ☐ definite limitations, half speed
40 ☐ not able to do

Level_____ / 3=_____

Problems with Sports

Describe the problems you would have with your knee after participating for one hour without guarding or l imitations in each of the three sports categories below. (____check here if you are using a brace.)

Strenuous Sport
(soccer, football, basketball, volleyball)
check one box:
100 ☐ no problems
☐ moderate problems during or after game
☐ severe problems; cannot participate

Moderate Sport
(tennis, racquetball)
check one box:
80 ☐ no problems
☐ moderate problems during or after game
☐ severe problems; cannot participate

Light Sport
(golf, bowling, hiking)
check one box:
60 ☐ no problems
50 ☐ moderate problems during or after game
30 ☐ severe problems; cannot participate

Total Points _____

SPORTS ACTIVITY AND FUNCTION FORM

CINTI KNEE RATING SYSTEM

Courtesy of Frank R. Noyes, M.D.

TABLE 6-7 *Modified Noyes knee questionnaire*

Please answer every section, and mark in each section only the one statement which applies to you. We realize that two statements in any one section may relate to you, but just mark the <u>one</u> which most closely describes your problem.

Pain

20___ I experience no pain in my knee.
16___ I have occasional pain with strenuous sports or heavy work. I don't think that my knee is entirely normal. Limitations are mild and tolerable.
12___ There is occasional pain in my knee with light recreational sports or moderate work.
8___ I have pain brought on by sports, light recreational activities, or moderate work. Occasional pain is brought on by daily activities such as standing or kneeling.
4___ The pain I have in my knee is a significant problem with activities as simple as walking. The pain is relieved by rest. I can't participate in sports.
0___ I have pain in my knee at all times, even during walking, standing, or light work.

Intensity:	A. ( ) Mild	B. ( ) Moderate	C. ( ) Severe	
Frequency:	A. ( ) Constant	B. ( ) Intermittent		
Location:	A. ( ) Medial (inner side)		B. ( ) Lateral (outer side)	
	C. ( ) Anterior (front)		D. ( ) Posterior (back)	
	E. ( ) Diffuse (all over)			
Occurs:	A. ( ) Kneel	B. ( ) Stand	C. ( ) Sit	D. ( ) Stairs
Type:	A. ( ) Sharp	B. ( ) Aching	C. ( ) Throbbing	D. ( ) Burn

Swelling

10___ I experience no swelling in my knee.
8___ I have occasional swelling in my knee with strenuous sports or heavy work.
6___ There is occasional swelling with light recreational activities, or moderate work; it limits my vigorous activities, sports, or heavy labor.
4___ Swelling limits my participation in sports and moderate work. Occurs infrequently with simple walking or light work, about three times a year.
2___ My knee swells after simple walking activities and light work. The swelling is relieved by rest.
0___ **I have severe swelling with simple walking activitie. The swelling is not relieved by rest.**

Stability

20___ My knee does not give out.
16___ My knee gives out only with strenuous sports or heavy work.
12___ My knee gives out occasionally with light recreational activities or moderate work; it limits my vigorous activities, sports, or heavy labor.
8___ Because my knee gives out, it limits all sports and moderate work. It occasionally gives out with walking or light work.
4___ My knee gives out frequently with simple activities such as walking. I must guard my knee at all times.
0___ I have severe problems with my knee giving out. I can't turn or twist without my knee giving way.

Stiffness:	A. ( ) None	B. ( ) Occasional	C. ( ) Frequent	
Grinding :	A. ( ) None	B. ( ) Mild	C. ( ) Moderate	D. ( ) Severe
Locking :	A. ( ) None	B. ( ) Occasional	C. ( ) Frequent	

(Continues)

TABLE 6-7 *(Continued)*

Overall Activity Level

20___ No limitations. I have a normal knee, and I am able to do everything including strenuous sports and/or heavy labor.

16___ I can partake in sports including strenuous ones, but at a lower level. I must guard my knee and limit the amount of heavy labor or sports.

12___ Light recreational activities are possible with RARE symptoms. I am limited to light work.

8___ No sports or recreational activities are possible. Walking activities are possible with RARE symptoms. I am limited to light work.

4___ Walking activities and daily living cause moderate problems and persistent symptoms.

0___ Walking and other daily activities cause severe problems.

Walking

10___ Normal, unlimited.
8___ Slight, mild problems.
6___ Moderate problem, flat surface up to half a mile.
4___ Severe problems, only 2-3 blocks.
2___ Severe problems, need cane or crutches.

Stairs

5___ Normal, unlimited.
4___ Slight, mild problems.
3___ Moderate problems, only 10-15 steps possible.
2___ Severe problems, require a bannister for support.
1___ Severe problems, only 1-5 steps with support.

Running

10___ Normal, unlimited, fully competitive.
8___ Slight, mild problems, run at half speed.
6___ Moderate problems, only 1-2 miles possible.
4___ Severe problems, only 1-3 blocks possible.
2___ Severe problems, only a few steps.

Jumping and Twisting

5___ Normal, unlimited, fully competitive.
4___ Slight, mild problems, some guarding.
3___ Moderate problems, gave up strenuous sports.
2___ Severe problems, affects all sports, always guarding.
1___ Severe problems, only light activity possible (golf/swim).

If I had to give my knee a grade from 1 to 100, with 100 being the best, I would give my knee a _____.

(Modified from Noyes FR et al.[163])

and activities of daily living. Levels 6–10 involve participation in sports such as skiing, basketball, tennis, and soccer. Levels 4–5 include heavy work, jogging, and cycling. Levels 1–3 include light work, walking, and swimming. The Tegner score was developed to be used in conjunction with the modified Lysholm score. In an ACL-deficient population, significant differences in Lysholm scores were obtained, depending on the Tegner activity level. Outcome information becomes more meaningful if average knee function score (modified Lysholm) is correlated to mean activity level (Tegner), and relevant surgical, clinical, and rehabilitation information. A primary ACL-repair group with a relatively high modified Lysholm score (86), significant increases in sagittal ligament laxity (+3 mm), and changes in mean Tegner activity level from level 7 (recreation team sports) preinjury to level 5 (recreational individual sports) can easily be compared with the outcomes of an ACL-deficient or ACL-reconstructed patient group.

A 1991 survey of British orthopaedic surgeons found that over half used no knee rating system, 48 percent used the Lysholm, 40 percent used the Cincinnati, and 11 percent used the Hospital for Special Surgery/Marshall questionnaire in their assessment of knee patients.[167] Comparison of Lysholm and Tegner with the Hospital for Special Surgery (HSS)/Marshall questionnaire found that Lysholm and Tegner numerical scores provided greater information than the HSS/Marshall system.[160] Comparison of Lysholm with the Cincinnati knee scale revealed a linear relation between the two (coefficient of correlation 0.87).[162] Patients scored higher on the Lysholm than the Cincinnati (Lysholm = 30 + 0.72 Cincinnati). The authors felt the difference in scores was due to the greater emphasis on functional disability (six of eight questions) in the Cincinnati system (versus three of eight in the Lysholm). Although not referenced, it appears that the authors used the modified Noyes portion of the Cincinnati system.

The modified Noyes questionnaire is a shortened form of the Cincinnati-Noyes Knee rating system. The modified portion is a 100-point patient-rated system with questions about symptoms (pain, swelling, stability) and function (activity level, walking, stairs, running, jumping and twisting). The Cincinnati system more specifically addresses sports activities and function by including questions concerning exposure (frequency of participation and potential exposure rate for reinjury) and intensity (occupational, light recreational, vigorous recreational, competitive, professional). The meticulous data collection possible in the Cincinnati system also assists the clinician in detecting knee abusers. Inconsistencies may become apparent in their answers. A simple 0 to 100 self-rating visual analog allows another comparison with any of the scoring systems. Patients who are wildly different in their visual analog and questionnaire scores may be symptom magnifiers or abusers.

Sgaglione et al.[168] compared the Lysholm, Hospital for Special Surgery, Tegner, and Cincinnati knee rating system. They found that the use of ligament rating scales tended to inflate the results of reconstructed knees, particularly when the scores were converted to categories (excellent, good, etc.). This was probably due to the inclusion of low activity level subjects with high activity level subjects. This distinction has been noted by other authors.[151] Patients tended to score higher and show better improvement on the HSS, Tegner, and modified Lysholm scales than on the Cincinnati system. The Lysholm and Tegner scores rely on patient assessment of function, while the HSS system is more heavily weighted toward objective assessment.[168] The Cincinnati system more precisely defines the outcome, while tending to be more demanding in its requirements for excellent results.

Rating scales are used most often for patients with ACL reconstructions, but can be used with other ligamentous injuries. Reider et al.[169] used the HSS scale to evaluate athletes with grade III MCL sprains treated with early functional rehabilitation. They found an average score of 45.9/50 after 5-year follow-up. The reinjury rate was three percent.

Knee rating systems can also be used to compare the results of rehabilitation protocols. Bynum et al.[170] compared open versus closed chain rehabilitation protocols following ACL reconstruction with a variety of evaluation tools, including the Lysholm rating scale and the Tegner activity scale. No difference in results was found between the two groups. It was determined that the closed chain protocol (using the Sport Cord system) was superior to the open chain protocol since KT 1000 results were better (although the reported difference of 1.1 mm is within the sensitivity of the KT) and closed chain patients had six percent fewer complaints of patellofemoral pain. The closed chain group also reported slightly better satisfaction, but there were no differences in return to full activity. Both protocols allowed unrestricted sports at 12 months, although the closed chain protocol called for sport-specific drill at 16 weeks, while the open chain protocol allowed drills at 28–32 weeks.[170]

The best way to measure knee outcome remains to be seen. Seto et al.[171] combined aspects of Lysholm and Noyes to make a new functional activity and sports participation scale. No significant relation was found between objective instability measures and functional activity score. There was a positive correlation between functional activity score and ability to participate in sports.

A review of the literature regarding foot-ankle rating systems revealed a greater emphasis on objective assessment rather than patient ratings.[161] Measurements such as ROM at the foot-ankle show low reliability, however. Kaikkonen et al.[172] reported on a scoring system that they felt showed excellent reproducibility and significant correlation to subjective functional assessment and opinion about recovery (Table 6-9). Their system combines patient rating with clinical examination findings, making it more time-consuming to administer. (The nine categories include symptoms, questions about walking, running, stair-climbing, single-leg heel raising, single-leg toe raising, stork balance, dorsiflexion ROM measurement, and ligamentous laxity). The scale successfully differentiates between poor and reference results, as well as excellent and poor results. It is not sensitive enough to make a statistical distinction between those patients rated as excellent and those rated as good. Olerud and Molander developed a subjective

TABLE 6-8 *Ankle scoring scale*

1. Subjective assessment of the injured ankle[a]	
No symptoms of any kind	15
Mild symptoms	10
Severe symptoms	5
2. Can you walk normally?	
Yes	15
No	0
3. Can you run normally?	
Yes	10
No	0
4. Climbing down stairs[b]	
Under 18 seconds	10
18–20 seconds	5
Over 20 seconds	0
5. Rising on heels with injured leg	
Over 40 times	10
30–39 times	5
Under 30 times	0
6. Rising on toes with injured leg	
Over 40 times	10
30–39 times	5
Under 30 times	0
7. Single-limb stance with injured leg	
Over 55 seconds	10
50–55 seconds	5
Under 50 seconds	0
8. Laxity of the ankle joint	
Stable (≤5 mm)	10
Moderate instability (6–10 mm)	5
Severe instability (>10 mm)	0
9. Dorsiflexion range of motion	
≥10 degrees	10
5–9 degrees	5
<5 degrees	0

[a] *Pain, swelling, stiffness, tenderness, or giving way during activities (Mild = only one of these symptoms is present; Moderate = 2 to 3 are present; Severe = 4 or more are present.)*
[b] *Two levels of staircase (length 12 m) with 44 steps (height 18 cm, depth 22 cm)*
Total: Excellent = 85–100, Good = 70–80, Fair 55–65, Poor ≤50.
(From Kaikkonen A et al,[172] with permission.)

TABLE 6-9 *Ankle fracture outcome scale*

PARAMETER	DEGREE	SCORE
Pain	None	25
	While walking on uneven surfaces	20
	While walking on even outdoors	10
	While walking indoors	5
	Constant and severe	0
Stiffness	None	10
	Stiffness	0
Swelling	None	10
	Only evenings	5
	Constant	0
Stair-climbing	No problems	10
	Impaired	5
	Impossible	0
Running	Possible	5
	Impossible	0
Jumping	Possible	5
	Impossible	0
Squatting	No problems	5
	Impossible	0
Supports	None	10
	Taping/wrapping	5
	Stick/crutch	0
Work/Activities of Daily Life	Unchanges	20
	Loss of tempo	15
	Change to simpler job or part-time work	10
	Severely impaired work capacity	0

(From O'Doherty D,[161] *with permission.)*

scale for outcome of ankle fractures (Table 6-10).[161,173] Their 100-point patient-rated systems contains three categories on symptoms: pain, swelling, and stiffness, and six categories on function: stairs, running, jumping, squatting, supports, and work/ADL. Other practitioners have adapted scores like the modified Noyes for the ankle, as questions about stability and giving way remain highly relevant.

References

1. Palmitier RA, An KN, Scott SG, et al: Kinetic chain exercise in knee rehabilitation. Sports Med 11:402–413, 1991

2. Shelbourne KD, Nitz PA: Accelerated rehabilitation after anterior cruciate ligament reconstruction. The effect of timing of reconstruction and rehabilitation. Am J Sports Med 18:292–299, 1990

3. Noyes FR, Butler DL, Paulos LE, et al: Intra-articular cruciate reconstruction. I: Perspectives on graft strength, vascularization, and immediate motion after replacement. Clin Orthop Rel Res 172:71–76, 1983

4. Andrews JH, Sanders Ra, Morin B: Surgical treatment of anterolateral rotatory instability. A follow-up study. Am J Sports Med 13:112–119, 1985

5. Teitge RA, Indelicato PA, Kerlan RK: Iliotibial band transfer for anterolateral rotatory instability of the knee: summary of 54 cases. Am J Sports Med 8:223–227, 1980

6. Feagin JA, Curl WW: Isolated tear of the anterior cruciate ligament: 5-year follow-up study. Am J Sports Med 4:95–100, 1976

7. Sommerlath K, Lysholm J, Gillquist J: The long-term course after treatment of acute anterior cruciate ligament ruptures: a 9 to 16 year followup. Am J Sports Med 19:156–162, 1991

8. Salter RB, Simmonds DF, Malcolm BW: The biological effects of continuous passive motion on the healing of full thickness defects of articular cartilage. J Bone Joint Surg 62A:1231–1251, 1980

9. Noyes FR, Mangines RE, Barber S: Early knee motion after open and arthroscopic ACL rehabilitation. Am J Sports Med 15:149–160, 1987

10. Clancy WG: Intra-articular reconstruction of the anterior cruciate ligament. Orthop Clin North Am 16:181–190, 1985

11. Hughston JC: Complications of anterior cruciate ligament surgery. Orthop Clin North Am 16:237–240, 1985

12. Lephart SM, Perrin DH, Fu FH et al: Relationship between selected physical characteristics and functional capacity in the anterior cruciate ligament-insufficient athlete. J Orthop Phys Ther 16:174–181, 1992

13. Freeman MAR, Dean MRE, Hanham IWF: The etiology and prevention of functional instability of the foot. J Bone Joint Surg 47B:678–685, 1965

14. Tropp H: Pronator muscle weakness in functional instability of the ankle. Int J Sports Med 7:291–294, 1986

15. Fridén T, Zätterström R, Lindstrand A, et al: A stabilometric technique for evaluation of lower

limb instabilities. Am J Sports Med 17:118–122, 1989

16. Yack HJ, Riley LM, Whieldon TR: Anterior tibial translation during progressive loading of the ACL-deficient knee during weight-bearing and nonweight-bearing isometric exercise. J Orthop Sports Phys Ther 20:247–253, 1994

17. Shelbourne KD, Whitaker HJ, McCarroll JR et al: Anterior cruciate ligament injury: evaluation of intra-articular reconstruction of acute tears without repair: two to seven year follow-up of 155 athletes. Am J Sports Med 18:484–489, 1990

18. Wilk KE, Andrews JR: Current concepts in the treatment of anterior cruciate ligament disruption. J Orthop Sports Phys Ther 15:279–293, 1992

19. Mandelbaum BR, Myerson MS, Forster R: Achilles tendon ruptures: a new method of repair, early range of motion, and functional rehabilitation. Am J Sports Med 23:392–395, 1995

20. Troop RL, Losse GM, Lane JG et al: Early motion after repair of Achilles tendon ruptures. Foot Ankle 16:705–709, 1995

21. Brownstein BA, Bronner S: Patellar fracture associated with accelerated ACL rehabilitation, abstracted. J Orthop Sports Phys Ther 25:142, 1996

22. Donatelli RA: Normal anatomy and biomechanics. p 3. In Donatelli RA (ed): The Biomechanics of the Foot and Ankle. FA Davis Co, Philadelphia, PA 1990

23. Gray G: Functional kinetic chain rehabilitation: overuse and inflammatory conditions and their management . . . a strategy of oxymorons. Sports Med Update 24–30, 1995

24. Root ML, Orien WP, Weed JH, et al: Biomechanical Examination of the Foot, Vol I. Clinical Biomechanics Corp, Los Angeles, CA 1971

25. McPoil TG: Evaluation and Management of the Foot and Ankle. Course notes, 1990

26. Michaud TC: Abnormal motion during gait. p. 57. In Michaud TC: Foot Orthoses and Other Forms of Conservative Foot Care. Williams & Wilkins, Baltimore, MD 1993

27. Gross MT: Lower quarter screening for skeletal malalignment—suggestions for orthotics and shoewear. J Orthop Phys Ther 21:389–405, 1995

28. Perry J: Gait Analysis: Normal and Pathological Function. Slack Inc, Thorofare, NJ 1992

29. Godges JJ, MacRae H, Longdon C et al: The effects of two static stretching procedures on hip range of motion and gait economy. J Orthop Sports Phys Ther 10:350–357, 1989

30. Waters RL, Barnes G, Husserl T et al: Comparable energy expenditure after arthrodesis of the hip and ankle. J Bone Joint Surg 70A:1032–1037, 1988

31. Inman VT, Ralston HJ, Todd F: Human Walking. Williams & Wilkins, Baltimore, MD 1981

32. Saunders JBCM, Inman VT, Eberhart HD: The major determinations in normal and pathological gait. J Bone Joint Surg 35A:543–558, 1953

33. Elveru RA, Rothstein JM, Lamb RL: Goniometric reliability in a clinical setting: subtalar and ankle joint measurements. Phys Ther 68: 672–677, 1988

34. Lattanza L, Gray GW, Kantner RM: Closed versus open chain measurements of subtalar joint eversion: implications for clinical practice. J Orthop Sports Phys Ther 9:310–314, 1988

35. Smith-Oricchio K, Harris BA: Interrater reliability of subtalar neutral, calcaneal inversion and eversion. J Orthop Sports Phys Ther 12:10–15, 1990

36. McPoil TG, Knecht HG, Schuit D: A survey of foot types in normal females between the ages of 18 and 30 years. J Orthop Sports Phys Ther 9:406–409, 1988

37. McPoil TG, Cornwall MW: The relationship between subtalar neutral position and rearfoot motion during walking. Foot Ankle 15:141–145, 1994

38. McPoil TG, Hunt GC: Evaluation and management of foot and ankle disorders: present problems and future directions. J Ortho Sports Phys Ther 21:381–388, 1995

39. Oatis CA: Biomechanics of the foot and ankle under static conditions. Phys Ther 68: 1815–1821, 1988

40. McPoil TG, Knecht HG: Biomechanics of the foot in walking: a function approach. J Orthop Sports Phys Ther 7:69–72, 1985

41. Winter DA, MacKinnon CD, Ruder GK et al: An integrated EMG/biomechanical model of upper body balance and posture during human gait. Prog Brain Res 97:359–367, 1993

42. Winter DA: Foot trajectory in human gait: a precise and multifactorial motor control task. Phys Ther 72:45–56, 1992

43. Mann RA, Moran GT, Dougherty SE: Comparative electromyography of the lower extremity in jogging, running, and sprinting. Am J Sports Med 14:501–510, 1986

44. Montgomery WH, Pink M, Perry J: Electromyographic analysis of hip and knee musculature

during running. Am J Sports Med 22:272–278, 1994

45. Reber L, Perry J, Pink M: Muscular control of the ankle during running. Am J Sports Med 21: 805–810, 1993

46. Rodgers MM: Dynamic foot biomechanics. J Orthop Sports Phys Ther 21:306–316, 1995

47. Shiavi R: Electromyographic patterns in normal adult locomotion. p. 97. In Smidt GL (ed): Gait in Rehabilitation. Churchill Livingstone, New York, 1990

48. Monad H: Contractility of muscle during prolonged static and repetitive dynamic activity. Ergonomics 28:81–89, 1985

49. Donatelli RA: Abnormal biomechanics. p. 32. In Donatelli RA (ed): The Biomechanics of the Foot and Ankle. FA Davis Co, Philadelphia, PA 1990

50. Bates BT: Foot function in running. p. 293. In Terauds J (ed): Biomechanics in Sports: Proceedings of the International Symposium of Biomechanics in Sports. Academic Publishers, Del Mar, CA 1983

51. Dillman CJ: Kinematic analyses of running. Exer Sport Sci Rev 3:193–218, 1974

52. Cavanagh PR, Lafortune MA: Ground reaction forces in distance running. J Biomechanics 13: 397–406, 1980

53. Berg K: Balance and its measure in the elderly: a review. Physiother Can 41:240–246, 1989

54. Tropp H, Ekstrandt J, Gillquist J: Stabilometry in functional instability of the ankle and its value in predicting injury. Med Sci Sports Exer 16: 64–66, 1984

55. Garn SN, Newton R: Kinesthetic awareness in subjects with multiple ankle sprains. Phys Ther 68:1667–1671, 1988

56. Lentell GL, Katzman LL, Walters MR: The relationship between muscle function and ankle stability. J Orthop Sports Phys Ther 11:605–615, 1990

57. Ryan L: Mechanical stability, muscle strength, and proprioception in the functionally unstable ankle. Aust J Physiother 40:41–47, 1994

58. Tropp H, Ekstrand J, Gillquist J: Factors affecting stabilometry recordings in single limb stance. Am J Sports Med 12:185–188, 1984

59. Fridén T, Zätterström R, Lindstrand A et al: Disability in anterior cruciate ligament insufficiency. Acta Orthop Scand 61:131–135, 1990

60. Löfvenberg R, Kärrholm J, Sundelin G, Ahlgren O: Prolonged reaction time in patients with

chronic lateral instability of the ankle. Am J Sports Med 23:414–417, 1995

61. Sojka P, Johansson H, Sjolander P et al: Fusimotor neurons can be reflexively influenced by activity in receptor afferents from the posterior cruciate ligament. Brain Res 483:177–183, 1989

62. Johansson H, Sjolander P, Sojka P: Activity in receptor afferents from the anterior cruciate ligament evokes reflex effects of fusimotor neurons. Neurosci Res 8:54–59, 1990

63. Zätterström R, Fridén T, Lindstrand A et al: The effect of physiotherapy on standing balance in chronic anterior cruciate ligament insufficiency. Am J Sports Med 22:531–535, 1994

64. Cornwall MW, Murrell P: Postural sway following inversion sprain of the ankle. J Am Podiatr Assoc 81:243–247, 1991

65. Konradsen L, Bohsen Ravn J: Prolonged peroneal reaction time in ankle instability. Int J Sports Med 12:290–292, 1991

66. Nawoczenski DA, Owen MG, Ecker ML et al: Objective evaluation of peroneal response to sudden inversion stress. J Orthop Phys Ther 7: 107–109, 1985

67. Nitz AJ, Dobner JJ, Kersey D: Nerve injury and grades II and III ankle sprains. Am J Sports Med 13:177–182. 1985

68. Kleinrensink GJ, Stoeckart R, Meulstee J et al: Lowered motor conduction velocity of the peroneal nerve after inversion trauma. Med Sci Sports Exerc 26:877–883, 1994

69. Wilkerson GB, Nitz AJ: Dynamic ankle stability: mechanical and neuromuscular interrelationships. J Sport Rehab 3:43–57, 1994

70. O'Connor B, Visco D, Brandt K et al: Neurogenic acceleration of osteoarthritis. J Bone Joint Surg 74A:367–376, 1992

71. Levine JD, Dardick SJ, Basbaum AI et al: Reflex neurogenic inflammation: I. Contribution of the peripheral nervous system to spatially remote inflammatory responses that follow injury. J Neurosc 5:1380–1386, 1985

72. McPoil TG, Schuit D, Knecht HG: A comparison of three positions to evaluate tibial varum. J Am Podiatr Med Assoc 78:22–28, 1988

73. Garbalosa JC, McClure MH, Catlin PA et al: The frontal plane relationship of the forefoot to the rearfoot in an asymptomatic population. J Orthop Sports Phys Ther 20:200–206, 1994

74. Tiberio D: The effect of excessive subtalar joint pronation on patellofemoral mechanics: a theo-

retical model. J Orthop Phys Ther 9:160–165, 1987

75. McCulloch MU, Brunt D, Linden DV: The effect of foot orthotics and gait velocity on lower limb kinematics and temporal events of stance. J Orthop Phys Ther 17:2–10, 1993

76. Coplan JA: Rotational motion of the knee: a comparison of normal and pronating subjects. J Orthop Phys Ther 10:366–369, 1989

77. D'Amico JC, Rubin M: The influence of foot orthoses on the quadriceps angle. J Am Podiatr Med Assoc 76:337–339, 1976

78. Eng JJ, Pierrynowski MR: Evaluation of soft foot orthotics in the treatment of patellofemoral pain syndrome. Phys Ther 73:62–68, 1993

79. Rodgers MM, LeVeau BF: Effectiveness of foot orthotic devices used to modify pronation in runners. J Orthop Phys Ther 4:86–90, 1982

80. Nawoczenski DA, Cook TM, Saltzman CL: The effect of foot orthotics on three-dimensional kinematics of the leg and rearfoot during running. J Orthop Phys Ther 21:317–327, 1995

81. Zimmy ML, Schutte M, Dabezies E: Mechanoreceptors in the human cruciate ligament. Anat Rec 214:202–209, 1986

82. Sjolander P, Johansson H, Sojka P et al: Sensory nerve endings in the cat cruciate ligaments: a morphological investigation. Neurosci Lett 102: 33–38, 1989

83. Zimny ML, Wink CS: Receptors in the knee joint. J Electromyog Kinesiol 1:148–157, 1991

84. Solomonow M, Baratta R, Zhou BH et al: The synergistic action of the anterior cruciate ligament and thigh muscles in maintaining joint stability. Am J Sports Med 15:207–213, 1987

85. Freeman M, Wyke B: Articular reflexes at the ankle joint: an electromyographic study of normal and abnormal influences of ankle-joint mechanoreceptors upon reflex activity in the leg muscles. Br J Surg 54:990–1001, 1967

86. Baratta R, Solomonow M, Zhou BH et al: Muscular coactivation: the role of the antagonist musculature in maintaining knee stability. Am J Sports Med 16:113–122, 1988

87. Wojtys EM, Huston LJ: Neuromuscular performance in normal and anterior cruciate ligament-deficient lower extremities. Am J Sports Med 22: 89–104, 1994

88. Gauffin H, Tropp H: Altered movement and muscular-activation patterns during the one-legged jump in patients with an old anterior cruciate ligament rupture. Am J Sports Med 20:182–192, 1992

89. Hagood S, Solomonow M, Baratta R et al: The effect of joint velocity on the contribution of the antagonist musculature to knee stiffness and laxity. Am J Sports Med 18:182–187, 1990

90. Hirokawa S, Solomonow M, Luo Z et al: Muscular co-contraction and control of knee stability. J Electromyogr Kinesiol 1:199–208, 1991

91. Lutz GE, Palmitier RA, An KN et al: Comparison of tibiofemoral joint forces during open-kinetic-chain and closed-kinetic-chain exercises. J Bone Joint Surg 75A:732–739, 1993

92. Walla DJ, Albright JP, McAuley E et al: Hamstring control and the unstable anterior cruciate ligament-deficient knee. Am J Sports Med 13: 34–39, 1985

93. Beard DJ, Dodd CAF, Trundle HR et al: Proprioception enhancement for anterior cruciate ligament deficiency. J Bone Joint Surg 76B:654–659, 1994

94. Berchuck M, Andriacci TP, Bach BR et al: Gait adaptations by patients who have a deficient anterior cruciate ligament. J Bone Joint Surg 72A: 871–877, 1990

95. Noyes FR, Schipplein OD, Andriacchi TP et al: The anterior cruciate ligament-deficient knee with varus alignment: an analysis of gait adaptations and dynamic joint loadings. Am J Sports Med 20:707–716, 1992

96. Tibone JE, Antich TJ, Fanton GS et al: Functional analysis of anterior cruciate ligament instability. Am J Sports Med 14:276–284, 1986

97. Branch TP, Hunter R, Donath M: Dynamic EMG analysis of anterior cruciate deficient legs with and without bracing during cutting. Am J Sports Med 17:35–41, 1989

98. Ciccotti MG, Kerlan RK, Perry J et al: An electromyographic analysis of the knee during functional activities. II. The anterior cruciate ligament-deficient and -reconstructed profiles. Am J Sports Med 22:651–658, 1994

99. Andriacchi TP: Dynamics of pathological motion: applied to the anterior cruciate deficient knee. J Biomechanics, 23(suppl 1):99–105, 1990

100. Andriacchi TP, Birac D: Functional testing in the anterior cruciate ligament-deficient knee. Clin Orthop Rel Res 288:40–47, 1993

101. Gauffin H, Tropp H, Odenrick P: Effect of ankle disk training on postural control in patients with functional instability of the ankle joint. Int J Sports Med 9:141–144, 1988

102. Lass P, Kaalund S, leFevre S et al: Muscle coordination following rupture of the anterior cruciate ligament. Acta Orthop Scand 62:9–14, 1991

103. Sinkjaer T, Arendt-Nielsen L: Knee stability and muscle coordination in patients with anterior cruciate ligament injuries: an electromyographic approach. J Electromyog Kinesiol 1:209–217, 1991

104. Muneta T, Yamamoto H, Ishibashi T et al: Computerized tomographic analysis of tibial tubercle position in the painful female patellofemoral joint. Am J Sports Med 22:67–71, 1994

105. Insall J: Current concepts review: patellar pain. J Bone Joint Surg 64A:147–152, 1982

106. Caylor D, Fites R, Worrell TW: The relationship between quadriceps angle and anterior knee pain syndrome. J Orthop Sports Phys Ther 17:11–16, 1993

107. Reikeras O: Patellofemoral characteristics in patients with femoral anteversion. Skeletal Radiol 21:311–313, 1992

108. Puniello MS: Iliotibial band tightness and medial patellar glide in patients with patellofemoral dysfunction. J Orthop Phys Ther 17:144–148, 1993

109. Guzzanti V, Gigante A, Di Lazzaro A et al: Patellofemoral malalignment in adolescents: computerized tomographic assessment with or without quadriceps contraction. Am J Sports Med 22:55–60, 1994

110. Grelsamer RP, Proctor CS, Bazos AN: Evaluation of patellar shape in the sagittal plane: a clinical analysis. Am J Sports Med 22:61–66, 1994

111. Grabiner MD, Koh TJ, Draganich LF: Neuromechanics of the patellofemoral joint. Med Sci Sports Exerc 26:10–21, 1994

112. Steinkamp LA, Dillingham MF, Markel MD et al: Biomechanical considerations in patellofemoral joint rehabilitation. Am J Sports Med 21:438–444, 1993

113. Karst GM, Willett GM: Onset timing of electromyographic activity in the vastus medialis oblique and vastus lateralis muscles in subjects with or without patellofemoral pain syndrome. Phys Ther 75:813–823, 1995

114. Dillon PZ, Updyke WF, Allen WC: Gait analysis with reference to chondromalacia patellae. J Orthop Phys Ther 5:127–131, 1983

115. Hébert LJ, Gravel D, Arsenault AB et al: Patellofemoral pain syndrome: the possible role of an inadequate neuromuscular mechanism. Clinical Biomechanics 9:93–97, 1994

116. Reynolds L, Levin TA, Medeiros JM et al: EMG activity of the vastus medialis oblique and the vastus lateralis in their role in patellar alignment. Am J Phys Med 63:61–70, 1983

117. Mariani P, Canuso I: An electromyographic investigation of subluxation of the patella. J Bone Joint Surg (Br) 61B:169–171, 1979

118. Voight ML, Wieder DL: Comparative reflex response times of vastus medialis obliquus and vastus lateralis in normal subjects and subjects with extensor mechanism dysfunction. Am J Sports Med 19:131–137, 1991

119. Bennett JG, Stauber WT: Evaluation and treatment of anterior knee pain using eccentric exercise. Med Sci Sports Exerc 18:526–530, 1986

120. Wyke B: The neurology of joints. Ann R Coll Surg Eng 41:25–50, 1967

121. Janda V: Muscles, motor regulation and back problems. p. 27. In Korr IM (ed): The Neurologic Mechanisms in Manipulative Therapy. Plenum Publishing Corp, New York 1978

122. Bullock-Saxton JE, Bullock MI: Changes in hip and knee muscle strength associated with ankle injury. N Z J Physiother 21:10–14, 1993

123. Bullock-Saxton JE: Local sensation changes and altered hip muscle function following severe ankle sprain. Phys Ther 74:17–31, 1994

124. Nicholas JA, Strizak AM, Veras G: A study of thigh muscle weakness in different pathological states of the lower extremity. Am J Sports Med 4:241–248, 1976

125. Kegerreis S: The construction and implementation of functional progression as a component of athletic rehabilitation. J Orthop Phys Ther 5:14–19, 1983

126. Kegerreis S, Malone T, McCarroll J: Functional progression: an aid to athletic rehabilitation. Phys Sports Med 12:67–71, 1984

127. Rivera JE: Open versus closed kinetic chain rehabilitation of the lower extremity: a functional and biomechanical analysis. J Sport Rehab 3:154–167, 1994

128. Tippett SR, Voight NL: Functional Progressions for Sport Rehabilitation. Human Kinetics, Champaign, IL 1995

129. Tiberio D: Functional rehab in ankle injuries. Rehab Management 7:31–33, 1994

130. Thurston AJ: Spinal and pelvic kinematics in osteoarthrosis of the hip joint. Spine 10:467–471, 1985

131. Andriacchi TP, Galante JO, Fermier RW: The in-

fluence of total knee-replacement design on walking and stair climbing. J Bone Joint Surg 64A:1328–1335, 1982

132. Knutzen KM, Price A: Lower extremity static and dynamic relationships with rearfoot motion in gait. J Am Podiatr Med Assoc 84:171–180, 1994

133. Rowinski MJ: Afferent neurobiology of the joint. p. 49. In Gould JA (ed): Orthopaedic and Sports Physical Therapy. 2nd Ed. C.V. Mosby, St. Louis, 1990

134. Nyland J, Brosky T, Currier D et al: Review of the afferent neural system of the knee and its contribution to motor learning. J Orthop Sports Phys Ther 19:2–11, 1994

135. Skinner HB, Barrack RL: Joint position sense in the normal and pathologic knee joint. J Electromyog Kinesiol 1:180–190, 1991

136. Hoffman M, Payne VG: The effects of proprioceptive ankle disk training on healthy subjects. J Orthop Sports Phys Ther 21:90–93, 1995

137. Tropp H, Askling C: Effects of ankle disc training on muscular strength and postural control. Clin Bio 3:88–91, 1988

138. Balogun JA, Adesinasi CO, Marzouk DK: The effect of a wobbleboard exercise training program on static balance performance and strength of lower extremity muscles. Physiother Can 44:23–30, 1992

139. Bullock-Saxton JE, Janda V, Bullock MI: Reflex activation of gluteal muscles in walking. Spine 18:704–708, 1993

140. Thorstensson A: How is the normal locomotor program modified to produce backward walking? Exp Brain Res 61:664–668, 1986

141. Flynn TW, Soutas-Little RW: Mechanical power and muscle action during forward and backward running. J Orthop Sports Phys Ther 17:108–112, 1993

142. Brunnstrom S: Movement Therapy in Hemiplegia: A Neurophysiologic Approach. 1st Ed. Harper and Row, New York, 1970

143. Bobath B: Adult Hemiplegia: Evaluation and Treatment. William Heinemann Medical Books Ltd, London, 1970

144. Myatt G, Baxter R, Dougherty R et al: The cardiopulmonary cost of backward walking at selected speeds. J Orthop Sports Phys Ther 21:132–138, 1995

145. Threlkeld AJ, Horn TS, Wojtowicz GM et al: Kinematics, ground reaction force and muscle balance produced by backward running. J Orthop Sports Phys Ther 11:56–63, 1989

146. Flynn TW, Soutas-Little RW: Patellofemoral joint compressive forces in forward and backward running. J Orthop Sports Phys Ther 21:277–282, 1995

147. Voight ML, Draovitch P: Pliometrics. p. 45. In Albert M (ed): Eccentric Muscle Training in Sports and Orthopaedics. Churchill Livingstone, New York 1991

148. Kottke F, Halpern D, Easton JK et al: The training of coordination. Arch Phys Med Rehab 59:267–272, 1978

149. Yamamoto SK, Hartman CW, Feagin JA et al: Functional rehabilitation of the knee: a preliminary study. J Sports Med 3:288–291, 1976

150. Miller RK, Carr AJ: The knee. p. 228. In Pynsent PB, Fairbank JCT, Carr A (eds): Outcome Measures in Orthopaedics. Butterworth-Heinemann Ltd, Oxford, 1993

151. Noyes FR, Barber SD, Mooar LA: A rationale for assessing sports activity levels and limitations in knee disorders. Clin Orthop Rel Res 246:238–249, 1989

152. Tegner Y, Lysholm J: Rating systems in the evaluation of knee ligament injuries. Clin Orthop Rel Res 198:43–49, 1985

153. Hu HS, Whitney SL, Irrgang J et al: Test-retest reliability of the one-legged vertical jump test and the one-legged standing hop test (Abstract for Poster Presentation, APTA Combined Sections Meeting, 1992). J Orthop Sports Phys Ther 15:51, 1992

154. Booher LD, Hench KM, Worrell TW et al: Reliability of three single-leg hop tests. J Sport Rehab 2:165–170, 1993

155. Bandy WD, Rusche KR, Tekulve FY: Reliability and limb symmetry for five unilateral functional tests of the lower extremity. Isokinetics Exerc 4:108–111, 1994

156. Barber SD, Noyes FR, Mangine RE et al: Quantitative assessment of functional limitations in normal and anterior cruciate ligament-deficient knees. Clin Orthop Rel Res 255:204–214, 1990

157. Noyes FR, Barber SD, Mangine RE: Abnormal lower limb symmetry determined by function hop tests after anterior cruciate ligament rupture. Am J Sports Med 19:513–518, 1991

158. Lunsford BR, Perry J: The standing heel-raise test for ankle plantar flexion: criterion for normal. Phys Ther 75:694–698, 1995

159. Anderson MA, Gieck JH, Perrin D et al: The relationships among isometric, isotonic, and isokinetic concentric and eccentric quadriceps and

hamstring force and three components of athletic performance. J Orthop Sports Phys Ther 14: 114–120, 1991

160. Tegner Y, Lysholm J, Lysholm M et al: A performance test to monitor rehabilitation and evaluate anterior cruciate ligament injuries. Am J Sports Med 14:156–159, 1986

161. O'Doherty D: The foot and ankle. p. 245. In Pynsent PB, Fairbank JCT, Carr A (eds): Outcome Measures in Orthopaedics. Butterworth-Heinemann Ltd, Oxford, 1993

162. Lysholm J, Gillquist J: Evaluation of knee ligament surgery results with special emphasis on use of a scoring scale. Am J Sports Med 10: 150–154, 1982

163. Wilk KE, Romaniello WT, Soscia SM et al: The relationship between subjective knee scores, isokinetic testing, and functional testing in the ACL-reconstructed knee. J Orthop Sports Phys Ther 20:60–73, 1994

164. Kannus P, Niittymäki S: Which factors predict outcome in the nonoperative treatment of patellofemoral pain syndrome? A prospective follow-up study. Med Sci Sports Exerc 26:289–296, 1994

165. Chesworth BM, Culham EG, Tata GE et al: Validation of outcome measures in patients with patellofemoral syndrome. J Orthop Sports Phys Ther 11:302–308, 1989

166. McMullen W, Roncarati A, Koval P: Static and isokinetic treatments of chondromalacia patella: a comparative investigation. J Orthop Sports Phys Ther 12:256–266, 1990

167. Bollen S, Seedhom BB: A comparison of the Lysholm and Cincinnati knee scoring questionnaires. Am J Sports Med 19(2):189–190, 1991

168. Sgaglione NA, Del Pizzo W, Fox JM et al: Critical analysis of knee ligament rating systems. Am J Sports Med 23:660–667, 1995

169. Reider B, Sathy MR, Talkington J et al: Treatment of isolated medial collateral ligament injuries in athletes with early functional rehabilitation. Am J Sports Med 22:470–477, 1993

170. Bynum EB, Barrack RL, Alexander AH: Open versus closed chain kinetic exercises after anterior cruciate ligament reconstruction. A prospective randomized study. Am J Sports Med 23: 401–406, 1995

171. Seto JL, Orofino AS, Morrissey MC et al: Assessment of quadriceps/hamstring strength, knee ligament stability, functional and sports activity levels five years after anterior cruciate ligament reconstruction. Am J Sports Med 16:170–180, 1988

172. Kaikkonen A, Kannus P, Järvinen M: A performance test protocol and scoring scale for the evaluation of ankle injuries. Am J Sports Med 22:462–469, 1994

173. Olerud C, Molander H: A scoring scale for symptom evaluation after ankle fracture. Arch Orthop Trauma Surg 103:190–194, 1984

7

Movement Skills in Sports

BRUCE   BROWNSTEIN

This book focuses on two aspects of human activity—function and movement. It is clear that the two concepts are linked. The greater the availability of movement, the greater the possible function. Loss of mobility (an aspect of movement) as defined by range of motion (ROM) is one of the great limiters of function in activities of daily living (ADLs) (see ch. 9). One of the primary goals of physical therapy treatments is to increase motion. This expands the movement possibilities available to the individual, leading to better function. In the older adult, the basic tools of movement require a blend of mobility, strength, and somatosensory input. These are the areas that are primarily affected by aging, injury, and deconditioning. Balance, agility, coordination, and other sports skills require that these tools be used to the fullest. In the athlete, maximal performance is the usually the goal. Blending the different skills acquired through natural capacity, training, and motivation enables the trained athlete to utilize and place demands on the musculoskeletal system that sometimes seem impossible.

Sports Skills

What are the skills that underlie sporting activities? According to Adams, a skill ". . . is learned, and it is differentiated from capacity and ability because an individual may have the capacity and ability to perform a skill but cannot do it because it has not been learned."[1] Skill implies superior performance along with greater repeatability of performance. Adams quotes T. H. Pear, a British psychologist, as giving a definition of skill as " . . . the integration of well-adjusted muscular performances." The addition of the word "muscular" differentiates between intellectual capacity—such as decision-making—from physical, motor, or psychomotor performance.[1] Developing skill involves a combination of physical capacity, perceptual processes, and learning.[2]

Nicholas et al.[3] attempted to describe a classification system for movement skills in sports. They developed a list of six fundamental categories of movement. The categories are (in order of usage in sports) throwing, stance, jumping, kicking, running, and walking. Walking and running are classically differentiated by the incorporation of float, a phase of gait when both legs are off the ground during running. Stance includes maintenance of a specific posture over a period of time. Jumping, kicking, and throwing are defined as ballistic movements involving these traditional motions. Throwing includes catching, swinging activities (batting, golf, etc.), upper extremity motions in swimming, and pushing activities such as the shotput. It is not a surprise that throwing was considered the most common activity since it includes all movements of the upper extremity during sports. Nor is it a revelation that walking is the least common skill since sports activities tend to be high energy, high velocity activities. It is interesting that stance, including postural skills, is the number two category in this classification. Yet most sports research has focused on measurement of the bal-

TABLE 7-1 *Performance traits of athletes*

PHYSICAL	NEUROMUSCULAR	COGNITIVE	ENVIRONMENTAL
Muscle strength	Balance	Alertness	Equipment
Endurance	Agility	Motivation	Playing Conditions
Body type	Coordination	Intelligence	
Flexibility	Timing	Creativity	
Speed	Reaction Time	Discipline	
	Rhythm	Practice	
	Accuracy	Steadiness	

(Adapted from Nicholas JA et al,[3] with permission.)

listic activities and sports techniques, rather than the movement skills that underlie them.[4]

Nicholas et al. also included a description of performance traits that included 13 neuromuscular, five psychomotor, and three environmental.[3,5] These traits are rearranged into four categories and presented in Table 7-1. Some overlap between categories may exist for some traits. For example, strength, speed, and endurance may be defined in either physical or neuromuscular terms. For this discussion, these traits are considered physical traits since they are more dependant upon physiologic characteristics of the muscle rather than somatosensory input and control systems.

Although the assignment of various skills to different sports was subjective, the work by Nicholas et al. remains unique. This work, whose accuracy would have been enhanced by present day sports analysis techniques, was not clouded by the wealth of information that those techniques have produced. The aims of this chapter are to highlight some of the skills that are part of sports and to review some of the literature concerning muscle function in sports.

Strength and Stretch-Shortening

Strength is more a physical capacity than a skill. Strength testing, in its many forms, rarely has a strong causal relation to sports performance.[6–8] Yet strength testing remains a basic part of as-

sessment.[9,10] Strength is a strong contributor to many athletic tasks.[10] Perhaps the best use of strength testing is to identify deficits that may not limit performance but may place an athlete at risk of injury. This is one of the purposes of functional testing protocols.[11] Isokinetic dynamometry can be used as a screening tool as well (see ch. 3), but probably not as an indicator of function or skill. Some sports activities require that muscles function at relatively high activity levels for long periods of time.[12,13] Strength testing can offer the first clue that a patient will have difficulty executing coordinated movements.

Ballistic sports imposes greater demand on the neuromuscular system of athletes than slower moving sports. Higher forces, larger accelerations, more muscles involved in control of forces are all part of ballistic movements. Greater muscle strength of athletes is augmented by more efficient use of the stretch-shortening cycle. The stretch-shortening cycle is used whenever a cocking phase or loading phase exists in the movement being generated. The key factor during this phase is the time in which the muscle is being stretched and its elastic capacity is being called upon.[14–17] Other factors include the velocity and force involved in the stretch.[14,15] Utilization of the stretch-shortening capacity of the neuromuscular system is implicit in rapid changes of direction (cutting), developing high levels of tension (jumping), and accelerating objects at high speeds (throwing). The ability of muscle to effectively use its stretch-shortening capability may also protect the joint from high forces involved in sports movements.

Balance and Posture

Controlling the center of gravity during movement and athletic activities is the primary concern of the postural control system.[18] The postural control system uses the movement strategies available to it to maintain balance during stance activities as well as to integrate the information from various sensory elements to prepare the muscular system for response to changes in the environment and base of support, either expected or unexpected. Results of several studies indicate that athletes utilize strategies that are a result of their training to maintain postural control.

Mouchnino et al.[19] studied the strategies used by trained dancers and untrained subjects in maintaining control of the center of gravity and orientation of the head during single leg raising in a standing position. They found that both groups of subjects were able to accomplish the task, but the groups used different movement strategies. The dancers were able to utilize a feed-forward strategy that maintained a vertical orientation of the trunk and head. Naive subjects were able to maintain head orientation, but were unable to control the trunk. The movement in this group appeared to be under feedback control, since the hip and trunk movements always lagged behind rotation of the leg on the ankle. Dancers, on the other hand, were able to control movements at the hip in advance of the motion around the ankle. The dancers' strategy was deemed to be more effective since it minimized the problem of calculating different frames of reference (head verticality, head with respect to trunk, and trunk verticality) and reduced the degrees of freedom problem since fewer computations are required to control the center of gravity. The authors hypothesized that the dancers' strategy was built up by training and indicated a more accurate internal representation of the center of gravity.

Dancers were also noted to have superior balance abilities than nondancers by Crotts et al.[20] They measured the ability of subjects to maintain stance on one leg under several different visual and support surface conditions. Dancers were able to balance significantly better than nondancers in a composite score of all test conditions as well as on individual tests under the most challenging conditions (no vision, foam surface). The authors echoed Mouchnino et al. by stating that the superior performance of the dancers was a result of training.

Gymnasts demonstrate similar superior equilibrium control when faced with tasks that challenge the postural control system. Rapid backward bending performed in standing was accomplished more efficiently and with less excursion of the center of gravity in gymnasts than in untrained subjects.[21] When the test was repeated while standing on a balance beam, the gymnasts again outperformed the nongymnasts. The authors also noted that the trained subjects were able to adapt their movement patterns more readily than naive subjects when constraints were placed on their movement. Untrained subjects did not show any variation in muscle activation when support conditions (narrow beam versus floor) for the postural task were changed.

Although dancers and gymnasts may have superior balance and postural skills compared to nonathletes as a result of their training in body orientation, postural control is also improved within participants of varying skill in some sports activities. Dancers of the professional caliber have better balance capacity than beginning dancers.[22] Weight shifting during the swing of beginning golfers using two different clubs—a driver and an eight iron—varies from that of experienced golfers.[23] Top level rifle shooters show less variation in speed and amplitude of center of force than national level shooters.[24] The national level shooters were better stabilizers than untrained shooters. This difference was more significant during the last phase of the shot. Also, in the untrained shooters, postural stability was better in trials that included the best shots than the trials that included the worst shots.

Injury has a negative effect on balance and control of posture. Zätterström, et al.[25] found that injury to the anterior cruciate ligament (ACL) resulted in decreased one-legged standing balance control for several months after injury. Normal values did not return fully until 12 months of retraining. Similar alterations have been noted in other functional activities following ACL injury (see section on Coordination).[26,27]

Other injuries have also been implicated in reduced balance skills in athletes. Golomer et al.[28] studied the balance performance of soccer players with acutely sprained ankles as well as basketball players with acute patella tendinitis. In both cases, selected balance measures showed greater displacements and decreased contribution of somatosensory elements (based upon frequency analysis). In the test with basketball players, no change was noted when balance was tested with eyes open. Differences were noted in the eyes closed situation. The authors hypothesized that pain was a contributing factor, since the tests were performed on acutely injured joints. Perhaps movement patterns were altered to accommodate pain reactions.[28] Altered muscle function,[29] increased reaction times,[30] and changes in proprioceptive input[31] can all contribute to poorer performance on balance tests following ankle sprains.

Similar proprioceptive changes and muscle pattern alteration has been seen as a result of injury to the lumbar spine.[32] Given the importance of the spinal musculature in postural movements and control,[33,34] injuries to the joints of the spine must be considered potentially detrimental to balance and postural skill in all athletes, particularly the industrial athlete.

Coordination of Movement

As a working definition, coordination is defined as the controlled activation of muscle to produce distinctive patterns of segmental motion.[35] Coordination also implies a fluidity of motion that is qualitative and can be appreciated through observation of skilled athletes and performers. For most sports activities, coordinated muscular function is achieved through a proximal to distal activation of muscle, with a similar process occurring in the generation of joint torque and velocity (See Fig. 7-1).[35a]

Putnam has studied the sequential motions of various sporting skills including striking, throwing, kicking, and the swing phase of walking and running.[35,36] In each of these activities, the movement sequence was initiated by proximal muscles. The proximal joints achieved maximum acceleration before the distal joints. In fact, the proximal joints generally began to decelerate before the achievement of maximal limb velocity. Putnam notes that there is an interaction that occurs between the most distal and proximal segment—shoulder-wrist, hip-ankle—that is inde-

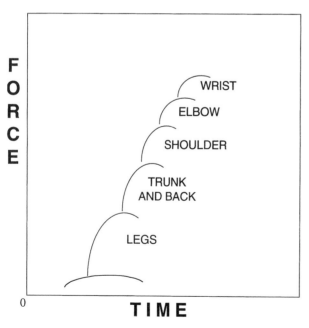

FIGURE 7-1 *Demonstration of proximal-distal summation of forces from the ground through the legs, trunk, shoulder, elbow, and wrist during a throwing or swinging task. Altered timing or force generation/transmission at any level may result in poor performance as well as pathology at any other level. Pathology is probably propagated from the ground to the wrist. (From Kibler WB,[112] with permission.)*

pendent of the middle segment, the elbow or knee.

The motions analyzed by Putnam share certain similarities. All these movements involve producing an optimal velocity of the free distal segment (which may or may not be holding an object) with accuracy. Chapman and Sanderson[4] found that the proximal-distal activation sequence produces optimal results in throwing and kicking when computer modeling techniques are used. Maximal performance followed a proximal to distal pattern, regardless of whether maximal velocity or maximal distance thrown was the end goal. Some alteration in the kinematics of the throw were noted, but not in the pattern of accelerations.

De Kooning et al.[37] found a proximal to distal coordination of leg muscles during speed skating. They noted that the velocity of the upper leg segment reached a maximum before the lower leg segment, confirming the proximal-distal sequence. Speed skating has constraints imposed by the frictive conditions of the ice and the skates themselves, producing a learned pattern of activation. No difference was noted in the timing sequence between elite and trained skaters. Elite skaters are, however, able to maintain optimal hip, knee, and trunk angles and produce more power.

The proximal to distal sequence is also found during the sprint push-off.[38] Muscle activation and power generation proceed in an olderly fashion from proximal to distal. Jacobs and van Ingen Schnau state that almost all the muscles of the leg produce positive power during the sprint push-off. Nitz et al. (see ch. 2) suggest that the proximal to distal sequence is characteristic of concentric, power-creating movements of the extremities. Indeed, the proximal to distal sequence is repeated in jumping.[39,40]

In contrast, Scholz et al.[41] found a distal to proximal sequence of activation of vastus lateralis with respect to erector spinae during repetitive lifting. This relationship was unchanged by the amount of load. These were the only two muscles that were monitored, and joint movements were not calculated. Subjects were instructed to lift with their legs, which may have

produced an adaptation in the usual proximal to distal sequence of explosive tasks[42] as a result of imposed constraints.[21]

Distal to proximal sequencing is observed when landing from a jump. McNitt-Gray[43,44] observed early activation of the ankle extensors followed by the knee and then hip extensors. Peak angular velocity also follows this pattern, but not net joint moments.[44] Joint moments peaked first at the knee, followed by the ankle and hip, which are linked together. This pattern is consistent for different drop heights and skill levels of subjects (gymnasts versus recreational athletes). Dyhre-Poulsen[45] found that the ankle muscles were activated before touch-down and initiated a distal to proximal sequence upon landing. The timing was not affected by skill level in the gymnasts studied. Similar results were found by McKinley and Pedotti.[46]

Emergence of Skill

The emergence of coordinated, skilled movements has not been widely studied. Bernstein[47] suggested that developing coordinated movements involves imposing constraints on the available movement choices. The rigid sequencing that occurs in repetitive sports-related movements implies that, under known conditions, the human successfully limits his choices to a narrow band of efficient movements. When the conditions are changed by altering the environment, the athlete chooses from a repertoire of movement strategies that have been learned over time, strategies that have proven effective in similar situations.[48]

Developing skilled movements involves creating a dynamic, controlled system that is responsive to various environmental and goal conditions.[49] Using kicking as a model, Anderson and Sidaway[50] analyzed the changes that occurred in novice soccer kickers after 20 sessions of practice. The results showed that, with practice, terminal velocity of the foot increased by 50 percent. Greater motion occurred at the hip and knee joints, and the kick motion began to acquire the stylized timing of trained kickers. Young and Marteniuk[51] undertook a similar study. They found that the interjoint power and force relationships became constrained with practice. The kicking motion became highly sequenced in a proximal to distal fashion, as previously described.

Motor learning and control theory lists several factors as being important in the development of sports skills. They are memory, transfer of existing skills, attention, knowledge of results, knowledge of process, and practice.[1,2,52,53] Imagery may play a role in sports performance, but the impact of imaging on learning sports skills is probably minor.[54]

Movement Strategies

A movement strategy is a multilink pattern of muscle activation to preserve the stability or capability of the body.[55] This includes maintaining a stable eye or head position, retaining knowledge of vertical and gravity, orientation of the limbs, maintaining center of gravity over a base of support, and retaining flexibility to modulate the muscular response.[55] The strategy may seek to preserve any of these variables first, eliciting a synergistic pattern related to the parameter being preserved. Horak and Nashner[56] suggest that the sensory input from the ankle may be the triggering response to these synergies. Keshner et al.[57] proposed that upper body proprioceptive responses of the head and neck may be just as important.

Using this definition, a movement strategy is any synergistic pattern that is used by the central nervous system (CNS) to maintain or change its orientation in order to perform a desired task, ranging from postural stabilization to landing from a gymnastic leap.

Response, Reaction and Movement Time

Reaction time (RT) is defined as the interval from the onset of a stimulus to the initiation of movement. Movement time (MT) begins when RT ends, and is measured from the end of RT to the completion of a task. Together, MT and RT equal response time.[58] In general, MT increases as a function of the complexity of the task and the accuracy needed during the task.[59] Reaction time and movement time are not correlated. Reaction time is further broken down into sensing time and decision time. The subject senses a stimulus and then must select the appropriate or best movement strategy to initiate a successful response. In terms of sports, this constitutes choosing the correct strategy to avoid an obstacle or to track and intercept a moving object.

Harbin et al. define the oculomotor response as RT plus MT and precision of movement.[58] They studied the ability of athletes of various sports and levels of competition to react to a visual stimulus and choose the correct movement strategy in response to the stimulus. They found no difference in oculomotor response between football and basketball players of equal skill levels. There were significant differences between athletes of the professional level and all others, indicating that RT is a skill that athletes at higher competitive levels refine. Harbin et al. also noted that response time declined significantly as the season progressed, and that athletes who suffered injuries tended to have lower response times than athletes who did not get injured.[58]

Taimela and Kujala[60] measured RTs in adolescent athletes as a function of participation in sports and of injury. They found that adolescent athletes who had injuries had slower RTs in simple tasks than those who did not have injuries. Adolescent athletes and nonathletes did not have significantly different RTs during simple tasks. This may have been a function of the age of the participants and the reaction test used to measure. This was a simple RT test requiring subjects to push a button after a light flashed.

The ability to quickly and accurately react is clearly a skill that athletes try to maximize. This is particularly true of the team sports such as baseball, football, soccer, hockey, as well as other individual competitive sports (tennis, squash). Research into the measurement and testing of this movement skill will probably be a rewarding area.

Visual Skills—Tracking, Catching, Orientation

Some of the roles of vision in movement are reviewed in Chapter 1. Vision as a sports skill involves tracking of objects and orientation of the body. Trained athletes often have different or more task-effective strategies for using visual information.[61–67] Orientation of the body and head is included in this section since vision is essential for maintaining awareness of the vertical position and identifying the location of the head in space.[68–70]

Rézette and Amblard[68] measured the importance of vision in orienting the body while subjects performed gymnastic leaps under varying lighting conditions. They concluded that visual cues during motion are necessary to allow the body to prepare and stabilize upon landing. This is a combination of orientation of the body and awareness of the location of the ground. It is interesting that two of the gymnasts were unable to complete the leaps in darkness due to vertigo, indicating that the vestibular system is linked to the visual in maintaining awareness of the vertical under certain conditions.[68] Vision seems to be primary to vestibular for these purposes.

Fairly complex computations based upon visual data must be undertaken in order to track, intercept, or catch a moving object.[61,70] These computations are made more difficult by the need to include time to initiate muscle contractions (approximately 100 msec) as well as make any last minute movement changes necessary to accomplish the task. Regardless, baseball players and other athletes who must run to catch a ball are capable of computing ball trajectories and accelerations by using both spatial cues as well as just velocity estimations of the ball. This is a characteristic of the visual system that is highly developed in athletes who need to track rapidly moving objects. Ishigaki and Miyao[65] determined that athletes were able to identify the physical characteristics of objects moving at higher velocities than nonathletes. They termed this ability visual acuity.

The ability to acquire a target, visually fixate,

and stabilize the head during a sports activity was measured by Ripoll et al.[66] They found that experienced basketball players were better able to locate the basket, orient the head, and maintain visual contact with the basket during a jump shot better than unexperienced players. Moreover, during free-throw shooting, experienced athletes focus on the basket better than unexperienced ones. Roll et al.[71] found that appropriate aiming was essential for successful completion of an aiming task.

Athletes also use different visual strategies to search their environment for cues. Search strategies are particularly important in sports that require tracking of rapidly moving people or objects (baseball, football, volleyball, racquet sports, soccer, etc.). Visual search strategies have been studied in volleyball,[72] soccer,[63] and racquet sports.[64,65] Athletes are able to scan their environment more rapidly, identify appropriate cues, and initiate a movement response faster and more accurately than nonathletes. This coordination between the visual and proprioceptive systems should be evaluated in the course of orthopaedic and sports physical therapy.

It is not surprising that athletes have different visual skills than nonathletes, given the link between vision and proprioception in targeting,[73] orientation,[67–70] and awareness of the environment during locomotion and complex tasks.[21,73,74] Their visual skills and the capability to trigger movement strategies are two of the factors that separate athletes from nonathletes in terms of performance. Functional training programs should take this into account and incorporate visual input into the functional training progressions of injured athletes. Visual-proprioceptive training exercises can be used in the treatment of nonathletes as well. The training of proprioceptive skills is accepted as a normal aspect of orthopedic and sports physical therapy. Movement skills implies that vision must be integrated into our approach to make proprioceptive training more functional. Training devices such as the Fastex (Cybex), which provide visual cues for movement and reaction time rehabilitation, will probably become more important as this aspect of movement recovery is explored in the rehabilitation of athletes.

Paradoxically, elite athletes are able to perform stylized activities better than less trained athletes in the absence of vision. Dancers and gymnasts are able to perform leaps and twists without visual cues. It appears that the visual cues provided during these activities are not essential to the completion of the movement. As mentioned earlier, however, landing from a leap or jump is much easier when vision is utilized. In these instances, elite athletes are better able to repeat a well practiced motion without visual cues. In another example, power lifters are able to reproduce the lifting technique with greater consistency and accuracy without vision.[75] Video analysis shows that highly trained lifters are able to reproduce accurately the kinematic parameters of a powerlift squat at 50 percent maximum weight when blindfolded.

Most athletes are aware of the importance of vision and visual control within their sport. Sports-related eye trauma makes up a significant percentage of severe eye injuries.[76] Protective eyewear is becoming more prevalent in high speed sports such as football, hockey, and racquetball. Yet, two sports in which objects can easily cause eye trauma, baseball and basketball, do not require eye protection. One concern that an athlete may have is the limitation of visual field by protective eyewear. Miller and Miller[76] found that the use of polycarbonate goggles does not affect the visual field of an athlete or their ability to identify targets of varying intensity and size.

Sports Movements

Certain movements are basic to many sports. Of interest here are the movements of jumping, cutting, catching, and throwing. These movement skills represent the primary movements involved in many injuries, particularly acute rather than overuse injuries. These are the movements that require a balance of physical and neuromuscular skills during their performance. Failure of one

of the systems (proprioceptive, muscular, visual) to function optimally may result in an injury. Running and walking have been extensively studied and are not included in the sports movement section.

CUTTING AND PIVOTING

Cutting refers to the mechanism by which running athletes change direction.[77] Cutting can also be applied to walking, but the forces involved are much lower and do not present a challenge to the neuromuscular system. Difficulty with cutting activities is one of the hallmarks of ACL-deficient knees.

The cutting mechanism has three components—deceleration, plant and cut, and take-off.[77] The deceleration phase is characterized by quadriceps contraction to slow the forward motion.[78] Planting and cutting is distinguished by rotation of the pelvis and torso over the knee and ankle. Finally, the take-off phase is characterized by acceleration in the chosen direction, with activity of gastrocnemius-soleus, quadriceps, and probably, hip extensors.

Andrews et al.[77] categorizes cutting as either side-step or crossover. No other classification of cutting is offered in the literature. This maneuver is more complex than that simple classification. A runner may cut-off of either foot in any direction. Schot et al.[79] found different forces exerted on a force plate depending upon the angle of the cut. Andriacchi[80] suggests that a motor program exists that may limit the cutting choices made by athletes with ligament deficiencies (Fig. 7–2). This raises questions as to how the CNS selects a cutting strategy in response to obstacles on a playing field. If the cutting mechanism is altered, as suggested by Andriacchi[80] and Shiavi et al.,[78] it remains to be seen if the normal mechanism can be reprogrammed. Research by Gauffin and Tropp[26] and Zätterström[25] suggests that muscle patterns altered by ACL injury can be rehabilitated, although timing alterations persist after rehabilitation.[81,82] External bracing does not alter the timing patterns in ACL deficient patients.[81] The electromyography (EMG) hallmark of ACL deficiency appears to be altered hamstring timing.[78,80–82] Bullock-Saxton et al.[83] have shown that muscles inhibited by injury can be retrained to function normally during gait activities. The challenge to physical therapists is to identify the movement changes that occur following injury and develop techniques to restore them. Sometimes, this requires learning a new strategy, one that enables the movement at high performance levels without risking injury.

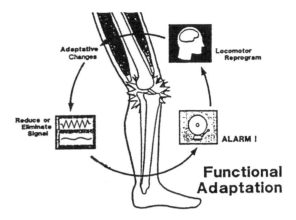

FIGURE 7-2 **(B)** *Proposed mechanism for generation of a new motor program that results in adaptive avoidance of quadriceps use during locomotion. The neural information presented by the knee joint is abnormal, forcing the CNS to take protective action. The new motor program must be counteracted by emphasizing normal use of lower extremity muscle and encouraging quadriceps function. (From Andriacchi TP,[80] with permission.)*

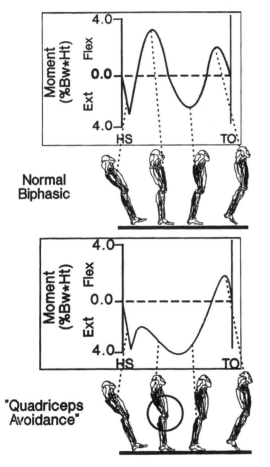

FIGURE 7-2 **(A)** *Illustration of the "quadriceps avoidance" gait. The normal knee forces are altered by the ACL deficient patient to avoid the movements that require quadriceps activity to counteract the knee flexion that would ordinarily occur in gait. It is hypothesized that reducing the need to use the quadriceps eliminates strain on the ACL. (From Andriacchi TP,[111] with permission.)*

JUMPING

Jumping is a common sports activity that is, in reality, a complex movement skill. Jumping consists of two broad phases—take-off and landing. Most injuries associated with jumping are a result of landing and attempting to move or pivot during or after landing.[84–86] Factors that contribute to injury include total force, landing surfaces, and symmetry of landing. Forces generated by landing also characterize many running injuries.

The impact force created by landing is related to jump height.[43,44] Landing strategies are altered by increased landing height. Trained gymnasts are able to anticipate the forces involved with increased heights and adjust their muscle response better than recreational athletes. Sports participants who suddenly find themselves higher in the air than usual (e.g., a skier going too fast over a mogul) may be at risk when landing, since they may not be able to adjust their landing strategy for the increased height, longer air time, and higher forces involved. A proposed mechanism is that the forces involved overwhelm the musculoskeletal system, whose landing strategy is geared toward a different set of anticipated mechanical variables.

The landing surface also plays a role in the strategy selected for landing. The shock-absorbing characteristics of the landing surface affect the forces imparted to the musculoskeletal system. McNitt-Gray et al.,[81] however, suggest that the presence of a mat does not necessarily imply that lower forces will be present upon landing, depending upon landing technique. The position of the body and the activity performed in the air may cause higher or lower impact forces and may affect the athlete's motor program upon landing.[46]

Gauffin and Tropp examined the landing patterns of ACL-deficient subjects during one-legged hop for distance.[26] They found that the ACL-deficient leg exhibited higher forces at touch-down particularly at the knee. Higher flexion angles for the hip and knee were noted. Electromyography (EMG) of the quadriceps had lower values in the injured leg, which may indicate an avoidance strategy.[80] Small deficits on isokinetic testing of the involved quadriceps were noted, but all subjects were participating in high levels of athletic activity. No data are offered on the strength of the hip or ankle, which may play a role in the landing strategy of the subject. Changes in hip[29] or ankle[30] muscle function as a result of ankle sprains can be as detrimental to controlling landing forces as ACL deficiency.

CATCHING

One of the most challenging sports activities is catching. It requires the ability to track a moving object, move to meet that object, and then place the hands precisely to catch the ball or hit it with a racquet. The visual tracking skills involved in catching a ball have been discussed earlier in this chapter.

The catcher uses information gathered from visual and spatial data to estimate the location and time of contact of the moving object (Fig. 7–3).[88] The expected location of the ball is then estimated with respect to the catcher, probably using the eye as a reference frame. As we will see, it may not be necessary to actually see the ball into the hands. It appears that using a glove improves catching without visual control. Bare-handed catchers (i.e., football players) are advised to use as much visual input as possible, including following the ball into the grasp.[89] The catcher must then transform that data into coordinates that can be used to orient the hand, shoulder, head, and eye. After that, positioning of the hands can be made for the catch and the hand muscles must be triggered to close the glove or grab the ball. It is not surprising that errors can often occur, particularly when the catcher is running and other participants are prepared to hit him as soon as the catch is made.

Fischman and Mucci[89] investigated the role of a glove in the catching task. They found that the glove made the catching task easier, regardless of whether visual feedback of the glove was present. They hypothesized that the glove reduced the positioning accuracy requirements and grasp timing normally needed for catching. When the glove was not used, peripheral vision of the limb was a necessary input for controlling grasp timing. In football, receivers do not use gloves, and peripheral vision is often occupied by the presence of defenders. The result is often that a ball hits a receiver in the hands, but is not caught due to poor timing of the grasp. Diggles et al.[90] found that athletes skilled in catching sports required less visual feedback than athletes unskilled in catching tasks.

Muscle Function in Sports

Surprisingly, comprehensive studies of muscle activity while performing sports techniques are relatively scarce, probably due to the technical problems associated with physiologic and biomechanical investigation of very dynamic activities. The biomechanics laboratory at the Kerlan-Jobe clinic has provided EMG and biomechanical analysis of a wide variety of sports, particu-

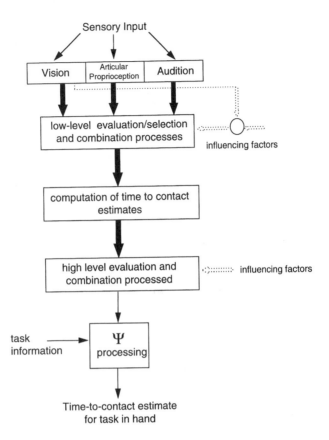

FIGURE 7-3 *Factors involved in a tracking task, such as catching or striking a ball. Note that computation and processing are influenced by cognitive (task) information and other factors at many levels. (From Treslian JR,[88] with permission.)*

larly with regard to shoulder function. For the most part, the lower extremities are involved with running, supporting the upper body, maintaining balance, and generating power that can be transmitted through the spine and utilized by the upper extremities for throwing, striking, and other skill activities. The following is a review of these studies, with supplemental information regarding the sports being investigated.

BASEBALL

Batting

Baseball has two skilled activities that have been studied, hitting and throwing. Catching has not been investigated in the field. Batting represents a combination of skills that includes balance, weight shifting, kinetic linkage, and tracking.[91] The end goal is to contact the ball with maximum velocity of the bat. Shaffer et al.[92] di-

vides the batting swing into four phases—wind-up, preswing, swing, and follow-through. (Fig. 7-4).

The wind-up phase is a time of relatively low muscle activity, as the bat and body are prepared to generate the forces to be used during the swing. Preswing is characterized by increasing hip (hamstring and gluteus maximus), trunk, and quadriceps (VMO) activity, as the body begins to generate the power used in the swing. Posterior deltoid and triceps activity were present during this phase. The swing phase is characterized by continued increase in vastus medialis oblique (VMO) activity, along with a strong weight shift toward the leading leg. Once weight shift is accomplished, the EMG activity in the back leg diminishes. Trunk activity in both the abdominals and erector spinae remains high, while deltoid, triceps, and serratus activity does not reach high relative values. This is probably

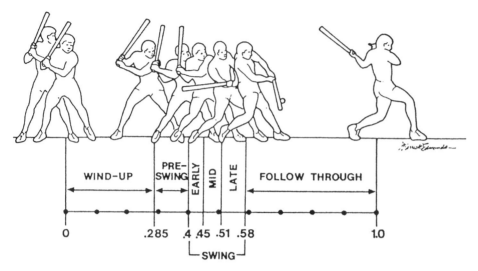

FIGURE 7-4 *Phases of the batting swing. (From Shaffer B et al.,[92] with permission.)*

representative of the importance of the legs and trunk in generating bat speed, while the role of the upper extremities is to place the bat and maintain position. The legs drive the body forward while the trunk muscles serve to provide rotation. Upper extremity muscle activity is highest at the later stages of the swing, marking the end of force progression from the legs to the trunk to the arms.

The coordination of muscle activation is in line with the mechanical aspects of batting. The body coordinates the movements of the lower extremities, trunk, and arms to generate bat speed by utilizing a kinetic linkage.[92] Higher velocities are achieved when timing between the links is optimized. Appropriate weight shift and control of balance is maintained by the nature of the stride, which occurs between wind-up and swing. This is one of the more variable components of hitting. Ideally, weight shift will occur only in lateral direction, but some anterior-posterior shifting is inevitable.

Pitching/Throwing

Pitching is comprised of the wind-up, cocking (early and late), acceleration (throwing), and follow-through phases (Fig. 7-5). Other types of throws have these phases, but may lack the stylized wind-up that is present in pitching. EMG analysis of pitching has been performed by Jobe et al.[93,94] and Gowan et al.[95]

The cocking phase is characterized by deltoid activity in the early stage, as the arm is elevated to 90 degrees. The activity of the deltoid decreases as cocking continues, while the rotator cuff increases its activity for stabilization and in preparation for acceleration. The serratus anterior and pectoralis major are also active in late cocking. Serratus anterior, pectoralis major, subscapularis, and latissimus dorsi are active in the acceleration phase. The posterior rotator cuff, posterior deltoid, and trapezius are the most active muscles in the follow-through phase.

Two important distinctions must be made. First, professional and amateur pitchers show different patterns of muscle use, indicating a skill level-related pattern of coordinated muscle use. Professionals appear to be more efficient and selective in the use of their rotator cuff and scapular stabilizers.[12] Throwers with instability demonstrate markedly different patterns of use with decreased activity of the scapula stabilizers, increased usage of the supraspinatus during cocking and acceleration, and decreased func-

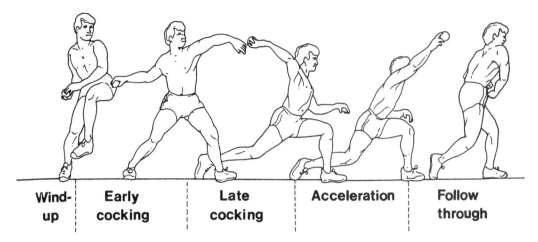

| Wind-up | Early cocking | Late cocking | Acceleration | Follow through |

FIGURE 7-5 *Phases of the baseball pitch. (From Glousman R,[12] with permission.)*

tion of the subscapularis and pectoralis major in protecting the anterior shoulder.[96] This type of altered function in the glenohumeral and scapular rotators is a consistent finding in patients with instability, regardless of direction.[97–99]

The importance of the coordinated nature of upper extremity muscles in throwing is emphasized by the lack of correlation between strength measures of the arm muscles and throwing speed. Pedegana et al.[100] and Bartlett et al.[101] found minor relationships between strength of selected muscles measured on a Cybex II dynamometer. Pedegana found a relationship between elbow and wrist extension and speed, while Bartlett noted a weak correlation between adductor strength and throwing speed. This underscores the notion that most of the velocity generated in the throw is a result of the kinetic chain forces generated in the lower extremities and trunk. The major purpose of the arm may be to position the hand in space while imparting the generated forces to the ball. The upper extremity is also responsible for controlling the timing of the force progression (Fig. 7-1). Injury to the stabilizers of the joint or overuse syndromes will interfere with this timing mechanism, reducing performance both in terms of velocity of the throw and accuracy.

Throwing is not limited to baseball. Throwing is a basic motion in football (quarterback), javelin, hammer, water polo, jai alai, and bowling. These sports differ from baseball in that the exact motion varies. Some throwing activities do not have the same overhead motions. Water polo does not utilize ground reaction force to generate ball speed. All throwing activities involve some involvement of cocking, acceleration, and follow-through. Therapists should analyze each sport in terms of the forces involved in the throw and where they are generated. The pitch in baseball and the serve in tennis represent two extremes of overhead motions. These two movements present the athlete with the combined need for coordinated movement and generation and control of high forces.

TENNIS

The phases of the tennis serve and stroke are similar to that of throwing. The serve has the same phases as throwing, except that cocking is not divided into two stages (Fig. 7-6A). This is due to the contribution of the trunk in both lateral flexion and rotation.[102] The groundstrokes do not have a cocking phase since the shoulder has minimal elevation during these activities.

Since cocking is absent in groundstrokes, the muscle function during forehand and backhand movements is fairly simple. Subscapularis, pectoralis major, biceps brachii, and serratus ante-

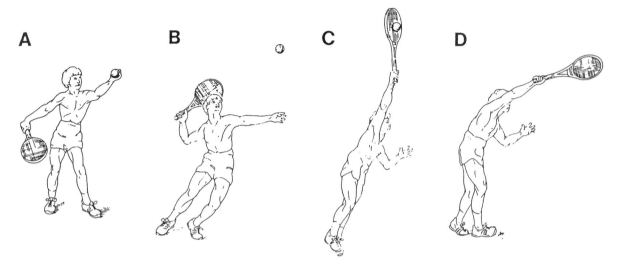

FIGURE 7-6 *Phases of the tennis serve. Note the absence of a biphasic cocking stage. (From Ryu RK et al.,[102] with permission.)*

rior are active in the acceleration phase of the forehand, while the middle deltoid, infraspinatus, and supraspinatus contribute to acceleration during the backhand. The external rotators are responsible for deceleration during the forehand. The subscapularis accomplishes this task during the backhand. Once again, the role of the upper extremity is to position and control the racquet while transferring power from the legs and trunk.

The serve involves greater forces and movement of the arm. Coordinated function of the upper and lower extremities with the trunk produces the power behind a tennis serve. Increased activity of the trunk is used to bring the arm into proper position, without the robust deltoid and rotator cuff activity noted during the cocking phase of throwing. The subscapularis is active in decelerating the cocking motion and, together with pectoralis major, rapidly internally rotates and adducts the humerus to keep pace with the trunk motions. Serratus anterior is active in maintaining the scapula position on the thoracic wall, which contributes to efficient function of the subscapularis and serves as a platform for the humerus.

One of the major differences between throw-ing and the tennis serve is the nature of the aiming activities involved. In throwing, only one type of aiming control is required—delivering the ball to a target. Serving incorporates some elements of catching, in that the racquet must be aimed to contact the thrown ball at an optimal point in space. The sensorimotor elements that function during reaching are probably active at this time. From a movement skills viewpoint, serving is probably more difficult than throwing; there are more elements that must be controlled and computed. The ball toss must be performed accurately; otherwise, the serve will be less effective, since the trunk and arm positions must be adjusted to match the ball position.[103]

GOLF

The phases of the golf swing include the take-away, forward swing, acceleration, and follow-through (early and late). Figure 7-7 illustrates the golf swing phases.[104] Golf uses the upper extremities in a similar fashion to batting, in that both arms are moving through essentially the same motions. The lateral trunk flexion that characterizes tennis serving and pitching is not present in golf. Neither are the extreme shoulder

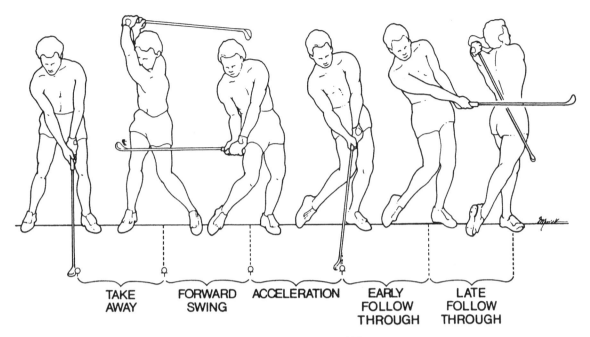

FIGURE 7-7 *Phases of the golf swing. (From Jobe FW et al.,[104] with permission.)*

accelerations generated in throwing and serving. This may account for the relatively low muscle activity in the rotator cuff, although the subscapularis may be very active throughout the golf swing.

The muscle activity generated in the arms is almost symmetrical for each of the phases.[104,105] Little deltoid activity is present, related to the minimal elevation of the humerus that occurs. Rotator cuff activity is present in all phases, particularly in the subscapularis in all phases but swing,[104] and the infraspinatus during follow-through. Jobe et al.[104] found no difference between men and women in the relative activation of any muscles measured during the swing.

The golf swing does not have the forceful drive of the legs that is present in batting, but coordination of the legs and trunk to maintain postural stability and achieve adequate trunk rotation is essential to maximal velocity of the club head. In the golf swing, contributions of the pectoralis major and latissimus dorsi may contribute more to the velocity of club than these muscles do in acceleration during the tennis serve or batting.

Swimming

Swimming strokes are comprised of two phases, pull-through and recovery, both of which have an early and late stage (Fig. 7-8).[13,106,107] Swimming represents an entirely different mechanical situation than dry land sports. The action of the legs goes into propulsion, rather than creating reaction forces to be utilized by the trunk and arms. The upper extremities also play

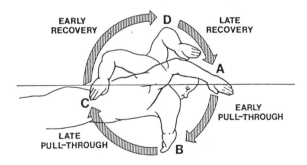

FIGURE 7-8 *Phases of the freestyle swimming crawl stroke. (From Pink M et al.,[13] with permission.)*

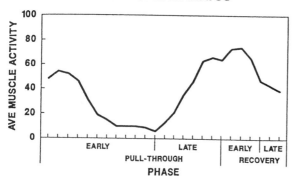

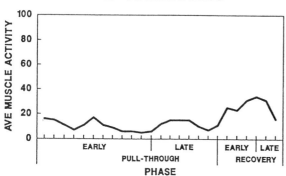

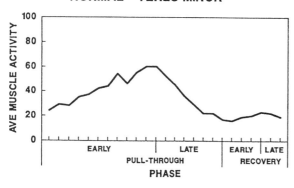

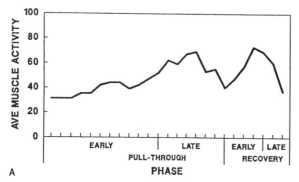

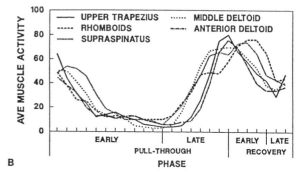

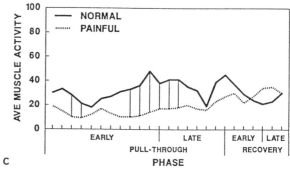

FIGURE 7-9 **(A)** *Muscle activity of the normal rotator cuff during the freestyle crawl stroke. Note that each muscle has peaks at different times during the stroke cycle. (From Pink M et al.,[13] with permission.)* **(B)** *Muscles acting in phase during the freestyle stroke cycle. These are considered to be the prime movers. Note that the group includes scapula stabilizers/rotators (rhomboid and upper trapezius), a glenohumeral stabilizer (supraspinatus) and glenohumeral movers (middle and anterior deltoid). (From Pink M et al.,[13] with permission.)* **(C)** *Comparison of electromyographic activity of the scapular stabilizers in normal and painful freestyle swimming. There is a change both in timing and amplitude of the activity. These muscles show the greatest change in activity along with the deltoid group, which did not show timing changes. The change in EMG of the rotator cuff in painful swimming is minimal (From Scovazzo ML et al.,[107] with permission.)*

a major role in propulsion, with latissimus dorsi and pectoralis major contributing to propulsion during the pull-through phase. Interestingly, latissimus and pectoralis major do not peak simultaneously. Pectoralis major peaks in early pull-through while latissimus peaks in late pull-through. This may be an example of what Perry terms reciprocal phasing.[108]

The middle and anterior deltoid are necessary to elevate the arm during the recovery (early) phase. All three portions increase their activity at the end of pull-through in preparation for recovery. The rotator cuff muscles do not function as a unit; rather, they show discrete patterns.[13] Each muscle peaks at different times during the freestyle stroke (Fig. 7-9). Infraspinatus peaks during late recovery and is relatively inactive during the stroke cycle. Subscapularis is relatively active throughout the stroke cycle, with peaks during late pull-through and early recovery. Teres minor is most active during the pull-through phase. Supraspinatus shows the

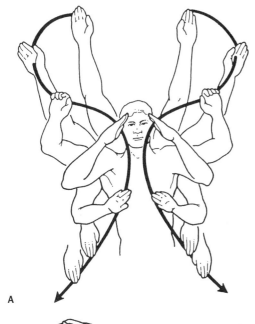

A

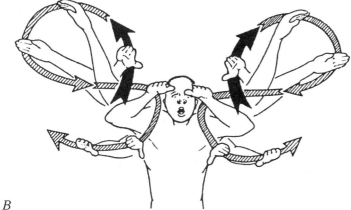

B

FIGURE 7-10 *Comparison of the S-shaped pull between the freestyle* **(A)** *and the butterfly* **(B)**. *The movements are accomplished by action of the teres minor and pectoralis major in early pull-through, followed by the latissimus dorsi, posterior deltoid, middle, and then anterior deltoid, carrying the arm into the recovery phase. Both strokes retain similar timing in the functions of these muscles. (From Pink M et al.,[13] and Pink M et al.,[109] with permission.)*

greatest swings of activity, going from almost zero activity in the middle of the pull-through to 80 percent of maximal voluntary contraction (MVC) in early recovery.

Some of the muscles function in phase with each other. The patterns of upper trapezius, rhomboids, supraspinatus, middle deltoid, and anterior deltoid are almost identical. Their maximal activities correspond with hand entry into and exit from the water. The timing and rhythm of the muscle patterns provides a unique S-shaped path in the water during pull-through followed by a circular shoulder movement during recovery.

The timing and pattern of activity is disrupted in the painful shoulder. Rarely do the muscles of a painful shoulder generate the same peaks as in the normal shoulder, and the peaks that are produced are out of phase with the normal pattern of activity. In freestyle swimming, serratus anterior is notably affected, resulting in inadequate scapular stabilization. Rhomboids fire abnormally to compensate for serratus, but they do not have the same function, resulting in altered scapular mechanics. The pattern of the rotator cuff is relatively unaffected, as are the propulsive muscles. Failure of the scapular muscles to function normally results in changed glenohumeral mechanics, and can result in impingement.[107]

The butterfly stroke movement pattern is affected by pain slightly differently from the freestyle.[109,110] The rotator cuff shows a marked change in the manner in which it functions, particularly the teres minor, which is severely inhibited. Serratus is again affected strongly, particularly during the pull-through phase. In the butterfly, serratus is apparently compensated for by latissimus dorsi. The differences between the freestyle and butterfly are probably explained by the symmetry of the two strokes. Both shoulders are in phase during the butterfly, while they are out of phase in freestyle. The compensation or protective strategy is based upon the capacity of muscles to stabilize the scapula. In butterfly, both rhomboids are contracting together and reach higher peaks than in butterfly. The S-pattern of movement in the two strokes is different

(Fig. 7-10), which also influences which muscles are available for contribution. The timing and progression of activity are similar, however.

Conclusion

The muscles of the arm generate precise, coordinated patterns of activity that are associated with skilled movements in athletes. This is accompanied by a transfer of force from the legs through the trunk and into the arms during dry land sports. Recognition of altered muscle patterns must occur when pain is present. Treatment progressions that move from isolated strengthening to precise patterning of activity should be utilized in rehabilitation. Careful examination of movement patterns during rehabilitation and in the early phases of reconditioning should be made to ensure that skilled, coordinated movement is being recreated.

References

1. Adams JA: Historical review and appraisal of research in the learning, retention, and transfer of human motor skills. Psychol Bull 101:41–74, 1987
2. Annett J: The learning of motor skills: sports science and ergonomics perspectives. Ergonomics 37:5–16, 1993
3. Nicholas JA, Grossman RB, Hershman EB: The importance of a simplified classification of motion in sports relation to performance. Orthop Clin North Am 8:499–532, 1977
4. Chapman AE, Sanderson DJ: Muscular coordination in sporting skills. p. 608. In Winters JM, Woo SL-Y (eds): Multiple Muscle Systems: Biomechanics and Movement Organization. Springer Verlag, New York, 1990
5. Nicholas JA: Risk factors in sports medicine and the orthopedic system: an overview. J Sports Med 3:243–259, 1976
6. Considine W, Sullivan W: Relationship of selected tests of leg strength and leg power on college men. Res Quart Exer Sport 44:404–415, 1973

7. Mayhew JL, Piper FC, Schwegler TM et al: Contributions of speed, agility, and body composition to anaerobic power measurement in college football players. J Appl Sports Sci Res 3: 101–106, 1989

8. Murphy AI, Wilson GJ, Pryor JF: The use of isoinertial force mass relationship in the prediction of dynamic human performance. Eur J Appl Physiol 69:250–257, 1994

9. Sapega AA: Muscle performance evaluation in orthopaedic practice. J Bone Joint Surg 72A: 1562–1574, 1990

10. Abernethy P, Wilson G, Logan P: Strength and power assessment. Issues controversies and challenges. Sports Med 19:401–417, 1995

11. Tippett SR, Voight ML. Functional Progressions for Sports Rehabilitation. Human Kinetics Champaign, Ill. 1995

12. Glousman R: Electromyographic analysis and its role in the athletic shoulder. Clin Orth Rel Res 288:27–34, 1993

13. Pink M, Perry J, Browne A et al: The normal shoulder during freestyle swimming. An electromyographic and cinematographic analysis of twelve muscles. Am J Sports Med 19:569–576, 1991

14. Asmussen E, Bonde-Petersen F: Storage of elastic energy in skeletal muscles in man. Acta Physiol Scand 91:385–392, 1974

15. Bosco C, Komi P: Potentiation of the mechanical behavior of the human skeletal muscle through prestretching. Acta Physiol Scand 106:467–472, 1979

16. Chu D: Jumping into Plyometrics. Leisure Press, Champaign, IL, 1992

17. Wilk KE, Voight ML, Keirns MA et al: Stretch shortening drills for the upper extremities; theory and application. J Orthop Sports Phys Ther 17:225–237, 1993

18. Massion J: Postural control system. Curr Opinion Neurobiol 4:877–887, 1994

19. Mouchnino L, Aurenty R, Massion J et al: Coordination between equilibrium and head-trunk orientation during leg movement: a new strategy built up by training. J Neurophysiol 67: 1587–1598, 1992

20. Crotts D, Thompson B, Nahom M et al: Balance abilities of professional dancers on select balance tests. J Orthop Sports Phys Ther 23:12–17, 1996

21. Pedotti A, Crenna P, Deat A et al: Postural synergies in axial movements: short-and long-term adaptation. Exp Brain Res 74:3–10, 1989

22. Shick J, Stoner LJ, Jette N: Relationship between modern dance experience and balance performance. Res Q Exercise Sport 54:79–82, 1983

23. Koslow R: Patterns of weight shift in the swings of beginning golfers. Percept Mot Skills 79: 1296–1298, 1994

24. Era P, Konttinen N, Mehto P et al: Postural-stability and skilled performance—a study on top-level and naive rifle shooters. J Biomechanics 29: 301–306, 1996

25. Zätterström R, Fridén T, Lindstrand A et al: The effect of physiotherapy on standing balance in chronic anterior cruciate ligament insufficiency. Am J Sports Med 22:531–536, 1994

26. Gauffin H, Tropp H: Altered movement patterns and muscular-activation patterns during one-legged jump in patients with old anterior cruciate ligament rupture. Am J Sports Med 20: 182–192, 1992

27. Timoney JM, Inman WS, Quesada PM et al: Return of normal gait patterns after anterior cruciate ligament reconstruction. Am J Sports Med 21:887–889, 1993

28. Golomer E, Dupui P, Bessou P: Spectral frequency analysis of dynamic balance in healthy and injured athletes. Arch Int Physiol Biochem Biophys 102:225–229, 1994

29. Bullock-Saxton JE, Janda V, Bullock MI: The influence of ankle sprain injury on muscle activation during hip extension. Int J Sports Med 15: 330–334, 1994

30. Konradsen L, Ravn JB: Prolonged peroneal reaction time in ankle instability. Int J Sports Med 12:290–292, 1991

31. Konradsen L, Ravn JB, Sørensen AI: Proprioception at the ankle: the effect of anaesthetic blockade of ligament receptors. J Bone Joint Surg 75B: 433–436, 1993

32. Parkhurst TM, Burnett CN: Injury and proprioception in the lower back. J Orthop Sports Phys Ther 19:282–295, 1994

33. Andersson GBJ, Winters JM: Role of muscle in postural tasks: spinal loading and postural stability. p. 375. In Winters JM, Woo SL-Y (eds): Multiple Muscle Systems: Biomechanics and Movement Organization. Springer Verlag, New York, 1990

34. Gracovetsky S: Musculoskeletal function of the spine. p. 410. In Winters JM, Woo SL-Y (eds): Multiple Muscle Systems: Biomechanics and

Movement Organization. Springer Verlag, New York, 1990

35. Putnam CA: A segment interaction analysis of proximal to distal sequential segment motion patterns. Med Sci Sports Exer 23:130–144, 1991

36. Putnam CA: Sequential motions of body segments in striking and throwing skills: descriptions and explanations. J Biomechanics 26(suppl 1):125–135, 1993

37. De Kooning JJ, de Groot G, van Ingen Schnau GJ: Coordination of leg muscles during speed skating. J Biomechanics 24:137–146, 1991

38. Jacobs R, van Ingen Schnau GJ: Intermuscular coordination in a sprint push-off. J Biomechanics 25:953–965, 1992

39. Bobbert MF, van Ingen Schnau GJ: Coordination in vertical jumping. J Biomechanics 21: 241–262, 1988

40. Pandy MG, Zajc FE: Optimal muscular coordination strategies for jumping. J Bioemechanics 24:1–10, 1991

41. Scholz JP, Millford JP, McMillan AG: Neuromuscular coordination of squat lifting I: effect of load magnitude. Phys Ther 75:119–132, 1995

42. Gregoire L, Veeger HE, Huijing PA et al: Role of mono- and bi-articular muscles in explosive movements. Int J Sports Med 5:301–305, 1984

43. McNitt-Gray JL: Kinematics and impulse characteristics of drop landings from three heights. Int J Sport Biomech 7:201–204, 1991

44. McNitt-Gray JL: Kinetics of the lower extremities during drop landing from three heights. J Biomechanics 26:1037–1046, 1993

45. Dyhre-Poulsen P: An analysis of split leaps and gymnastic skill by physiological recordings. Eur J Appl Physiol 56:390–397, 1987

46. McKinley P, Pedotti A: Motor strategies in landing from a jump: the role of skill in task execution. Exp Brain Res 90:427–440, 1992

47. Bernstein NA: The Coordination and Regulation of Movements. Pergamon Press, Oxford, 1967

48. Sporns O, Edelman GM: Solving Bernstein's problem: a proposal for the development of coordinated movement by selection. Child Development 64:960–981, 1993

49. Vereijken B, van Emmerik REA, Whiting HTA et al: Free(z)ing degrees of freedom in skill acquisition. J Motor Behavior 24:133–142, 1992

50. Anderson DI, Sidaway B: Coordination changes associated with practice of a soccer kick. Res Q Exerc Sport 65:93–99, 1994

51. Young RP, Marteniuk RG: Changes in inter-joint relationships of muscle movements and powers accompanying the acquisition of a multi-articular kicking task. J Biomechanics 28:701–713, 1995

52. Shea JB, Hunt JP: Motor control. Clin Sports Med 3:171–183, 1984

53. Gentile AM: Skill acquisition. p. 93. In Carr JH, Sheperd RB (eds): Movement Science. Foundations for Physical Therapy in Rehabilitation. Aspen Publishers, Rockville, MD, 1987

54. Howe BL: Imagery and sports performance. Sports Med 11:1–5, 1991

55. Keshner EA, Allum JHJ: Muscle patterns coordinating postural stability. p. 480. In Winters JM, Woo SL-Y (eds): Multiple Muscle Systems: Biomechanics and Movement Organization. Springer Verlag, New York, 1990

56. Horak FB, Nashner LM: Central programming of postural movements: adaptations to altered support-surface configurations. J Neurophysiol 55:1369–1381, 1986

57. Keshner EA, Woollacott MH, Debu B: Neck and trunk muscle responses during postural perturbations in humans. Exp Brain Res 71:455–466, 1988

58. Harbin G, Durst L, Harbin D: Evaluation of oculomotor response in relationship to performance. Med Sci Sports Exer 21:258–262, 1989

59. Shumway-Cook A, Woollacott M: Motor Control. Theory and Practical Applications. Williams and Wilkins, Baltimore, 1995

60. Taimela S, Kujala UH: Reaction times with reference to musculoskeletal complaints in adolescence. Percept Mot Skills 75:1075–1082, 1992

61. McBeath MK, Shaffer DM, Kaiser MK: How baseball players determine where to run to catch fly balls. Science 268:569–573, 1995

62. Vom Hofe A, Fery YA: Is spatial judgement of ball trajectories a highly differentiated or hierarchically organized skill? Percept Mot Skills 76: 1091–1096, 1993

63. Williams AM, Davids K, Burwitz L et al: Visual search strategies in experienced and inexperienced soccer players. Res Q Exerc Sport. 65: 127–135, 1994

64. Ripoll H: Uncertainty and visual strategies in table tennis. Percept Mot Skills 68:507–512, 1989

65. Ishigaki H, Miyao M: Differences in dynamic visual acuity between athletes and nonathletes. Percept Mot Skills 77:835–839, 1993

66. Ripoll H, Bard C, Paillard J: Stabilization of the

head and eyes on target as a factor in successful basketball shooting. Hum Movement Sci 5: 47–58, 1986

67. Starkes JL, Gabrielle L, Young L: Performance of the vertical position in synchronized swimming as a function of skill, proprioceptive and visual feedback. Percept Mot Skills 69:225–226, 1989

68. Rézette D, Amblard B: Orientation versus motion visual cues to control sensorimotor skills in some acrobatic leaps. Hum Movement Sci 4: 297–306, 1985

69. Jeannerod M: The interaction of visual and proprioceptive cues in controlling reaching movements. p. 227. In Humphrey DR, Freund H-J (eds): Motor Control: Concepts and Issues. John Wiley & Sons, New York, 1991

70. Lacquaniti F, Carrozzo M, Borghese N: The role of vision in tuning anticipatory motor responses of the limbs. p. 379. In Berthoz A (ed): Multisensory Control of Movement. Oxford University Press, Oxford, 1993

71. Roll R, Bard C, Paillard J: Head orienting contributes to the directional accuracy of aiming at distant targets. Hum Movement Sci 5:359–371, 1986

72. Starkes JL, Edwards P, Dissanayake P et al: A new technology and field test of advance cue usage in volleyball. Res Q Exerc Sports 66: 162–167, 1995

73. Berthoz A, Pozzo T: Head and body coordination during locomotion and complex movements. p. 147. In: Swinnen SP, Massion J, Heuer H et al (eds): Interlimb Coordination: Neural, Dynamical, and Cognitive Constraints. Academic Press, San Diego, 1995

74. Thomson JA: How do we use visual information to control locomotion? TINS 3:247–250, 1980

75. Bennett S, Davids K: The manipulation of vision during the powerlift squat: exploring the boundaries of the specificity of learning hypothesis. Res Q Exerc Sports 66:210–218, 1995

76. Miller BA, Miller SJ: Visual fields with protective eyewear. J Orthop Sports Phys Ther 18:470–472, 1993

77. Andrews JR, McLeod WD, Ward T et al: The cutting mechanism. Am J Sports Med 5:111–121, 1977

78. Shiavi R, Limbird T, Borra H et al: Electromyography profiles of knee joint musculature during pivoting: changes induced by anterior cruciate ligament deficiency. J Electromyog Kinesiol 1: 49–57, 1991

79. Schot P, Dart J, Schuh M: Biomechanical analysis of two change-of-direction maneuvers while running. J Orthop Sports Phys Ther 22:254–258, 1995

80. Andriacchi TP: Dynamics of pathological motion: applied to the anterior cruciate deficient knee. J Biomechanics 23(suppl 1):99–105, 1990

81. Branch TP, Hunter R, Donath M: Dynamic EMG analysis of anterior cruciate deficient legs with and without bracing during cutting. Am J Sports Med 17:35–41, 1989

82. Kälund S, Sinkjaer T, Arendt-Nielsen L et al: Altered timing of hamstring muscle action in anterior cruciate ligament deficient patients. Am J Sports Med 18:245–248, 1990

83. Bullock-Saxton JE, Janda V, Bullock M: Reflex activation of gluteal muscles in walking with balance shoes: an approach to restoration of muscle function for chronic low back pain patients. Spine 18:704–708, 1993

84. Gerberich SG, Luhmann S, Finke C et al: Analysis of severe injuries associated with volleyball activities. Phys Sports Med 15:75–79, 1987

85. Gray J, Taunton JE, McKenzie DC et al: A survey of injuries to the anterior cruciate ligament of the knee in female basketball players. Int J Sports Med 6:314–316, 1985

86. Dufek JS, Bates BT. Biomechanical factors associated with injury during landing in jump sports. Int J Sports Med 12:326–337, 1991

87. McNitt-Gray JL, Yokoi T, Millward C: Landing strategies used by gymnasts on different surfaces. J Appl Biomechanics 10:237–252, 1994

88. Tresilian JR: Perceptual and motor processes in interceptive timing. Hum Movement Sci 13: 335–373, 1994

89. Fischman MG, Mucci WG: Influence of a baseball glove on the nature of errors produced in simple one-hand catching. Res Q Exerc Sport 60: 251–255, 1989

90. Diggles VA, Grabiner MD, Garhammer J: Skill level and efficacy of effector visual feedback in ball catching. Percept Mot Skills 64:987–993, 1987

91. Welch CM, Banks SA, Cook FF et al: Hitting a baseball: a biomechanical description. J Orthop Sports Phys Ther 22:193–201, 1995

92. Shaffer B, Jobe FW, Pink M et al: Baseball batting. An electromyographic study. Clin Orthop Rel Res 292:285–293, 1993

93. Jobe FW, Tibone JE, Perry J et al: An EMG analysis of the shoulder in throwing and pitching. A preliminary report. Am J Sports Med 11:3–5, 1983

94. Jobe FW, Moynes DR, Tibone JE et al: An EMG analysis of the shoulder in pitching. A second report. Am J Sports Med 12:218–220, 1984

95. Gowan ID, Jobe FW, Tibone JE et al: A comparative electromyographic analysis of the shoulder during pitching. Professional versus amateur pitchers. Am J Sports Med 15:586–590, 1987

96. Glousman RE, Jobe FW, Tibone JE et al: Dynamic EMG analysis of the throwing shoulder with glenohumeral instability. J Bone Joint Surg 70A:220–226, 1988

97. Broström, L-Å, Kronberg M, Nemeth G: Muscle activity during shoulder dislocation. Acta Orthop Scand 60:639–641, 1989

98. Kronberg M, Broström L-Å, Nemeth G: Differences in shoulder muscle activity between patients with generalized joint laxity and normal controls. Clin Orthop Rel Res 289:181–192, 1991

99. Pande P, Hawkins R, Peat M: Electromyography in voluntary posterior instability of the shoulder. Am J Sports Med 17:644–648, 1989

100. Pedegana LR, Elsner RC, Roberts D et al: Relationship of upper extremity strength to throwing speed. Am J Sports Med 10:352–354, 1982

101. Bartlett LR, Storey MD, Simons BD: Measurement of upper extremity torque production and its relationship to throwing speed in the competitive athlete. Am J Sports Med 17:89–91, 1989

102. Ryu RKN, McCormick J, Jobe FW et al: An electromyographic analysis of shoulder function in tennis players. Am J Sports Med 16:481–485, 1988

103. Elliott BC: Biomechanics of the serve in tennis. A biomedical perspective. Sports Med 6:295–294, 1988

104. Jobe FW, Perry J, Pink M: Electromyographic shoulder activity in men and women professional golfers. Am J Sports Med 17:782–787, 1989

105. Jobe FW, Moynes DR, Antonelli DJ. Rotator cuff function during a golf swing. Am J Sports Med 14:388–392, 1986

106. Nuber GW, Jobe FW, Perry J et al: Fine wire electromyography analysis of muscles of the shoulder during swimming. Am J Sports Med 14:7–11, 1986

107. Scovazzo ML, Browne A, Pink M et al: The painful shoulder during freestyle swimming. An electromyographic and cinematographic analysis of twelve muscles. Am J Sports Med 19:577–582, 1991

108. Perry J: Anatomy and biomechanics of the shoulder in throwing, swimming, gymnastics, and tennis. Clin Sports Med 2:247–270, 1983

109. Pink M, Jobe FW, Perry J et al: The normal shoulder during the butterfly stroke. Clin Orthop Rel Res 288:48–59, 1993

110. Pink M, Jobe FW, Perry J et al: The painful shoulder during the butterfly stroke. Clin Orthop Rel Res 288:60–72, 1993

111. Andriacchi TP, Birac D: Function testing in the anterior cruciate ligament-deficient knee. Clin Orthop Rel Res 288:40–47, 1993

112. Kibler WB: Evaluation of sports demands as a diagnostic tool in shoulder disorders. p. 379. In Matsen FA, Fu FH, Hawkins RJ (eds): The Shoulder: A Balance of Mobility and Stability. AAOS, Rosemont, IL, 1994

8

Movement and Function in Dance

MARIJEANNE LIEDERBACH

One of the most interesting aspects of dance is its fundamental difference from sports and the impact of that difference on functional movement and the restoration of skill following injury. There are three basic factors that distinguish dance from sport:

- Expressivity
- Extreme ankle and hip range of motion
- Lack of specificity and periodization in training

Distinctions of Dance

EXPRESSIVITY

Dancers and athletes share highly refined motor skills and an acquired finesse for detailed coordination and precision with timing. In dance, dramatic skills from the paradigms of theater and music are also applied to movement. Although some sports, like figure skating, gymnastics, and synchronized swimming also use theatrical elements, the athletes and coaches in those sports use theatricality for the purpose of promoting the presentation of movement skill accomplishment. In dance, by contrast, the use of theatrical elements is intended for development of expressivity and might ultimately override presentation

of movement skills in order to fulfill dramatic purpose.

EXTREME ANKLE AND HIP RANGE OF MOTION

With the exception of gymnasts, who often use dance as a training modality, dancers are required to achieve range of motion (ROM) at the ankle and hip that far exceeds the expectations of most other athletes:

1. Ballet requires its female participants to accomplish weight-bearing stances on the tips of the tarsal phalanges with greater than 90 degrees of ankle/foot plantar flexion, known as "relevé en pointe" (Fig. 8-1). Modern dancers assume a "demi-pointe relevé," requiring the same maximal foot and ankle plantar flexion, but with 90 degrees of dorsiflexion at the metatarsophalangeal (MTP) joints (Fig. 8-2).
2. Classical dancers are required to assume standing postures of bilateral external rotation of the lower extremities, known as "turnout," that approximate or meet a 180-degree angle.

LACK OF SPECIFICITY AND PERIODIZATION IN TRAINING

Dancers maintain regular daily training schedules[1] which intensify when they go into performance cycles. During those times, their work-

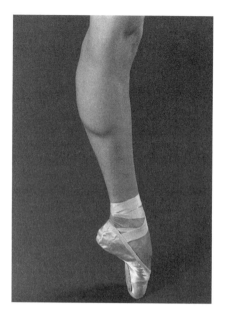

FIGURE 8-1 *Relevé en pointe.*

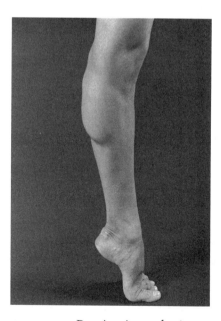

FIGURE 8-2 *Demi-pointe relevé.*

loads require significantly higher heart rates[2] and an increase of approximately 4 more hours of work per day.[3] Unlike athletes, however, dancers don't have predictable annual seasons where periods of rest follow the increased bouts of intensity, or a regulated training schedule that would provide a sense of goal orientation. Except in rare instances, they do not have reliable, objective measures of success such as trophies, game scores, or cash prizes indicating job security or personal success.[4] The closest a dancer usually gets to a sense of discernible achievement is through acceptance into an elite company or appointment of a coveted role within a company's repertory. Those rewards, however, are often short-term and unreliable in nature, and do not provide a sense of guaranteed status; they are typically governed by highly subjective and/or circumstantial criteria.

Serious ballet training typically begins by the age of 8 for females and 12 for males, and continues until age 17–20, at which time the dancer hopes to join a professional company. Some forms of dance, such as ballet, are strictly codified and are often representational and linear in their compositional structures. Other forms are more spontaneously inventive, abstract, and nonsequiturial in design and expression, making them more difficult to evaluate and replicate from the movement scientist's point of view.

Classical ballet dancers may train in one or more style of ballet, and in other dance disciplines such as modern, jazz, and ethnic dance. There are many different styles of modern dance technique, each of which embodies a unique vocabulary of movement with a particular stylistic emphasis on its dynamic and aesthetic approach.

A typical ballet class is 90 minutes in duration and always follows the same basic structure. Approximately 30 minutes is spent standing next to and holding lightly onto a barre, where exercises of increasingly complex and expansive leg motions that progressively integrate head, arm, and torso movements are practiced. This is followed by 1 hour in the center floor area of the studio, where slow, unsupported movement phrases, known as "adagio," are practiced. Then, quick, precise jumps that involve intricate footwork, known as "petit allegro," and turns are trained. Finally, big, traveling leaps, or "grand allegro," are practiced and the class ends with bows, called "reverence."

A survey of 3,000 dancers treated at a hospital-based orthopaedic dance clinic in New York City revealed that dancers, when asked to describe themselves as either students primarily of ballet, modern, both, or other, described themselves as serious students of *both* ballet and modern dance technique 92 percent of the time.[5]

Although this extent of cross-training exists among dancers, there is a glaring lack of specific training within dance for (1) the movements expected by choreographers who are responsible for evolving the art form with unique and inventive styling, and (2) the cardiovascular and musculoskeletal workloads dancers encounter during performance. These are two of many variables to be presented in this chapter that factor into the epidemiology of dance injuries.

Technical Aspects of Dance

DANCE-SPECIFIC MOTIONS

Performance demands in ballet differ between the sexes. Generally speaking, the women are asked to execute more precarious balance maneuvers (reduced surface area of the pointe shoe as opposed to the full-foot stances or demi-pointe relevé afforded the men) and rapid footwork. Men, in return, have traditionally been required to do more of the lifting and bravura-style jumping and leaping.

Nicholas et al.[6] created a motion scoring system to enable clinicians and educators to better understand the demands of varying sports and movement activities. They identified six fundamental movement categories: stance, walking, running, kicking, jumping, and throwing. Within dance, the motion categories relied on most were stance, kicking, and jumping, followed by running and throwing activities, with minimal involvement of walking activities.

In addition to these motions, dance movement also includes multiple variations of turning skills. Both genders are trained in turn skills, which can happen on one foot or two, knees, buttocks, shoulders, hands, or head, and can happen in either clockwise or counterclockwise direction, known in ballet as "en dehors" (outside) or "en dedans" (inside) turns. Turns can also take the form of inverted spins, like a somersault-type motion on the floor or with a partner. An investigation of the specific use of each of these motion categories in dance is merited.

Stance

The location of the center of gravity (COG) and its relationship to the base of support (BOS) differs between dance forms. For example, while all ballet exercises are done from stance, most modern dance techniques include sitting postures as part of their movement exercises. Evaluating the differences in relationship of COG to BOS between ballet and modern dance, Gray and Skrinar[7] studied the transfer of the COG from the warm-up portion of a dance class to the center floor section of the same class. They determined that both ballet and modern dance styles use support postures in their warm-up sections that are significantly dissimilar to their dancing sections. Specifically, ballet emphasizes a very narrow BOS for warm-up (as described in the next paragraph) while modern dance emphasizes a grounded BOS (Fig. 8-3). However, both styles of dance utilized a medium BOS for most of the actual dancing activities.

There are five basic stances within which ballet exercises are learned. They are known as first through fifth positions (Fig. 8-4). In these positions, maximal external rotation of the lower extremities is expected at all times, except in unusual choreographic applications. The feet positions vary in terms of width and direction of the BOS. Fourth and second positions have the widest base of support, coronally and sagitally, respectively, while first and fifth positions have the narrowest base of support. In addition to these turned-out positions, modern dance techniques typically incorporate a more anatomically neutral version of the same basic ballet stances, known as "parallel" positions, as well as numerous sitting and lying positions.

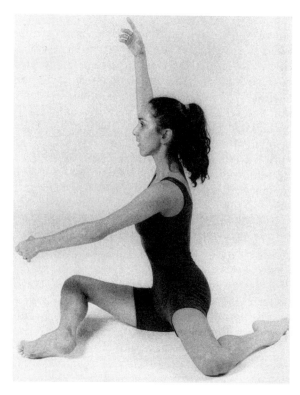

FIGURE 8-3 *Grounded base of support.*

Some choreography poses the lower body in opposition to the upper body as the stable versus mobile segments, or vice versa (Fig. 8-5). The spine and/or pelvis also may be emphasized as the stable base of support while all four limbs are free to gesture (Fig. 8-6).

Walking and Running

Dancers use walks and runs in class and on stage as transition steps to link other movement actions or phrases. The ambulations usually are carried out in a stylized manner, with lateral thigh rotation maintained and the heel strike phase often neglected. Toe-walking and toe-running are considered quieter, swifter, and more in keeping with the illusion of ease.

Kicking

Ballet exercises progress from two- to one-leg stance activities. In advanced ballet exercises, there is an increased use of unilateral lower ex-

tremity (LE) stance where the contralateral limb is mobile and gestural. These leg gestures can take the form of a kick to the front, side, or back of the dancer's body in a regularly practiced pattern known as "en croix," literally, "a cross." A kick performed with the knee in extension throughout is called a "battement." When a kick is begun with knee extension, but then folds back into the body's center through knee flexion (passé), it is called an "envelopé." Finally, when a large leg lift passes through passé to reach a knee-extended position, it is call a "developpé." Two other regularly practiced large leg gestures are "cloche," a sequential sagittal plane, arc swing of the leg forward and back, and "grand ronde de jambe en l'air," a circumducted hip action of the gesturing LE, where the limb is circled from front to back of the body (or vice versa) with a fully extended knee, while the hip is in ≥90 degrees of flexion.

The kicks in dance are performed while maintaining an erect and fixed trunk posture. The pelvis has been shown to be the accommodating region during "grand battement devant" (high kicks to the front), where the pelvis posteriorly rotates 30 degrees to allow the dancer to maintain an erect torso and a fully extended support limb.[8]

Jumping

Jumps are highly stylized and can take off from and/or land on one or both feet and can include complicated gestural footwork and/or airborne rotations. Difficulty level is determined by the motion of the turn (i.e., whether or not it contains angular as well as linear components), and whether one or two feet are utilized in take-off and landing. A simple "sauté" jump, for example, takes off from two feet and lands on two feet. The displacement is vertical and linear. An advanced version of this jump is the "tour en l'air," which takes off from two feet as does the sauté, but incorporates turns in the air. Depending on the choreography, this jump will end with a landing either on two feet, as in the simple sauté, or often on one foot while the opposite leg proceeds into a knee-flexed landing position. An example of a jump that also involves kicking motion—ac-

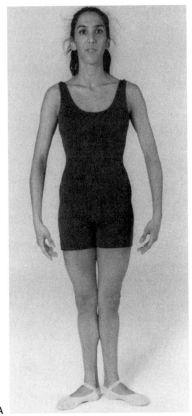

FIGURE 8-4 *(A) First position.*

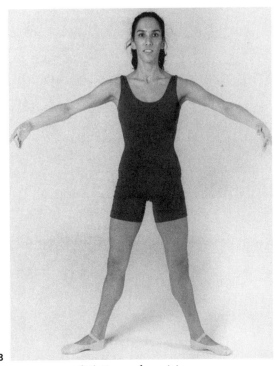

FIGURE 8-4 *(B) Second position.*

cording to the above classification system—and that takes off from and lands on one foot is the "jeté." This jump contains linear displacement with a horizontal as well as a vertical component and follows a projectile pathway. The advanced version of this jump incorporates an angular component and is known as the "tour jeté." Proficiency in jumps is determined by the height of the jump and the precision of location and control on the landing.

Throwing

When dancers gesture with their arms, the upper extremity (UE) action is referred to as "port-de-bras." Just as with the feet in ballet, there are specifically placed, port-de-bras patterns for the arms. When the dancer incorporates flexion, lateral flexion, or extension of the

spine into the port-de-bras movements, it becomes known as "port-de-corps." Partnering, or lifting, is considered a variation of throwing mechanics (Fig. 8-7). Because the purpose of dance movement is to convey expression, the UEs in dance are used in neither a purely postural mode nor a purely manipulative mode, as described by Gentile.[9] The arms are used in a manipulative function during partnering for lifts and turns, but for the most part are trained to serve in an expressive manner that renders them something other than postural in their function. Typically, the arms are carried to the side of the dancer's body (approximately 75–90 degrees abduction) in approximately 45 degrees of internal rotation with slight elbow flexion and a relaxed hand position. The dancer is trained to maintain the arm positions with minimal effort of the deltoid, rotator cuff, and scapular muscles, while recruiting

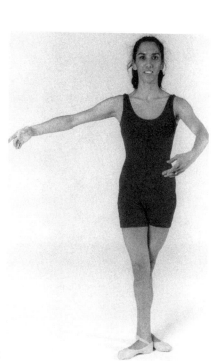

FIGURE 8-4 *(C) Third position.*

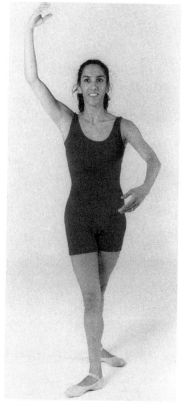

FIGURE 8-4 *(D) Fourth position.*

as little work as possible from other superficial back muscles and utilizing as little spinal ROM as needed.

Turning

Turns vary in difficulty depending on the number of rotations required and on the position of the legs and feet at the beginning of the turn, as well as on the action of the gesturing limb during the execution of the turn(s). Some turns, such as the pirouette, are initiated in an impulse fashion, where a force sizable enough to overcome the dancer's inertia is imparted to the floor over a very brief contact time. This LE activity is synchronized with precise coordination of UE activity. Ranney[10] compared the upper extremity action in dance turns to upper extremity action in the turns accomplished by other types of ath-

letes. He concluded that athletes are able to more freely utilize their arms to initiate and/or affect their turns throughout the entire duration of a turn, whereas the aesthetic dictates of ballet limits port-de-bras motion to the time synchronized to just at or just after takeoff.

Other turns, such as chainé and piqué, are stepped into; both legs are used in an alternating step fashion while the arms initiate and control the rotation by timed opening and closing. Another turn, the fouetté, requires coordinated leg extension, abduction, and flexion with opening and closing arm action to create its spin on the opposite stance limb.

Change in rotational motion depends upon a net torque, and torque depends on the magnitude of the applied force, the location of the applied force relative to the axis of rotation of the turning object, and the direction of the applied

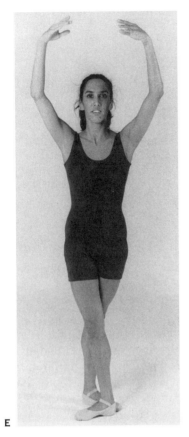

E

FIGURE 8-4 *(E) Fifth position.*

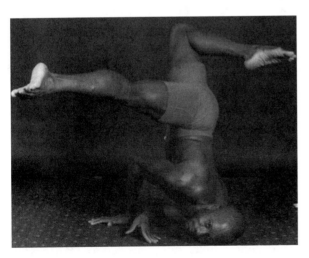

FIGURE 8-5 *Upper body as base of support.*

force. Laws[11] describes the pirouette as "a rotation of the body around a vertical axis over one supporting foot on the floor." He further writes, "any pirouette must commence with some preparation position followed by a torque exerted against the floor. Since the floor is the only source of forces or torques other than gravity (when there is no contact with a partner or barre), the torque of the floor against the dancer [is what] causes the angular acceleration that produces the turning motion. In a 'set-up' position for any turn, the body must be prepared to exert opposite horizontal forces with the two feet (a force 'couple') in order to apply the necessary torque." To set up for the initiation of a turn, the dancer does a plié (a bend of the knees) followed by a rapid extension of the knees while directing the center of mass (torso and pelvis) into the opposite direction of the foot force on the floor. Simultaneously, the dancer pushes rapidly onto the balls of the feet, which accomplishes two things. First, the rise onto the balls of the feet generates up to 10 times the dancer's body weight of force to the floor.[12] Second, the action of rising from flat foot to the ball of the foot reduces the foot's surface contact with the floor, redistributing the dancer's mass. Opposition to the turn maneuver is reduced via moment arm changes at the foot and ankle. This series of rapid preparatory actions directs the energy generated from applied and reaction forces into displacement and work. The larger the impulse, either from greater or more rapidly applied force, the larger the velocity response. The larger the velocity and the greater the mass of the dancer, the greater the angular momentum created. Therefore, the force required of the dancer to accomplish turns must be enough to not only overcome inertia, but to produce a net torque for acceleration.

In order to turn, the dancer must maintain a fixed position of the trunk and head[13] while the legs and arms initiate and control the motion. The dancer must rotate around a central, vertical axis of rotation. The dancer's ability to maintain a balanced, erect posture and fixed (rigid) square torso while maintaining precise placement over the base of support helps to conserve the energy of the turn. The force initiating

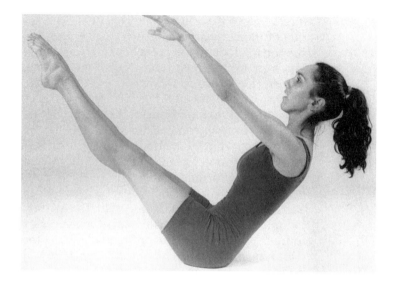

FIGURE 8-6 *Pelvis as base of support.*

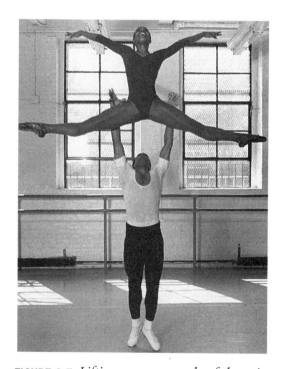

FIGURE 8-7 *Lifting as an example of throwing mechanics. (Photograph © Marbeth, 1996. Used with permission.)*

the turn depends upon the length of the distance from its point of application to the axis of movement (moment arm) and is usually applied by the gesture limb.[14] Turns initiated from second position will require less force than identical turns begun in first position. Similarly, turns from fourth position require less force than turns from third and fifth position. This is important to keep in mind as the dancer progresses back into his or her technique classes following injury.

Once a turn has actually begun, that is, the impulse has been imparted to the floor (action-reaction) and the momentum has been created, the dancer can then help to sustain the turn by appropriate positioning of the limbs. The dancer's ability to remain posturally erect with the arms and legs closely approximated at this point of the turn will decrease the moment of inertia, thereby enhancing momentum ($L = I\omega$).

Cognitive and Neuromuscular Aspects of Dance

LEARNING

It is worth repeating that the purpose of dance is different than the purpose of sport. Dance is an art form with the purpose of expression. Athletic endeavors find purpose in skill alone. The years of training a dancer undertakes in acquiring skill are all aimed toward optimization and precision of movement where *accomplishing* a movement skill is less the object, in and of itself, than the inner kinesthetic *awareness* of whether or not that movement skill is being performed efficiently. Elite athletes also strive to gain this level of "feel" for their movement, but in dancers, it is this level of physical awareness (cognitive recognition of somatic impulses and signals) and its subsequent technical acuity that frees the dancer to pursue the artistry of dance beyond physical mastery. It is then that the dancer can use the trained body to represent something sublime, something poetic; another physical language for the sake of art. The shape and skills are means to an end. The learning process is often central (imagistic thought) before peripheral (physical execution) and the process creates an inner sensibility that dancers call "muscle memory."

A scientific basis for this sensibility may be described by the results of two studies that examined level of skill as it pertains to replicability of movement tasks. Clarkson et al.[15] studied 23 classical ballet dancers and 19 physically active controls for movement patterns and reaction time with three dance movement sequences: (1) plié-demi-pointe relevé-plié, (2) plié-sauté (jump)-plié and (3) plié-relevé en pointe-plié. (See Posture and Alignment section for full description of these tasks.) The nondancers performed the first two tasks after laboratory instruction, but did not participate in the third task, since it was a skill requiring advanced training. The authors corrected for weight differences in their subjects and then analyzed the movements for timing differences. They found no differences between groups for execution of the relevé, but found that the dancers were able to perform the sauté (a small vertical jump from turned-out first position) significantly faster than the nondancers. While the nondancers had varying plié depths before and after their two tests, the dancers were able to replicate their plié position before and after every test, leading the authors to conclude that the regular, specific, and repeated movement pattern of the plié in

dance classes trained a "set" or determined depth of plié regardless of the transitory action preceding or following it. The authors further speculated that through this consistent movement training, the dancers influenced a proprioceptive feedback mechanism that allowed them to consistently reach their set demi-plié. This neuromuscular set, in turn, affects the timing and aesthetic appeal of the other dance movements connected to it by transition and, probably, other isolated dance tasks through a similar training effect. For example, Mouchnino[16] found that when comparing the transfer of weight from two legs to one in a group of trained dancers compared to naive subjects, the dancers arrived at the new position more efficiently and with more fixed sequencing than the naive subjects.

Dance is a discipline having an organized set of theories, concepts, principles, and skills. It involves both aesthetic (expression/experience) and utilitarian (discipline/exercise) learning and, like other educational disciplines, has a distinctive history, learning sequence, language, cultural basis, and conceptual content. Dance involves experiential action through the physicality of moving the body through time and space, encouraging learning on the task/concentration and skill-specific level as well as via sensory feedback mechanisms. The study of dance involves the acquisition of concepts, facts, and skills, which, on an explicit and verbal level, involves conscious awareness and decision-making. This level of activity promotes intellectual outcomes that utilize the cognitive domain. On the tacit or non verbal level, it involves expressive forms of communication and concerns itself with attitudes and interests in the affective domain, encouraging sensitivity and intuitive knowledge based on human experience and associative/behavioral habits.[17]

Traditionally, dance is taught to students through a process of imitation. Puretz[18] describes one mode of teaching as *bilateral transfer*, where movement is taught via a "transfer of motor patterns from one side of the body to the other through practice on only the one side," and provided evidence from earlier work that positive transfer exists not only from hand to hand, but also from hand to foot. (Dancers literally will "mark" a movement sequence with their hands before executing it with their lower extremities.) Direction of transfer is most successful when movement is taught from nondominant (or nonpreferred) to dominant side[19] and when it is taught in the frontal rather than sagittal plane.[20]

Shea and Hunt[21] discussed the importance of learning, attention, memory, and transfer in skill acquisition on ability to learn. Dancers learn by visual inspection of a moving model (imitation of video image or teacher demonstration), or by verbal cueing of teachers relying on known technical terms or imagistic spatial descriptors. Skrinar[22] reporting on the influence of instructional cues, concluded that a combination of visual, verbal, and kinesthetic cues was the most effective method of teaching movement rather than any one type of cue used in isolation. Facilitating touch—which tactilely describes direction and optimal effort of movement—is also a very common teaching tool utilized by dance educators. Dance classes are usually conducted in front of full-length mirrors that allow the dancers to correlate their own visual image with kinesthetic feedback.

Learning is associated with temporality. The dancer is sometimes asked to discover and learn dance movement through a process of real-time kinesthetic improvisation and experimentation in response to music, space, and/or verbal cues from a director who is looking for a particular movement quality, pattern, level, or directional facing. Conversely, in more structured forms of dance technique, the learning occurs through observation and replication of established movement and depends on memory. Once the dancer leaves the controlled studio environment for the more open environment of the stage, she must also deal with temporality on another level. In this case, externally paced movements such as other dancers in the space and the musical tempos set by a conductor directing a live orchestra must be attended and accommodated.[9]

Puretz[18] describes two biologically and physically distinct memory systems cited in the literature that she believes are used in dance education. She presents evidence that these systems reside in the brain and function under different biochemical controls. One system, the declarative knowledge system, controls the assimilation of facts and the other, the proceruaal knowledge system, controls the assimilation of skills. The latter system is the primary system used in dance and relies on a mechanism of memory storage and retrieval with a process that encodes movement material.

Overt (physical practice) and covert rehearsal processes (cognitive practice) are equally effective in terms of successful replication of the original task.[18] Both processes result in improved short- and long-term memory since there is no significant decrement in ability to replicate dance movement up to one week after the learning had occurred. This suggests that once movement is learned with the procedural knowledge system, it is rarely forgotten. The motor complexities of dance with respect to its length of movement sequencing and patterns require other factors along with learning, such as perceptual-motor organization, attention vigilance, contextual circumstances, premovement organization or strategy formations, and knowledge of movement relationships.

Bowman[22a] studied how field-dependent and field-independent learning styles play a role in the way that beginning dancers learn movement phrases. Field dependence refers to an inability to identify items when they are outside the expected setting and field independence is a strong ability to locate items outside the expected context.[22a] The most successful beginning dancers were field-independent.[22a]

Corsi-Cabrera[22b], on the other hand, found that neither level of skill nor exposure to training in dancers correlated with ability to manipulate an abstractly represented space. Barrell and Trippe[22c] reported opposite findings to those of Bowman. They reported that professional male ballet dancers were less field-independent than control subjects. One explanation may be that as skill level demands increase in dance, focus on field-dependent items may become more important for joint position sense and postural control.[22d,22e] The need for rapidly calibrating adjustments to perceptual and motor inputs also increases as skill demands increase.[22f]

Gender differences in training exposure may also account for the contrary findings. Several authors have noted that male dancers train up to 11 years less than women.[67,71,82,88] Hellerman et al[88] asked five dance professors to rank college and regional dance students from highest to lowest on technical skill. The authors analyzed the subjects according to age, training exposure, and gender, but were unable to find a significant relationship between any single or combination of variables. They speculated that the men were either more motivated, faster learners, or began their dance training at a technically higher level than the women, perhaps from previous involvement in other sports activities.

SKILL

Movement skill implies not only mastered learning of complex neuromuscular actions as evidenced by superior performance, but also the ability of a performer to demonstrate less variability between trials of that action than that of the same performer in a pretrained state or of a novice, control performer.[9] In dance, skill is partly dependent upon the ability to reliably replicate specific postures and to voluntarily control linear and angular motions. Gentile[9] states that there are two conditions that appear to enhance motor learning: (1) a regulated environment permitting low interference from the attention to the task, and (2) the availability of knowledge of results to the performer. The complex, alternatingly stable/mobile and acceleratory actions that are trained in dance typically occur under these conditions. They are practiced regularly, leading to an ability by the dancer to purposefully restrict his or her degrees of movement freedom in an effort to economize action and increase efficiency.[23,24] Reaction times and specific locations, directions, and durations of applied forces between the body and the environment are learned and repeated daily over many years. A few studies that provide clues to the appearance of ease that skilled dancers bring to their performances are described below.

Ryman[25] analyzed six jumps of an elite ballerina and made the following conclusions, which have been corroborated by other authors:[26,27]

1. The height of the jump is greatest following moderate rather than maximal knee flexion due to mechanical advantage at the knee joint.

2. Suspension during the flight phase, known in dance as "ballón," is not real but an illusion due to relative timing-to-height of the head, COG, and arms.

3. In jumps that also include rotational motion, the turns are initiated before the body leaves the ground, not at the height of the jump as is commonly taught. Angular momentum created on the push-off is maintained, and velocity of rotation is altered after leaving the ground by the manipulation of various body segments, such as a singular, rapid approximation of the arms or feet. This gives the illusion that the turn is just starting when, in fact, it starts with push-off.

POSTURE AND ALIGNMENT

As described by Winter et al.,[28] the subsystems that make up the postural control system include the sensory system made up of the vestibular, visual, and proprioceptive systems; the CNS; and the musculoskeletal system. The proprioceptive system provides information about the state of the effector system (length and force output of the muscles, relative orientation of body segments) and information about the environment (temperature, contact surface condition, pressure distribution, presence of noxious stimuli). The vestibular system provides information about body orientation in the inertial frame of reference and accelerations of the body. The visual system has also been categorized as a proprioceptive system because it not only provides information about the environment but also about the orientation and movement of the body and because of this, is referred to as "exproprioception." The postural effects of visual stimulus, training, and balance will be explored more fully in subsequent sections of this chapter.

All dancers begin their training with a sense of postural alignment that will become the "home base" for all dance exercises. Classical ballet refers to "line" as the balanced and proportioned alignment of static and dynamic posture. This may refer to the line of erect stance in first position, for example, or the line of a large, unilaterally extended leg gesture such as an arabesque (Fig. 5-1). As a universally codified movement form, ballet commands the most adherence to line because it impacts on aesthetic form to a much greater extent than in other dance styles. One of the first things a ballet student learns is how to stand in first position with correct postural alignment. The student is typically instructed to stand side view to a mirror and visually inspect correct versus incorrect alignment. Correct alignment in ballet mimics the plumb-line evaluation used in universal posture screening tests, where the plumb-line passes by the ear, mid-shoulder, greater trochanter, midline of the knee, and lateral malleolus. The exception for the ballet dancer is that the lower extremities are externally rotated and so, in evaluating a proper functional stance, the plumb-line passes over the talocrural or midfoot region rather than the lateral malleoli in the first and second positions. In third, fourth, and fifth positions the plumb-line passes between the feet.

Part of this basic dance posture—the hip turnout—if properly taught, is accomplished by the deep external rotators of the hip: the obturators internus and externus, the gemelli superior and inferior, the piriformis, and the quadratus femoris. In response the activation of those muscles, the knee, in stance and in movement, is trained to remain over the second metatarsal/cuneiform ray at all times.

Among the first movement skills a dancer is taught following correct stance is the "plié" (hip and knee flexion, with ankle and MTP dorsiflexion). There are two types of pliés: demi- and grand (Fig. 8-8). Demi-plié is used frequently in dance, both as a preparatory action for turns and jumps and as a transition step for linking longer movement phrases. When the dancer is taught to plié, the same spinal alignment that was taught in standing is dynamically enforced. This same principle is true for the relevé (hip in neutral with knee extension, ankle plantar flexion,

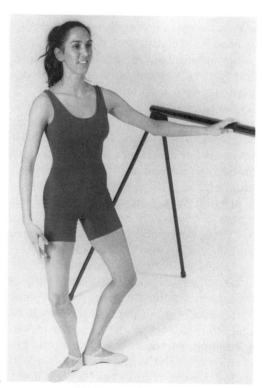

A

FIGURE 8-8 *(A) Demi-plié.*

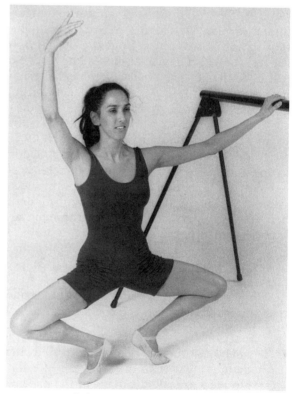

B

FIGURE 8-8 *(B) Grand plié.*

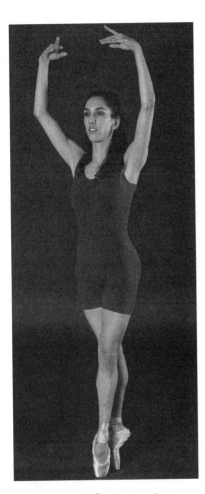

FIGURE 8-9 *Relevé en pointe.*

and MTP dorsiflexion in demi-pointe relevé—or with MTP plantar flexion if relevé en pointe, Fig. 8-9) and all subsequent movements that follow a progression to highly coordinated multijoint sequences of varying difficulty.

In addition to the movement principles mentioned above, an early postural alignment technique encountered by dancers in training is a spinal stabilization concept where instruction is given for the dancer to maintain a "square" torso, such that the shoulders align, anteriorly-posteriorly, over the hips at all times. Once the dancer has trained long and regularly enough to have achieved automatization of this postural control in all of the classroom exercises, technique training will advance to include stylistic inclinations

of the square posture by utilizing two spinal rotation concepts referred to as "opposition" and "épaulement."[13]

Opposition refers to contralateral balance of upper and lower extremities. The dancer must be in correct alignment with hips and shoulders level and lying parallel to each other, facing the same plane and directed to one point in the personal square, where the leg in front should be balanced by the opposite arm coming forward.[13] Next, a dancer will learn a related postural embellishment known as épaulement. Derived from the literal French translation of épauler, "to shoulder," épaulement refers to an expressive nuance of oppositional posture that many teachers refer to as "shading." Davie (in Lawson[13]) describes épaulement as "a rotary movement of the shoulders made in sympathy with a simultaneous movement of the arms and/or legs, the extent of which must be finely judged, and which depends on context since it is really reflective of a subjective state of mind." The shading of épaulement is taught to give a more freely flowing quality to the moving dancer's line than the purely classical placement offered by the fundamental alignment principles. De Valois (in Lawson[13]) instructs further about the functional use of épaulement as follows: "the dancer must determine the relationship of the arms and legs to the central point of balance and see that the laws of opposition and épaulement are logically used. Is the weight correctly centered? Are the legs and arms so counterbalanced that they help equalize the pressure of weight on the supporting leg? . . . . Is it easy to move from that step or pose to another as weight is transferred without twisting some part of the body and thus spoiling the line of movement?" It is important for the clinician to know that the use of opposition and épaulement affect rotation of the head as well as cervical through proximal lumbar spine segments. The spinal rotation and counterrotation taking place activates the deep abdominal and back muscles that act as both prime movers and spinal stabilizers. Épaulement has been taken to a highly stylized level in ballet. Modern and jazz dancers also use its principles.

Once these postural cues are learned by the dancer, they serve as the baseline shape of all accumulating movement skills. Eventually, this sense of correct placement becomes kinesthetic second nature to the dancer in static positions and throughout dynamic movement. One would expect that this increase in kinesthetic awareness is due, in part, to the known effects of regularly practiced motor patterns,[15,16] especially in the presence of cognitive attention, which uses imagery[29–31] and to extra-articular adaptations to movement demands which heighten the sensitivity to joint motion.[10,20]

Posture is also important for a dancer in its association to artistic expression. To successfully portray a character, feeling, or mood, a dancer will use posture and gesture as vehicles of expression. As an example of the theatrical power of posture, Gelabert[32] describes the role of the male lead in the ballet *Giselle*. Albrecht, visiting the grave of his love interest, "displays his grief as he walks slowly, measuring each step, lowering the head and sinking the shoulders, projecting sadness and remorse. The descriptive mood of this scene is created by the body language of emotion and not by dancing." Similarly, observing a dancer's posture in the clinical setting may provide clues not only about anatomic and functional asymmetries, but also about the dancer's psychological state. An elaborate system of dance notation, known as Labanalysis, includes methods for coding postural assessment in order to understand psychological or emotional intent.[33]

Posture, of course, is not just a static phenomenon; dance training demands precise and specific, held starting positions and explores any and every conceivable dynamic posture of gross and morphing shapes in space. Regardless of the numerous variations postural themes can take, the concept of correct alignment based on a square torso as home base is always fundamental to dance movement.

BALANCE

Balance is one of several important components of successful movement performance in dance. Dancers rely on a keen sense of balance to sustain extremely small bases of support for extended periods of time as well as to move rapidly and expansively between spatial postures—often shifting direction, timing, and level multiple times within just one movement phrase. It is not clear whether the highly skilled levels of balance demonstrated by dancers is a function of training or selectivity.

Gruen[20] compared professional dancers and nondancers in one physical measure of balance. Dancers, regardless of years of training, had better balance scores, supporting the selectivity school of thought. Other studies draw different conclusions. Shick et al.[34] measured 75 modern dancers on a stabilometer as well as on flat foot (described as "stork" position) to see if their ability to balance would reliably predict their performance level and learning time. The results showed a positive relationship between dynamic balance on the stabiliometer and performance level, but not on the static test (stork position), so that, overall, only 58 percent of the subjects could be correctly classified to level by balance ability. Bushey[35] studied the relation between subjective measures of modern dance performance level with objective measures of agility, balance, strength, power, and flexibility, and found no significant relations.

A study by Crotts et al.,[36] which supports the training school of thought, compared 15 experienced dancers to 15 healthy, age- and vision-matched physical therapy students for differences in balance performance using a modified Foam and Dome test. Subjects maintained one-legged balance under six different combinations of visual and support conditions. Dancers performed significantly better than controls in the most challenging of the balance conditions, but it was unclear if this was due to the dancer's ability to more rapidly assess internal postural and external environmental cues from prior experience, or from better overall endurance conditioning, since the most difficult test condition was not order-randomized and was tested last, resulting in subjective reports of fatigue from all the subjects.

Some studies have shown that movement practices that require diminished bases of support (e.g., balance beam or water skis) develop balance skills through acclimatization to those smaller surfaces.[37] Dancers, because of working in relevé, as well as on single-leg stances, would seem to qualify for this adaptation criteria. It is also known that dependence on proprioception increases, not only as a result of regular movement practice, but also as a result of working in diminished light environments.[38] Since dancers work under stage lights that vary from very dim to blinding (spotlights), it seems likely that some of their balance skills may come from this acclimatization as well.

The visual component of balance is specifically trained in dancers. They are taught to visually fixate or "spot" during turns to prevent dizziness or loss of balance. Irrgang et al.[39] call this a "suppression of induced vestibular nystagmus from angular acceleration."

Interestingly, balance does not appear to be directly related to strength. In a study that evaluated seven men before and after 14 days of bed rest with varying levels of inactivity, Haines[40] showed that balance impairment was not due to loss of muscular strength in the legs, but to changes in neurally coded information of postural control centers. Lentell[41] also reported no relation between muscular weakness and ankle instability. Hughson[42] studied balance in two groups of dancers following exercise programs with a BAPS board and theraband, respectively. She reported no differences within or between groups in balance function after 15 days of training.

MOVEMENT STRATEGIES RELATED TO POSUTRAL TRAINING AND BALANCE IN DANCE

Several studies have attempted to measure or discuss the dynamic component of posture in dance and the influence of long-term dance training on posture in general. Woodhull-McNeal et al.[43] studied 13 female college-level dancers with a minimum of 10 years of ballet or modern dance training for changes in linearity of posture in various stance positions. The dancers stood in parallel first position, and in three of the classical ballet stances: first, third, and fifth positions. The authors photographed and measured five bony landmarks: ankle, knee, hip, shoulder, and ear, as well as pelvic tilt. The subjects stood on a reaction board that was designed to enable the researchers to calculate anterior-posterior locations of COG. The photographs were digitized and analyzed for anterior-posterior landmarks relative to the ankle. They found that the ear was significantly forward of the COG for all positions; the hip and shoulder locations did not differ from COG; and the COG remained over the ankle only in the turned-out first position. They ascribed this to the fact that in the turned-out first position the base of support is very short in the sagittal plane, and so, the COG must shift backward to be within the base of support. In the other three positions, the COG was significantly forward of the malleoli. The COG above the hip did not differ between positions, but anterior pelvic tilt was significantly greater in fifth position than in the other stances, and progressively increased as base of support externally rotated and approximated.

A dancer, especially in relevé, must also make multiple small adjustments at the feet, ankles, and hips to maintain static and dynamic balance. Medial and lateral sway of the body during unilateral, flatfooted stance is countered by pronation and supination at the subtalar joint.[39,44] With reduced stance surface area, as in relevé, trunk and upper body muscles also play a role in balance stability.[45] Earlier recruitment and increased cocontraction of the trunk and neck muscles have been measured in dancers performing relevé, suggesting that a stiffer spinal musculature is required for more precarious base postures.[45,46]

Werner[46] compared the postural responses of skilled ballet dancers to nondancers for quiet stance and then further studied the dancers for response to perturbed relevé. In quiet stance, she found a similar pattern between the two groups; a distal to proximal, dorsal pattern ankle strategy[45] occurred, with the only difference being that neck muscles fired earlier in the dancers. In perturbed relevé tests among the dancers, abdominal activity preceded quadriceps, gastrocnemius, hamstring, and trunk extensors, respectively, and suggested that a mix of hip and ankle strategy existed, with hip as the dominant strategy site. An increase in the response frequency of abdominal, neck extensor, and flexor muscles was also noted. Ninety-five percent of trials resulted in a cocontraction of the neck antagonists.

These findings are likely a response to torso stabilization issues, to the slightly-forward COG/BOS relations relied on in the regularly practiced stance postures, and/or the positioning of the head. Dancers are trained not only to maintain their head-torso alignment at all times as part of their daily training, but are given verbal cues to lift the back of their heads from the region of their occipital protuberance, keeping their eye focus forward and outward. Eye focus is variable depending on the style and intent of a specific piece of choreography, but is almost never left undirected.

Lopez-Ortiz[14] looked at dancers performing pirouette turns relative to skill level. She found that as skill level increased, the "toppling effect" of a turn, that is, the deviation of center of mass from vertical axis of rotation, decreased. This suggests that the more skilled dancers are better able to stabilize their trunk, thus maintaining an erect and fixed posture to stabilize the vertical axis, providing the necessary centripetal force for the turns, although the author did not specify whether this improved stabilization is the result of alignment alone, balance ability, concentration, visual dynamics, strength, or some other variable. She also found that the more skilled dancers generated their greatest force in the initiation phase of a turn and were capable of controlling greater angular momentum near the end of the turn through progressive deceleration, while the less skilled dancers showed an opposite pattern. This work reinforces findings by Mouchnino et al.,[16] who found that skilled dancers employ a "translation strategy" of control for shifts in COG compared to an "inclination strategy" employed by naive subjects. In that study, a dynamic assessment of lower extremity weight shift tasks showed that dancers were more able to maintain verticality of their head-trunk axis compared to nondancers.[16]

Ubiquitous firing of the abdominal muscles in dancers demonstrates a training response resulting from the requirements for stiffness and stability in the torso during dance.[46] In ballet, the abdominal muscles work primarily in isometric and eccentric modes to maintain the square torso and to oppose the back extensors during various leg gestures. Modern dance techniques incorporate sitting, lying, and flexed trunk postures and activities into training and choreography. This involves the abdominals in concentric functions as well.

STYLIZATION, PERCEPTION, AND ACTION

Dance is concerned not only with accuracy of ROM, but with *effort* (the qualities and energies of movement: flow, weight, space, and time) and *shape* (the relationship between the body and the physical, as well as kinespheric space the body occupies) of assuming ROM that depends on self- and other-directed perceptions.[49] In addition to the level and positional differences between dance forms described for posture and skilled movement, different qualitative information is also cued by teachers of a given discipline, which, in turn, impact on perception and, therefore, action.[47] Ballet tends to emphasize cues that encourage the dancer to achieve a perception of lightness on his or her feet and a sense of lift in the torso. Ballet dancers are trained to move with that specific motor perception, as well as to be on the balls of their feet, ready for quick changes in direction, not unlike a tennis player. Many modern dance techniques, by contrast, emphasize a perception of weightedness into the floor, and therefore employ postures with concomitantly lower COGs.

Different dance forms will also vary in their preferred styles of movement tempo and flow, ranging from a sense of sustained, continuous, or smooth movement to one of rapid, staccato style. Some styles of dance may rely more on contracted rather than expanded body shapes. These position, velocity, and direction cues, in addition to the regularity with which they are practiced, will all uniquely and summarily affect perception and modify motor actions through CNS influence.[47,48] (For a detailed and eloquent exploration of movement shape, movement quality, and its analysis, see Bartinieff and Lewis.[49])

Given the ideal body placements and dynamic coordination expected of dancers, Marr[50] writes that most injuries are "caused by lack of understanding of the principles of placement and body mechanics," and that the first thing to teach the dance student is "to think [so] the student can consciously direct his body to hold correct posture in stillness and movement." In her own intuitive way, Marr is describing a well-respected phenomenon in neuropsychology commonly referred to as "attention vigilance."[31,51] By requiring the dancer to cognitively attend a movement task through both anatomic information and instruction for effort level, a psychosomatic integration is developed and, as a result, a greater degree of kinesthetic control and awareness is achieved.[29]

Over the years, many well-respected dance and movement teachers have discussed posture as it relates to technical proficiency, efficiency, and injury prevention.[52-55] Most agree that in attaining a sense of effortlessness or the automatization of the ability to maintain dance postures, changes occur in neuromuscular patterns. Gardner[55] stated that postural reflexes impede, rather than assist the execution of some movements in dance and must, therefore, be inhibited during the learning process. Recent studies regarding spinal stretch reflex adaptations support this assertion.

REFLEX ADAPTATIONS

Goode and Van Hoeven[56] reported diminished patellar and Achilles tendon tap (quick stretch) responses in trained dancers. This phenomenon was most common in female dancers who had trained in pointe work for 8–10 years. They felt that the loss of tendon reflex as well as lowered H-reflex recovery curve height was adaptive secondary to changes in muscle spindle output from extreme stretching of the extensor tendons and muscles.

Koceja et al.[57] compared seven skilled dancers with an average of 8 years of dance training to seven sedentary untrained subjects, in order to observe the effects of a conditioning reflex protocol on the force-time characteristics of the Achilles tendon tap reflex. The dancers exhibited 29 percent less unilateral isometric force and 60 percent longer half-relaxation times than the untrained subjects. Dancers also displayed marked short-latency facilitation and long-latency inhibition in the reflex force characteristics of a contralateral conditioning stimulus. Nielsen et al.[58] had a similar finding in internationally ranked professional ballet dancers.

The authors describe the soleus H-reflex as a monosynaptic reflex elicited by electrical stimulation of Ia afferents in the posterior tibial nerve. The size of the reflex is a measure of the central gain of the monosynaptic stretch reflex and it is determined by transmission across the synapses of the Ia afferents and the excitability of the motoneuronal pool.

Rochcongar et al.[59] found that H-reflex is smaller in anaerobically trained athletes than in those aerobically trained. (The anaerobic nature of ballet training is discussed later in this chapter.) He suggests that the small size of the reflex in the anaerobically trained subjects can be explained by a larger percentage of type II muscle fibers in those subjects. This is consistent with the findings of Heckman,[60] who noted that type I fibers are more easily excited by a volley in Ia afferents. However, the soleus is 90 percent type I tissue, and fiber profiles in dancers reveal a larger percentage of type I fibers.[61] The theory of Neilson et al.,[58] which surmises that the modifications are more likely caused by differences in the transmission across the synapses of the Ia afferents, becomes provocative. A pronounced presynaptic inhibition of Ia afferents could cause both small reflexes and small disynaptic reciprocal inhibition as seen in the ballet dancers. In this context, it is of particular interest that the ballet dancers have to perform a cocontraction of antagonistic muscles to maintain balance during the classical ballet postures and that a pronounced increase of presynaptic inhibition and decrease of disynaptic reciprocal inhibition has been reported during such contractions.[62]

Wolpaw[48] notes that modifications of the spinal stretch reflex (SSR) pathway probably play a role in acquisition of motor skills and that it is likely that improvement in more complex performance demands involves more or less simultaneous alterations in many neuromuscular influences which, over time, gradually modify sites throughout the CNS. He explains, "the necessary response to the H-reflex (or SSR) conditioning paradigm is simply a mode-appropriate change in reflex size, which could theoretically be achieved by merely increasing or decreasing the strength of the Ia synapse. From the perspective of the CNS, the problem presented by the conditioning paradigm is considerably more complicated. The CNS must adapt to acquire a new skill (i.e. a larger or smaller H-reflex) while still maintaining performance of previously learned skills that depend on the same neural elements. The Ia afferent, the motoneuron and the synapse between them participate in all behaviors involving the muscles they control or monitor. As a result, any change in these neural elements is likely to affect many motor skills. Plasticity is therefore essential if the CNS is to continue to perform all its behaviors satisfactorily."

In light of the discussion in the learning section of this chapter, future research about the impact of these changes on joint angle sense, timing, and functional strength in dancers would be extremely valuable.

PROPRIOCEPTION

Irrgang[39] states that proprioception is the ability to receive input from muscles, tendons, and joints and to process that information in a meaningful way in the CNS in order to locate limbs in space and adequately control posture. He corroborates Glencross and Thronton's[63] findings, where 33 mixed gender subjects under the age of 25 were studied for reproducibility of joint angle ranges according to ankle injury status. They found that reproducibility error rose with both frequency and severity of injury.

Their findings also support the conclusions of Marteniuk's[64] work on joint angle reproducibility, which stated that the largest of movements produced the greatest degrees of error. They suggested that "large ROMs require large scale firing of receptors" and are proportionate to the range covered. Dance is generally expansive in its ROM demands. Mountcastle[65] reports increased discharge in thalamic cells when extremes of range were reached. He speculates that if the total number of receptors is affected due to injury, then fewer receptors are available for activation at terminal ranges, resulting in greater error for joint position sense.

Barrack et al.[66] studied 12 professional ballet dancers averaging 25 years of age and 14 years of training, and 12 active, age-matched controls for joint laxity and knee joint position sense. In this particular study, the dancers were significantly more lax and performed significantly worse on estimating joint angle. The authors hypothesized that either the withdrawal of visual information from the dancers affected their ability to reproduce joint angles, since they are so accustomed to training in front of mirrors, or their joint hypermobility may have been be a factor in the decreased position sense. Interestingly, in a modified study by the same authors 1 year later, dancers performed significantly better than nondancers for recognition of the initiation of joint motion without visual input. In this study, the authors speculated that the highly trained neuromusculoskeletal systems in the dancers accounted for this greater kinesthetic sense of onset of motion,[67] which, as we have seen, is more in keeping with the broader body of literature on movement responses of trained dancers.

LANGUAGE

Language is a huge field of study and its impact on learning is too broad to cover in this chapter. On a superficial level, dance terminology is based on the original French ballet vocabulary and it may take some time and observation for a clinician to understand the movement functions or complaints presented by the dancer according to this vernacular.

The power of language on movement learning is a more complex phenomenon. Communication with the dancer extends beyond verbal language. Armstrong[68] after Gardner,[69] describes seven different intellectual domains of learning and perception that influence communication. Dancers, when learning movement, tend to be visual, musical, spatial, and kinesthetic learners and perceivers, and may utilize those pathways over verbal, logical, or interpersonal styles. Although they may not be primary verbal learners, dancers must rely heavily on descriptive language for imagistic understanding of how to impose effort on movement in order to convey its dramatic intent. As such, carefully chosen language can be a powerful tool for the clinician when reeducating proper movement patterns.

Physiologic Aspects of Dance

Although dance is not a competitive sport, dancers are athletes as much as they are artists, and the physical demands they endure are as potentially traumatic as those athletes face. A widely cited study on the demands of dance is an article from 1975 by Dr. James Nicholas.[70] In that study, 61 sports and recreational activities were assessed and ranked for difficulty by summating Likart-type scores assigned to each activity in three general categories: neuromuscular, psychometric, and environmental factors. Ballet ranked second behind football as the most demanding of all sports and activities. Although the subjective nature of that study has not gone without criticism, and technologies for objective scientific measurement of motor skills within and between sports have evolved tremendously, dancers are, in fact, unique athletes. In addition to the requirements of hyperflexibility, exquisite balance, and coordination, they are subject to rigorous aesthetic demands such as extreme thinness, and expansive, externally rotated postures that have tremendous global physiologic, biomechanical, and psychological effects.

The scope of this chapter does not permit an in-depth exploration of the many excellent studies that have been carried out in the realm of dance physiology. Just as one cannot truly separate the musculoskeletal system from the nervous system except to enhance purposeful learning, it is imperative to remember that global metabolic functions play a constant and integrated role in all neuromusculoskeletal activity. It would be unwise to consider one system without understanding the whole. Therefore, some basic considerations are presented here.

CARDIOVASCULAR AND METABOLIC ADAPTATIONS

Numerous studies have demonstrated that dance training produces moderate levels of aerobic fitness,[71–74] and that ballet performance tends to be short-burst, high-intensity in nature, intermittently relying on near maximum aerobic and anaerobic energy yields.[73] Classroom training and rehearsal demands are metabolically relaxed in comparison to stage performance demands.[73,75] Anaerobically, lactate levels average 8 mmol/L and are similar between genders in maximal tests.[72,73,76] In these same tests, however, a significant gender difference is found. Women dancers have been shown to be able to sustain peak power outputs over the full duration of a 30-second power test compared to the men, who declined rapidly after reaching an early peak.[76]

FIBER TYPE AND STRENGTH

Dahlstrom[61] looked at muscle fiber type and area in the vastus lateralis of 13 elite female dancers and found a significantly higher percentage of type I fibers and lower percentage of both type IIA and IIB fibers compared with sedentary, untrained, or moderately trained age-matched women. Their percentages were similar to profiles of endurance trained female runners.

Strength has been measured on dancers with both Cybex and load cell devices. The results have been compared between genders and sports.[77] When strength is normalized by lean body mass, it is reported to be significantly greater in male dancers than female dancers in the upper extremities ($P < .001$), and proximal thigh region ($P < .05$), but not different at the ankle joint.

Compared to soccer and football players, ballet dancers have significantly weaker dorsiflexors than the athletes, both alone and in relation to plantar flexors and overall ankle strength.[78] Isokinetic torques for quadriceps and hamstring muscle groups in regional ballet dancers compared to numerous other sports groups found male dancers demonstrated strength values similar to men in other sports, female dancers were about 30 percent below norms for women in other sports,[79] and about the same as scores for nonactive females.[72] The subjects being compared in the last two studies were not normalized for lean body mass or body weight. This can be important in cross-sectional comparison since women dancers tend to have smaller surface areas and leaner compositions than athletes and female nondancers. Dancers score higher for torque values on eccentric tests rather than concentric tests, which makes sense, since eccentric loads more truly mimic the forces dancers encounter in their training environments.[80]

The ability to dance well is clearly not the result of any one factor, such as strength, but instead, is the result of synergistic and globally complex processes and, perhaps, the luck of heredity.

FLEXIBILITY

Twenty-nine elite, professional ballet dancers were measured for flexibility[71] using the Nicholas[70] screen and demonstrated a "generally loose" constitution. All of the dancers were able to execute an Adams forward-bend test with palms not only flat on the floor but with the heels of the hands 7 in. behind the heels of the feet (Fig. 8-10). They were also easily able to execute a ≥ 90 degrees externally rotated leg stance, and averaged 10 degrees of genu recurvatum, a finding corroborated by others.[81,82]

Several other studies have measured the flexibility and joint ROM status of dancers and concluded that the selection criteria and adaptations to training were remarkably different than in populations of "normals" and other athletes.

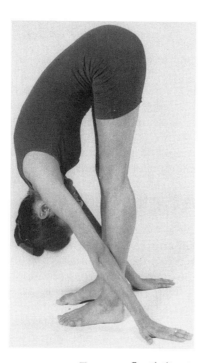

FIGURE 8-10 *Extreme flexibility in a dancer.*

Clippenger-Robertson[83] measured flexibility in 59 mixed level ballet students studying at the same professional ballet school and found that values for hip external rotation, abduction, flexion, and hyperextension, as well as spinal hyperextension, genu recurvatum, and sit-and-reach tests all significantly increased with training exposure and age. She also reported a nonsignificant trend for greater plantar flexion in the advanced level dancers as well as decreased dorsiflexion and hip internal rotation.

ANTHROPOMETRY AND SELECTIVITY

Biomechanical analysis is dependent upon measurement assessments of various body segments, links, masses, volumes, and inertias. As described by Freedson,[84] anthropometry serves "to improve understanding of human performance via precise quantification of body morphology, shape, size, composition, and proportion." Jensen[85] reminds us that "physical growth is a continuous process for each individual. The type and rate of growth of females is different from males and there are racial differences in physical growth. Consequently, we should be aware of differences between (and within) individuals."

Like elite athletes, in whom a discriminant analysis will separate somatotypes according to the sport played,[86] a homogeneic morphology is evident at the level of the professional dancer. Hamilton[87] has often commented on the "Darwinism of dance"; the dancers who make it to the top level have survived an inherent selectivity for the body type and personality able to adapt well to the aesthetic, psychologic, and physical training stresses along the way. The selection of dancers is highly subjective, based not on measures of time or distance, but on emotional and aesthetic attributes[88–91] and tends to be intensely discriminating. In national ballet schools only 5 percent of the children who begin their training at the age of eight graduate 9 years later.[92] Of approximately 20,000 dance students auditioning annually for company-affiliated schools, only 10 percent will be chosen for the school, with only 0.1 percent making it to the stage.[93] Data from profiling studies does indeed indicate a typical somatotype. In general, the typical dance archetype is described by low body weight and fat, long and slender legs, high-arched feet, and a general predisposition for articular and muscular flexibility.

BODY FAT, DISORDERED EATING, AND AMENORRHEA

There is a high incidence of eating disorders and menstrual dysfunction in the population of female dancers; as high as 78 percent compared to 2 percent in the general population, and between 10 and 60 percent (depending on the sport) among female athletes.[94] Amenorrhea is linked to decreased estrogen and loss of bone density and is thought to result from low caloric intake, strenuous exercise, and constant dieting to achieve a thin body shape.[94] Estrogen deficiency has a key role in the pathogenesis of osteoporosis while estrogen therapy is associated with increased peak bone mass, prevention of menopausal bone loss, as well as reduced risk of fracture.[95]

Weight-bearing exercise has been noted to partially offset the loss of bone seen in menopause despite hypoestrogenism and, in some cases, actually increases mass. Although numerous studies have shown that exercise increases bone mass, the intensity, frequency, duration of activity, and type of training that produces an increase are still controversial.[96] Cortical bone may be more responsive to loading than trabecular bone because it is either adjacent to or receives direct muscle insertions, while trabecular bone is central or medullary in position. Thus, cortical bone may be subject to greater deforming loads than trabecular bone during weight-bearing. Further, cortical bone may be less sensitive to hypogonadism than trabecular bone because it has a lower turnover. In fact, some studies on dancers have shown differences in regional bone mass and credited those findings to the virtue of this protective effect of direct loading through weight-bearing exercise.[97,98]

There is a moderate incidence of frank anorexia nervosa and bulimia among dancers.[94,99–101] A far more common practice, however, is what is known as "disordered eating," a phrase coined by the women's task force of the American College of Sports Medicine.[102] In this condition, the individual is described as practicing chronic restrictive and sometimes ritualistic, compulsive eating patterns. This is a condition the clinician should be aware of in terms of its potential effect on the dancer's full recovery from injury. Dancers have reported consuming as little as between 1,000 kcal and 1,800 kcal per day regularly, and in some cases since the age of 12, despite age-related or growth factor demands of physical development and despite several hours of dancing per day.[103–108]

The most technically talented dancer may not be accepted into a ballet company because of body size.[107] Female classical ballet dancers and modern dancers tend to be selected by averages of only 75 and 88 percent of expected body weight, respectively.[107,109] Aberrant nutritional patterns in dancers are associated with stress fractures before the development of bone density changes, suggesting that the quality of bone may be affected before changes are measurable.[96] Van Dijk[110] reported that a group of retired women ballet dancers had arthritic changes in their hip joints without symptomatic complaints. New work on bone mineral density in premenopausal ultramarathon runners demonstrates that low bone mineral density is related to a history of oligo/amenorrhea regardless of resumption of regular menstrual cycles, indicating that prolonged states of hypoestrogenism may negatively influence peak adult bone mass.[111]

Four studies have used hydrostatic methods to determine body composition in dancers (Table 8-1). Men average 5–7 percent fat and women between 11 and 17 percent.[103,104,112,113] In women dancers, the higher the level of skill ranking, the leaner the anthropometric measures. Two studies evaluated the link between anthropometric measures and perceptual assessments of performance. Ballet majors in a university dance department were measured for body fat and technical skill.[114] The dancers were subjectively divided into one of four group rankings based on their auditioner's assessments of technical proficiency and then measured for percentage of body fat. The average fat percentage ranged from 15.5 to 17.8 and was not significantly different between groups. The magnitude of ranges for fat values, however, diminished as level of rank increased. One could not tell from

TABLE 8-1 *Review of body fat measurements of dancers*

AUTHOR	NO. GENDER	AVERAGE AGE	HEIGHT	WEIGHT	LEAN MASS	FAT (%)	LEVEL	YEARS IN TRAINING	HOURS/DAY
Clarkson, 1985[113]	14 F	15 years	161 cm	48.4 kg	40.2 kg	16.4	preprofessional	9	—
Calabrese, 1983[103]	22 F	22 years	167 cm	53.0 kg	43.6 kg	16.9	professional-regional	10	4
Liederbach, 1986[71]	16 F	20 years	162 cm	49.0 kg	43.6 kg	11.1	professional-national	14	5
	13 M	21 years	180 cm	70.8 kg	66.1 kg	5.9	professional-national	9	5
Eisenman, 1995[114]	193 F	19 years	—	—	—	16.6	university	—	—

the data if this was a function of age,[115] preferential selection (aesthetic perception of the auditioners), or a determinant of some true performance capacity, since no objective measurements for skill or fitness level were obtained. Another study[116] looked at fat percentage measurements in relation to subjective ranking in professional ballet dancers by their company directors. No relation was found between rank and fat levels in men, but a significant negative correlation existed between fat percentage level and rank in the women. It appeared that women were judged for skill to some extent by percent body fat. Whether low body fat correlated better with skills such as balance, motivation from positive emotional feedback,[88] or the quality of movement accomplishment was not conclusive from this study, since neither further detail on how the ballet directors made their decisions nor objective data on functional skills were collected.

One important factor for the clinician to understand is that dancers are often driven more by how they look than how they are functioning during performance. Food can lose its worth as a fuel and ergogenic aid and become, instead, an irrational object representing something that they believe may lead to poor aesthetics. Female dancers often have an extreme fear of fat. Their subsequent eating habits may exclude fat completely from their diet or restrict overall calorie consumption to unbalanced and undernourishing or malnourishing levels, cascading into central fatigue, muscle failure, and injury.

Mechanisms of Injury

BIOMECHANICAL CONSIDERATIONS

There are different schools of thought concerning the ligamentous constitution most appropriate for dancing. Marr[50] has described the historical role of selectivity relative to ligamentous predisposition. In the Russian philosophy of selecting students, artistic directors have students assume various postures and select those with tight structures, the assumption being that looseness can trained. The Australians believe the direct opposite. There, dancers are selected for their loose body types, in the hope that training will tighten up their structures. Injury rates on Australian ballet dancers have been reported (Table 8-2), but, to this author's knowledge, no comparable data are available on Russian dancers. Hamilton[117] notes that even dancers with bodies extremely well suited for ballet will experience orthopaedic complaints, simply due to the nature of the movement demands.

Trunk and Pelvis

Recently published work that evaluates the first-year students at the Swedish Ballet School[118] reveals that dancers tend to be selected for axial hypermobility. In that study, dancers possessed less spinal kyphosis and lordosis than control subjects, and significantly more thoracic range of motion. Dancers who have reached elite levels of skill often present with reduced sagittal plane spinal curvatures. This is no doubt primar-

TABLE 8-2 *Review of types and location of injuries in dancers*

AUTHOR	LEVEL AND STYLE	NO. OF INJURIES	FREQUENCY OF INJURY SITE
Quirk 1984[197]	Mixed level ballet	2,113	22.3% ankle 20.1% foot 17.3% knee 11.4% other 8.6% hip 8.5% lower back 7.5% leg 4.3% thigh
Liederbach 1985[198]	Professional ballet	256	48.8% foot and ankle 18.4% leg 14.5% lower back 7.4% knee 7.0% hip 3.9% neck, upper back, upper extremity
Solomon 1986[199]	Professional modern	229	20.1% knee 19.6% ankle 15.3% lower back 14.5% upper back, neck, upper extremity 11.3% hip 7.0% leg 7.0% foot
Garrick 1993[200]	Professional ballet	309	37.2% foot and ankle 23.0% lower back 6.8% knee
Solomon 1995[149]	Professional ballet	70	29.0% ankle 18.0% foot 10.5% knee 9.0% hip/thigh 8.0% lumbar spine 8.0% cervical/thoracic spine 6.5% leg 6.0% shoulder 5.0% other

ily a function of selection, but is also reinforced with multiple years of dance training during which "flat backs" are encouraged. Orthopaedists refer to reduced cervical lordosis commonly seen on x-ray in dancers as "dancer's neck."

An extremely high incidence of scoliosis among both men and women in ballet[82,119] has been reported. Fifty percent of female dancers and 27 percent of male dancers in two elite ballet companies presented with scoliotic curves.[82] This compares with a general population rate of 4 per-cent.[121] Whether there is some soft tissue variation accompanying dancers with scoliosis that assists them in excelling in ballet (such as their ability to attain extreme flexibility), or whether it is simply some other coinciding event, such as the recommendation of a family physician that a parent and child attempt to control scoliosis through ballet lessons,[120] is purely speculative. Researchers investigating the etiology of idiopathic scoliosis have questioned whether or not collagen deficiencies or some mechanism for paraspinal muscle imbalance might be present and play a role in the development of scoliosis.[122-125] Rosenberg et al.[126] observed a similarity in the mesenchymal and embryologic development in ballerinas and patients with hypomastia and mitral valve prolapse, two groups in which the incidence of scoliosis is also quite high. A relationship between scoliosis, stress fracture rate, secondary amenorrhea, and delayed menarche has been reported in dancers.[119]

As discussed in the previous section, dancers are expected to maintain a square torso because it is thought to produce a more beautiful line as well as provide the greatest amount of stability for the difficult movements of the lower extremities. This demand for stability of the trunk against expansive movement ranges of the lower limbs results in functional hypermobility at the pelvis. Many dancers are able to assume extreme hip and lumbar spine hyperextensions against the square contralateral torso. For example, in an arabesque, the dancer is expected to maintain a square torso over the laterally rotated stance leg, clearly demonstrating that, as the skill requirements in dance training advance, so do the musculoskeletal requirements to maintain the baseline postures (Figs. 5-1, 5-6, 8-9, 8-17). In order for the dancer in arabesque to keep the torso square, a great deal of spinal rotation and extension must be employed in opposition to the gesturing limb. Accommodation for this ROM becomes available through vertebral rotation, mobility at the lumbosacral and sacroiliac (SI) joints, or sometimes, from spondylolysis.[81]

The majority of back injuries, like most other dance injuries, can be attributed to repetitive movement stress. Keller and West[127] attribute much of the mechanical back symptomology reported by dancers to the cumulative effects of spinal adjustments required to accommodate the constant technical demands for leveling and unleveling the pelvis while the center of gravity is shifting. They surmise that the asymmetrical loading of articular and soft tissue structures common in dance training, which is done repetitively and at extreme end-ranges of joint capacity, is a major risk factor in injury to the back. These risks are amplified during actions such as mps and overhead lifting.

Repetitive lumbar hyperextension in unilateral stance positions such as arabesque, and in bilateral stance positions such as port-de-corps to the back, place increased compression and shear forces on the posterior components of the spine with associated tensile forces anteriorly. This may contribute to lumbar stress fractures, facet joint impingement, and disc degeneration. The incidence of spondylolysis and spondylolisthesis in dancers (12–17 percent) resembles that of elite gymnasts, and is higher than the general population (6 percent).[125] Lower extremity weakness and/or injury also affects and is affected by lumbar spine and pelvic musculature.[129,130] Certainly, bone mineral density is a factor in the amenorrheic dancers, as well.

Marshall[131] reports that sacroiliac dysfunction is the most common lumbosacral pathology in professional classical dancers. He describes how, normally, the irregular articular surfaces of the S I joint and the posterior interosseus ligament as well as the anterior sacroiliac ligament and the iliolumbar, sacrospinous, and sacrotuberous ligaments, permit only limited gliding and rotary movements. Pathology at this region in dancers is related to both the torques inherent in the extreme movement demands of ballet technique as well as the ligamentous laxity most elite dancers possess.

The piriformis muscle can also cause low back, buttock, and leg pain. The piriformis originates from the anterior surface of the sacrum and attaches onto the greater trocanter. In the hip it functions as an external rotator and abductor. For dancers, it can become short and tight, due to chronic turnout postures. The sciatic nerve passes through (or under) the piriformis, and irritation to the nerve trunk may result from this prolonged positioning or from other biomechanical influences such as leg length discrepancy. Symptoms can occur in both genders and usually include tenderness on palpation and discomfort with stretch. A predisposing factor in this piriformis syndrome may be unilateral iliopsoas tightness or hip abductor weakness. Stability of the pelvis may be affected by these tight and short structures, resulting in overuse and spasm of the piriformis. By virtue of its muscular attachments, persistent piriformis spasm can limit pelvic and lumbar movement, in turn leading to gait deviations. In those dancers lacking spinal symmetry, one may suspect leg length discrepancies. Since scoliosis is so common among elite dancers, if leg length is a factor, usually the piriformis on the shorter leg side is involved.

Hip

Hip rotation is known to be greatest in infancy and declines during childhood.[132] The adaptations that occur in dancers to influence hip ROM are not yet fully understood. Watkins et al.[133] looked at 350 dancers of different ages and levels for turnout as measured by foot placement. The authors found that dancers 12 years and under had more turnout than college-age dancers. According to Sammarco,[134] up until the age of 11, a dancer has the opportunity to improve turnout to some extent by influencing the shape of the femoral neck angle. Thomassen,[135] however, feels that anteversion of the femoral neck cannot be altered, and that turnout can only be improved by stretching the iliofemoral ligament. And he contends that after the age of 15, it is not possible to improve rotation at all. Sammarco[134] states that after childhood, turnout is achieved by stretching the anterior hip capsule and that since the chemical structure of collagen permits relatively little elasticity, microscopic ruptures of the collagen fibers are responsible for any increase in external rotation during adolescence and adulthood. He also reports that the maintenance of static external rotation and abduction for several hours a day can lead to calcification in the capsule and acetabulum. This is an adaptation that leads to tension on the medial internal capsule with compression over the superior lateral acetabulum, in turn potentially leading to development of osteophytes on the femoral neck.

Clicks, pops, and snaps around the hip are common complaints of the dancer and are most often associated with the tensor fascia lata tendon passing over the greater trochanter or the iliopsoas tendon snapping over the anterior hip.[134] Renstrom[136] describes two types of hip snaps. The first type he describes occurs laterally from either a thickened posterior border of the iliotibial band or anterior border of the gluteus maximus moving over the greater trochanter, often producing secondary trochanteric bursitis. The second type is described as a more internal snapping, which results from the iliopsoas tendon passing over the iliopectineal eminence. Intra-articular causes of snapping hip symptoms include synovial chondromatosis, loose bodies, osteochondritis dissecans, osteocartilaginous exostosis, labral tear, or inverted labrum.

Bony and soft tissue constitution at the hip joint influence one's ability to achieve lower extremity external rotation, and dancers will vary in their ability to attain the desired range as demonstrated or described by the teacher. For the dancers whose turnout range at the hip is relatively restricted, compensatory mechanisms are frequently practiced in order to create an illusion of turnout. The most common of these mechanisms, especially in young dancers, is a strategy that includes decreased abdominal tone allowing for an increase in lumbar lordosis and anterior pelvic tilt. The result is a relaxation of the capsule and possible reorientation of the femoral heads to a more anteriorly translated position, thereby permitting greater lateral rotation of the hip.[137] Although the quest for perfect turnout may seem unreasonable to the clinician, it has been shown to permit increased abduction of the hip,[138] and so becomes very desirable to the dancer for advanced technical form and enhanced line.

Given the kinetic chain of events in this scenario and the stabilizing role of the abdominals in dance, it is not too surprising that some studies have documented poor isotonic abdominal strength scores in dancers.[139,140] It might be expected that a dancer utilizing the compensatory turnout strategy would not only score lower on tests of abdominal strength, but also demonstrate accompanying tightness in the iliopsoas and iliotibial band structures. Using a device designed to monitor pelvic motion as a measure of abdominal control, one study revealed that student dancers had significantly weaker abdominal strength scores than age-matched controls in Thomas tests and bilateral leg lowering tests.[139] Of related interest, Ellison et al.[141] looked at 150 non dance-trained persons in the general population and found that those with greater lateral hip rotation than medial hip rotation complained of low back pain more often than those with other hip rotation patterns.

Bauman[142] measured femoral neck anteversion angles in elite, classical dancers by analyzing the magnetic resonance images of both hips of 14 women. Two different formulas were used to calculate anteversion. The mean score of the 28 hips analyzed with the first formula was 11.9 degrees and 14.4 degrees on the second analysis. Standard reference texts often used by therapists define the "normal" range of anteversion angles as between 15 and 25 degrees.[143,144] According to Bauman's measurements, these dancers appeared to be below the traditionally defined "normal" measurements, leading one to suspect that it may account for their ability to manage extreme lateral hip rotation. However, his study also cited six other studies where the average anteversion angle of 1,436 anatomic specimens measured 11.4 degrees. Bauman's work indicates that magnetic resonance imaging technology redefines the traditional measures of "normal." We can infer that the functional external rotation dancers achieve is secondary to training-induced tissue changes and other movement strategies, since he concluded that the femoral neck anteversion in the measured group of dancers was similar to that of the general population.

Turnout in most dancers is actually accounted for by sequential contributions of segments in the spine, pelvis, and lower extremity. Approximately 60 percent of the lateral hip rotation in elite classical dancers comes from "above the knee," while the remaining 40 percent is provided "below the knee."[82,145]

Many authors[81–83,112,146–148] have reported increased measures of external hip rotation in dancers, the majority of whom conclude that dancer's hip ROM appears to be an adaptation to training. Garrick and Requa[146] studied 700 dancers for hip ROM and compared their findings to a large database of norms.[132] They found that the dancers' external hip rotation increased with age and technical proficiency and that the decline of internal rotation values cited as normal by Staheli[132] for late childhood and adult-

hood was not evident in the dancers, although they remained within normal ranges for internal rotation. That study and others[82,142] have concluded that overall ROM for the hip in dancers exceeds corresponding ranges for an age-matched, untrained population. Some studies report a reciprocal loss of some net internal rotation and attributed the adaptation to tight, highly developed hip external rotator muscles.[82,142]

Knee

The knee is exposed to considerable stress in dance. Some rotation of the lower limb is provided by rotation of the tibia[82] and a high frequency of eccentric loading is imparted to the quadriceps secondary to the repetitive landings from big jumps.[80] Some forms of modern dance technique appear to be harder on the knees than ballet training due to the fact that they include weight bearing activities directly on the knees.[149]

The knees of younger dancers tend to be at higher risk than older, more trained dancers,[150] due to the compensatory strategy used for limited external rotation of the hip. The dancer plants the feet in the desired angle of turn out and "screws home" the tibia on the femur (from a flexed to an extended knee in a closed chain stance) by pronating at the subtalar joints. This behavior increases the functional Q angle at the knees and predisposes the dancer to valgus stresses and patellofemoral syndromes.[150–154]

Typically, a 10–degree genu recurvatum exists in highly trained dancers,[81,82] and is thought by some to complement the look of the leg with its pointed foot. Genu recurvatum may be an indication of the general predisposition for ligamentous laxity in many dancers, or a necessary or useful compensation to maintain the COG over the equinus BOS.[82]

One study looking at the difference in electromyography (EMG) activity of the lower extremities in ballet versus modern trained dancers found that the ballet group possessed ≥ 10 degrees of genu recurvatum, where the modern dancers did not.[155] During stance and plié, the ballet dancers had greater anterior tibialis activ-

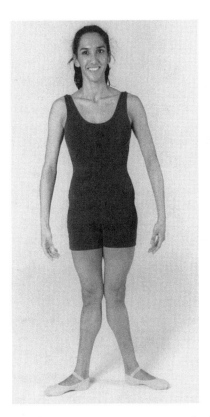

FIGURE 8-11 *Extreme genu recurvatum in first position.*

ity than the modern dancers in stance. This would likely be associated with their genu recurvatum, since this condition requires that the ankle assume a relatively plantar flexed orientation and the pelvis a relatively anteriorly tilted position (Fig. 8-11) to maintain verticality. The modern dancers, by contrast, had greater medial gastrocnemius activity in stance, denoting forward postural sway activity that one might expect with diminished BOS from the externally rotated legs.

Foot and Ankle

The ideal foot for ballet is described as a "square foot," which is flexible and in which the first and second metatarsals are the same length.[153,156] Aesthetically, the favored ballet foot is one with an appearance of a high arch for

pointe. Profiling data on elite dancers reveals a 90 percent prevalence of this apparent high-arched foot structure, with females being more homogeneous in type than males.[71] Dancers adapt to the needs for flexibility and control through hypermobility at the midtarsal joint, functional adaptations at the first and fifth rays, and powerful calf muscles.

Ninety degrees of plantar flexion is required at the ankle and midtarsal region of the foot in order for the dancer to accomplish pointe work[82] (Fig. 8-1). Likewise, 90 degrees of dorsiflexion at the MTPs is needed in order for the dancer to accomplish grand plié[157] (Fig. 8-8B), demi pointe (Fig. 8-2), and adequate propulsion for grand allegro skills. Hamilton et al.,[82] however, report decreased ankle dorsiflexion in their profile of elite professional ballet dancers, which they suspect is secondary to a capsular adaptation accommodating the increased need for ankle plantar flexion.

The pathomechanics of this functionally fixed equinus include adaptation for dorsiflexion at the midtarsal region and, therefore, extended pronation into gait cycle phases, exposing the dancer to excessive pressure and tensile forces on the medial column of the foot and, in turn, leading to increased compression forces at the lateral cuboid.[158,159] Late pronation allows for an unlocked forefoot near the toe-off phase of gait, where the angles of pull of the anterior tibialis and peroneal longus muscles are less optimal in their relationship to the first ray, preventing the ray from assuming its most effective position as a stable and rigid lever for propulsion.[158]

Contrary to what one might expect, the pedal intrinsic muscles in women ballet dancers tend to be weak. This may be due to the shoes they are required to wear in addition to the repetitive stress described above. Most dancers fit themselves for pointe shoes based on the visual appeal of a particular shoe, rather than for a truly proper fit. Very often the flex point of the shoe does not align with the first MTP joint, causing the dancer to place more compression stress and inordinate shear loads at this joint. The shoes may fit so tightly that they prevent the foot muscles and proprioceptors from being fully utilized

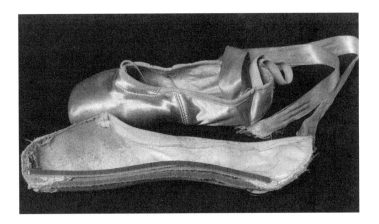

FIGURE 8-12 *Pointe shoe construction.*

because the foot is unable to articulate well in the shoe. Also, pointe shoes are made of inefficient shock-absorbing materials (cardboard and leather) and unforgiving vamps, so that impact loads are high (Fig. 8-12). Conversely, dancers who do not work in pointe shoes usually have highly developed intrinsic foot muscles, regardless of foot shape, assuming the absence of chronic injury.

Teitz et al.[66] looked at 13 ballet students in three groups according to toe length to determine relative pressures on the first and second toes on pointe. Toe length and padding affected the pressure on the second toe, but regardless of toe length, foot position, or padding, the first toe always bore the greatest pressure. Relevé with calcaneal eversion and forefoot abduction, a stylistic embellishment on the formal relevé position known as "winging" (Fig. 8-13), markedly increased the pressure at the first metatarsal phalangeal joint. Indeed, this foot posture also places the first ray at a mechanical disadvantage, requiring the flexor hallucis longus (FHL) and other supporting soft tissues to overcome inordinate tensile forces and encounter greater demands in order to flex the digits.

Other studies looking at the ankle mechanics of dancers yield dramatic findings. In a study of bone-on-bone forces during relevé en pointe, Galea[12] estimated the force at the ankle joint to be about 10 times body weight, comparable to that of a runner doing a 6-minute mile. In generating the power necessary to perform the relevé, muscle contraction greatly increases the amount

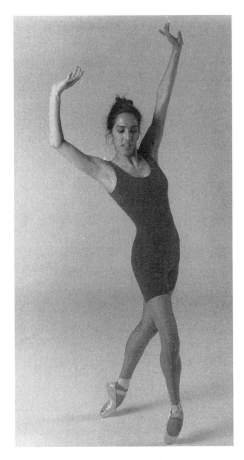

FIGURE 8-13 *Relevé with "winging".*

of compression forces acting at the joint surface. Unreported data from the same study indicate that the forces acting across the great toe joint are equivalent to more than twice body weight.

Sammarco and Miller[160] and Schneider et al.[161] suggest that forefoot deformity is correlated to dance movement. Conditions such as bunion deformity, hallux valgus, splay foot, hammer toes, and interdigital neuromas are common in ballet dancers. They suggest a relation between the unusual stresses and strains applied to the foot while performing pointe work. Several studies have attempted to assess stresses on the foot in functional dance activities. Kravitz et al.[162] electrodynographically measured foot forces of two ballet exercises, the relevé and the passé, in 16 dancers. The medial aspect of the first metatarsal head and hallux interphalangeal joint generated the greatest amount of pressure. Stacey[163] analyzed small ballet-specific jumps at three different speeds in three female ballet dancers in order to explore the relationship between electrical activity of selected lower leg muscles and foot contact force patterns. She found a significant relationship between medial foot impulse with EMG activity of the gastrocnemius and peroneus longus, suggesting stabilization activity against pronatory forces.

Two studies found an increased incidence of hallux changes in female ballet dancers compared to age and sex matched controls.[110,164] Ambre[164] measured the ROM of the first MTP joints in 20 female ballet dancers and found that their range was diminished regardless of age, perhaps due to a higher incidence of osteophytes on the margins of the metatarsal head than in nondancing controls. Van Dijk et al.[110] measured 19 retired professional dancers between the ages of 50 and 70 for ROM and roetgenographic examination of the MTP, ankle, and hip joints. He found statistically significant increases in hallux valgus deformity and first MTP dorsiflexion, with a decrease in toe plantar flexion. Dancers had increases in ankle inversion and eversion as well as in hip abduction, flexion, and external rotation compared to age-, sex-, and weight-matched controls. Einarsdottir et al.[165] looked at 64 active and 38 retired dancers from the Royal Swedish Ballet for incidence and severity of hal-

lux valgus deformity on radiograph. The authors concluded that age and gender, but not training exposure, influenced valgus angulation.

Since dancers spend so much time with a plantar flexed foot and ankle, they have been shown to develop a tight gastrocnemius-soleus complex with an accompanying loss of active dorsiflexion.[82] Limitation in functional dorsiflexion may contribute to subtalar pronation, known among dancers as "rolling in."[166] This condition also introduces the dancer to higher risks for flexor hallucis, Achilles, and posterior tibialis tendinitis,[46] cuboid problems,[167] and a myriad of compensatory responses along the kinetic chain. In addition, limitations in ankle plantar flexion or MTP dorsiflexion, especially in relevé, can cause calcaneal inversion with forefoot adduction or "sickling" and can increase risk of lateral ankle and foot trauma as well as suboptimal proximal compensations.

When the dancer is in relevé, the inherent anatomic stability of the talocrural joint (relatively close-packed in stance) is lost. Without anatomic stability, surrounding musculature—most notably the peroneal muscles—are forced to contract more forcefully to stabilize the foot.[168] Standing posture on pointe is further reported to change the biomechanics of the ankle invertors and evertors so that they become functional plantar flexors and dynamic stabilizers of the ankle.[169] The flexor hallucis longus tendon (Fig. 8-14) (referred to as the "dancer's Achilles heel") may become inflamed and lead to partial rupture. The erosion of this tendon within its osseofibrous tunnel, or stenosing tenosynovitis, can result in a condition commonly referred to as "trigger toe.[151,152,170,171] Crepitus may be palpated behind the medial malleolus and a visual triggering may be perceptible with flexion of the great toe when the ankle is pointed.[135]

A large portion of dance involves jumping activity. Improper mechanics on jump landings, such as double heel contact or no heel contact, has been attributed to shin pain.[172] Inefficient distribution of the forces throughout the foot and eccentric stretch velocities that are unable to assist the recoiling and elasticity of the lower extremity muscles have been cited as probable causes of the pain reactions.[163]

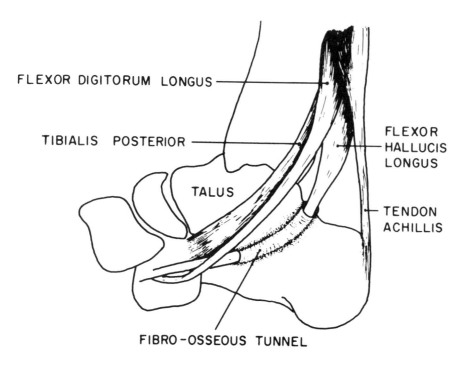

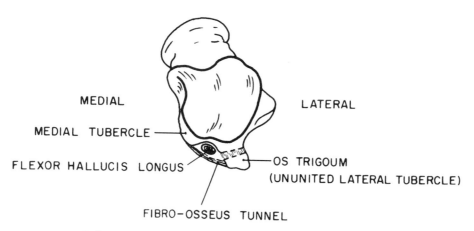

FIGURE 8-14 *Fibro-osseous tunnel of flexor hallucis longus. (From Hamilton,[207] with permission.)*

INJURY DISTRIBUTION

Injuries are common in dance. Between 50–80 percent of dancers report overuse syndromes sometime in their professional career[4] and up to 46 percent experience stress fractures.[119] Sixty-five percent of injuries are reported to result from overuse, and the other 35 percent result from trauma.[71,149] Significant differences in injury patterns were found in two elite ballet companies when age and onset of a professional career are considered. In one company, the incidence of stress fracture was higher among dancers of both genders who entered the professional company setting at a later age and was highest among women with amenorrhea. The frequency of injuries and time disabled were a function of exposure whereas severity of injury was a function of age.[4] In the second ballet company, subgroups of dancers ranked according to age and status revealed a generally unremarkable spread in their injury distribution tracking. One exception was noted in that a few of the dancers (10 percent of the company members) experienced more frequent injuries than the other 90 percent did.[149]

Ballet dancers suffer injuries to the foot and ankle more often than modern dancers. Modern dancers, in turn, tend to report injuries to their knees and backs more frequently (Table 8-2). Dance movement in classroom training is similar for both sexes, but footwear and choreographic demands differ in rehearsal and stage performance, particularly in ballet. Injuries vary, not only according to form, but to gender.

Gender-specific injury patterns were noted over a 9-year period in the Joffrey Ballet.[71] In that company, a 35 percent higher incidence of injury in the foot and ankle region was noted in female dancers. Men, on the other hand, had a higher incidence of back pain over the same time interval. Solomon et al.[149] reported that women suffered more than twice the number of foot and ankle injuries compared to men over 1-year period at the Boston Ballet, while male injuries were mainly knee, hip/thigh, cervicothoracic, and shoulder related.

Ballet does not specifically condition for the demands of lifting, and hence, the dancers who are required to execute the lifts are at risk of overload injuries. In addition, partnering practices in dance do not necessarily follow optimal lifting principles. Lycholat,[173] in a 1982 survey of three British ballet companies, reported that one-third of male back pain sufferers attributed their problems to lifting.

Men develop anterior ankle impingement more frequently than women dancers. Its occurrence is linked to years of landing from large jumps into the demi plié position where anterior articular margins of the tibia impinge on the talus and bone spurs develop. Anterior ankle impingement is associated with eccentric weakness of the calf and can lead to decreased ROM at the ankle and compensatory pronation or supination, depending on its location. This, in turn, can result in capsulitis of the first MTP joint.[153]

Women, working in the extreme plantar flexion of pointe, develop more posterior ankle impingements. The superior aspect of the posterior calcaneus impinges against the posterior articular margins of the tibia, producing an os trigonum (osteophyte of the posterior talus) (Fig. 8-15). This condition must be differentially diagnosed from Achilles tendinitis, plantar fascitis, and retrocalcaneal bursitis.

Other Components of Injury

PSYCHOSOCIAL CONSIDERATIONS

An understanding of the psychological culture within which a professional dancer rises is crucial to working with them in the rehabilitative context. As described by Kerr et al.[176] "a dancer is someone who trains daily for 10 years or more, investing time, money, and energy with the foreknowledge that gainful employment is questionable, and that even success guarantees little, [...in fact, a] good chance of living at the poverty level. Dancers have different values and priorities from persons in mainstream career cultures."

Dancers profile differently than athletes when it comes to the contribution of personality to injury. Hamilton et al.[4] suggest that this is due to the nature of dance, where "dancers have been programmed to compete continually with themselves rather than at specific intervals against an opposing team." They report that regardless of gender, the dancers with the greatest number of total injuries throughout their careers were significantly more enterprising than those with fewer injuries, according to measures on several self-report personality inventories. The dancers with stress fractures and other overuse syndromes were ascribed the personality type of the "overachiever." The authors concluded that the very personality factors that inspired the dedication and physical perfection required to make it to the elite levels of dance may be the same fac-

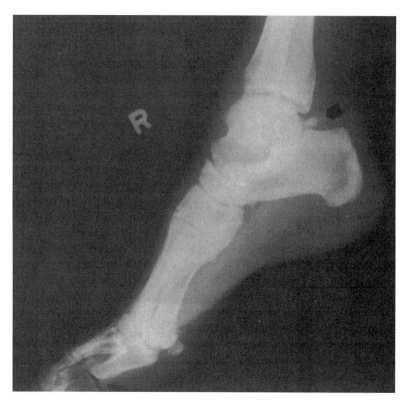

FIGURE 8-15 *Posterior impingement with os trigonum. (From Sammarco*[151]*, with permission.)*

tors contributing to overuse injuries in those dancers. Even at the elite levels, intense daily training continues and microtraumas ensue. When facilitating the restoration of function in the clinic, it is important for the clinician to be aware of the effort the dancer puts forth in any restorative exercises, in addition to the overall *effort exposure* (what else has the dancer done that day, week, year as well as how many years of their life they have been training). Values such as perfectionism and daily personal bests are engrained in the dancer. Relative rest and time-out from some activities in order to restore function *progressively* is anathema to their sense of professional responsibility as well as to the maintenance of their identity and self-worth.

Despite the emergence of dance medicine as a recognized subspecialty to orthopaedic sports medicine within the 1980s, the creation of dance-oriented medical organizations (PAMA, Performing Arts Medical Association, and

IADMS, International Association for Dance Medicine Sciences), and the formation of several special interest groups within organizations like the APTA and NATA, several studies have emphasized the lack of participation by dancers in seeking traditional medical treatment or in adhering to the recommendations prescribed at those consultations. Kerr et al.[174] describe a 97 percent injury rate among dancers, where only 20 percent of those injuries resulted in a physician visit. The authors postulated that, in addition to factors such as lack of money and time, dancers often complained that physicians saw their injury as an isolated event without the context of their entire lifestyle and training history.

Often, the intense concern of the dancer over an injury may put off a clinician not familiar with their mindset. The clinician may view the dancer as obsessive and unreasonable. As Hamilton[117] described it, "As with any professional athlete who depends on the maintenance of the body, the dancer becomes very conscious of injury. Like the racehorse, the dancer's life depends entirely on their physical condition, so psychologically they display great insecurity with regard to aches and pains. Every affliction, no matter how minor, becomes a catastrophic accident with thoughts of what if I can't dance flashing through their minds."

ENVIRONMENTAL CONSIDERATIONS

Most athletes have the benefit of being able to use shoes for injury prevention. Shoes not only protect the skin against bruising, but can provide stabilization, as well as absorb and return energy. Dancers are not so lucky. Modern dancers generally perform barefoot. Jazz dancers wear very soft oxford leather shoes allowing for maximal articulation of the foot, or character shoes which have heels anywhere between 2–6 in for Broadway show-style costume wear. Ballet dancers wear an even softer leather or canvas shoe, also for maximal foot articulation, or in the case of the women, a pointe shoe made of satin, cardboard, and glue (Fig. 8-13).

Performing surfaces, usually stages, are not always ideally built or maintained. They may be raked (sloped), splintering, or even made of cement. The ideal floor is of sprung wood construction, with marley or smooth wood surfacing. Stage lighting for dramatic effect can be very low or extremely bright, affecting the dancer's ability to visually regulate. Performances may take place outdoors where rain, humidity, or extreme temperatures may present injury or illness risks.

TRAINING METHODS

Methods of training dancers have come under criticism in recent years. Dance continues to be dictated by artistic, not scientific, traditions. Dance training does not incorporate modern conditioning principles that would better prepare dancers for the metabolic and specific strength stresses encountered during performance.[22]

Given the lack of reliable rest cycling and formal periodization to load build up, as well as the lack of cardiovascular endurance training inherent in dance training, its anaerobic nature, and the common practice of chronic calorie restric-

tion for maintenance of low body weight, the professional dancer is at high risk of fatigue injuries and illnesses at all times. The greatest number of injuries per year are reported during performance seasons when the dancers become most vulnerable to fatigue and burnout syndromes. Liederbach, Gleim, and Nicholas[3,174] measured urinary catecholamines and mood states in professional ballet dancers during a 5-week performance season and observed that both indices rose significantly over time into the season and coincided with onset of injury. Therefore, the practitioner should always be careful to monitor for overtraining status in dancers.

Monad et al.[175] found that muscles contracting at levels greater than 20 percent of their maximal contraction are susceptible to fatigue overload. Previous authors[176-178] have implicated muscle fatigue as the origin of tibial stress fractures, an injury common in ballet dancers (Fig. 8-16A). In women, this can be exacerbated by an oligo/amenorrheic status (Fig. 8-16B). All dancers are subject to lower extremity and spine fatigue reactions such as stress fractures, which are correlated with 5 or more hours of dance per

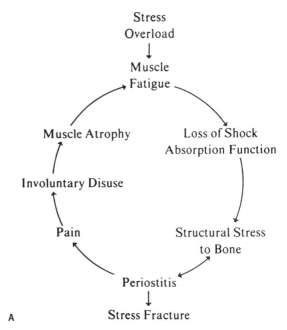

FIGURE 8-16 *(A) Etiologic theory of stress fractures. (From Clement[177], with permission)*

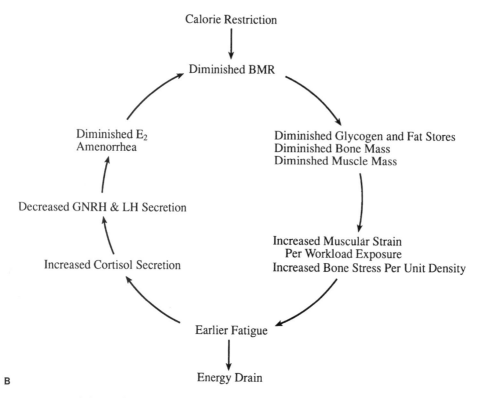

B

FIGURE 8-16 *(B) Etiologic theory of stress fractures in females.*

day.[179] The "dancer's fracture" is a spiral fracture of the shaft of the fifth metatarsal, and often occurs in an anterolateral inversion sprain from the pointe position. It may also be accompanied by distal fibular fracture, interosseous membrane irritation, or subluxation or dislocation of the peroneal tendons.[151,179] Fractures are also common in the tibia[161,180] second metatarsal,[169,181] pedal sesamoids[182] and the Lisfranc's joint.[183]

Long-term training produces changes in tissue composition that may result in less loading on the muscle spindle apparatus.[57] When this is not alternated with periods of appropriate rest and replenishment, damage may exceed recovery and anabolism. Noonan et al.[186] examined the effect of passive stretching on subclinical muscular injury. He presented data demonstrating changes in contractile function without measurable changes in muscle tension and discussed the athletic vulnerabilities from this form of muscular impairment. He stated that "just as a fracture in the tibia becomes a location at which

stresses are concentrated, a small defect in the muscle may act as an area where further muscle damage occurs with time and use, ultimately leading to total muscle rupture."

Steffen[185] studied the effects of fatigue on the performance of a vertical jump using force plate, EMG and cinematographic techniques in 9 advanced modern dancers. Jump height, joint angle, timing, and direction of jump were all affected by fatigue. Studies demonstrate significant relationships between fatigue, neuromuscular control, and coordination.[140] Among other variables, reflexes (already diminished in dancers) are known to diminish with fatigue.

Overall fitness training, therefore, is extremely important for dancers in the rehabilitation clinic to try to offset fatigue and repetitive stress issues. Dancers must train aerobically so that they may better physiologically manage the continual anaerobic cycling to which they are exposed. In addition, they should train specifically in anaerobic bursts for metabolic adaptability. Both forms of adjunct cardiovascular training can assist the dancers not only with weight control, but with the psychologic need for movement during required relative rest periods surrounding injury. Resistance training will not only maintain or promote strength and stability, but also potentially increase muscle metabolism, which will, in turn, demand greater energy expenditure, further assisting in weight control.

Technique training in dance remains constant while choreography does not. It is important to remember that dance as an art form exists in a cultural context, and adapts to changing social tides. A dance created in the 1990s is contextually and stylistically different than one that was created in the 1850s. Today's dancing is far more athletic than it was even two decades ago, and exhibits changes in gender responsibility. For example, women do much more of the lifting and large jumps today than they used to, exposing them to increased forces that they do not train for in technique class.

Although it is helpful to introduce fitness and strength concepts to the dancer in the clinic, generalized resistance training may provoke expressions of fear from the women dancers that the weights will either interfere with their technique or make their muscles bulky, causing them to gain weight and place them in jeopardy of not being able to maintain their contracted weight limits. It is important to take the time to educate the dancer about ability to develop functional strength without unduly influencing body shape and to discuss tissue density, which may reflect a change of body weight. Measurements of strength have been shown to improve first via neural recruitment followed by fiber hypertrophy. Lean body mass may change in some cases and it may be appropriate to intervene with the company director on this issue.

Dance-Specific Functional Movement Evaluation

Dance-specific evaluation should always be included in an initial or early evaluation. Basics of placement and technique should be well reeducated before skill reacquisition training and before resumption of class, rehearsal, and performance. Like other rehabilitation progressions, it is useful to master symmetrical and balanced postures before proceeding to off-balanced and form-specific movements. Therefore, alignment, muscular activation, and joint and postural stabilization is observed in the dancer's evaluation. Tables 8-3, 8-4, and 8-5 provide the clinician with a list of functional tasks they might find useful for picking up cues to the anatomic regions that dancers have been trained in or selected for that may leave them vulnerable to injury.

MOVEMENT EVALUATION CRITERIA

As stated earlier in the chapter, dancers do not have regulated training seasons. Hence, preinjury functional testing data are often not available on them. This can present a real problem for the clinician in terms of knowing to which objective criteria a given dancer's progression or current complaints should be compared.

Although the typical dance school or company lacks formal training cycles, there do exist fluxes in their workloads. For example, compared to the increased intensity of the performance season, the postperformance or posttour period is often relatively light, where the dancer will typically drop exposure to one class per day for technique maintenance. On the other hand, the preperformance cycle is quite rigorous because the dancer is not only learning new ballets, but is rehearsing them with "full-out" effort repetitively.

Although the unregulated, and often unpredictable, postperformance cycles are not truly representative of an off-season or preseason state, but merely of a more regular ongoing training status, they do, nevertheless, represent the best time for a clinician to gather baseline data. The clinician beginning coverage of a company or school, should be watchful for these relatively low-load cycles and set up a multistation functional screen to take place during that period. When this is not possible, the clinician will have to instead rely on the contralateral, uninjured side for functional criteria from which to make comparisons in the rehabilitation setting.

TABLE 8-3 *Static (postural) functional dance evaluation*

This table provides the basis for functional evaluation of static dance postures. Each position has specific criteria to assess in determining the ability of the dancer to achieve and maintain static postures. The evaluation criteria are to used as guidelines for observing the dancer with respect to key elements of each position/action.

DANCER POSITION/ACTION	CLINICIAN OBSERVATION	EVALUATION CRITERIA

Parallel first position stance	Sagittal View	COG to BOS relationship
		Compensatory strategy present
		    Fixed equinus? Midtarsal/first ray plantar flexed? longitudinal arches?
		    Genu recurvatum
		    Pelvic tilt
		    Hyper- or hypolordosis
		    Thoracolumbar to lumbosacral junctions?
		    Cervical/head posture/control

	Coronal (posterior) view	Symmetry
		    General LE weight-bearing
		    Calcaneal-crural alignment ("assumed" and STJ neutral stances)
		    Fore- to rearfoot relationship
		    Navicular tuberosity to floor
		    Popliteal and gluteal folds
		    PSIS, iliac crests, etc.
		    Scapular angles, acromion processes

Parallel foot plant while executing repetitive, transverse plane rhythmic pelvic rotations	Anterior	Pelvis on femur rotation relationship[127] Pelvic response? 1 degree spinal adaptation to rotation: Level? Transverse plane ROM symmetry? Primary LE adaptation to rotation: Subtalar? Midtarsal? Tibial? Integrity of whole LE? Inversion/eversion rocking with LE rotation?
	Sagittal	COP symmetry? Supernal compensations?
Adam's forward flexion	Posterior	Axial segment ROMs and sequencing Scoliosis? Soft tissue atrophy/hypertrophy?
	Sagittal	COP distribution? Location of COG over BOS? Change in genu recurvatum, fixed equinus
Port de bras, en bas to en haut (flexion) and en bas to seconde (abduction)	Posterior	Scapulothoracic balance? (upper-lower traprezius/serratus) Scapulothoracic symmetry? Shoulder impingement? Full abduction ROM? Scapular stabilization? Cervicothoracic spine dysfunction?
	Sagittal	Scapular protraction? Full flexion ROM? Thoracic extension?

(Continues)

TABLE 8-3 *(Continued)*

DANCER POSITION/ACTION	CLINICIAN OBSERVATION	EVALUATION CRITERIA
Static first postition parallel relevé (observe bi- and unilaterally)	Posterior	Calcaneal height? COP distribution? Strategic stabilization—where? Fore- to rear-foot relationship? ROM at ankle? Midtarsal? MTPs? Spinal adaptations? Weight shift assymetry right vs. left? Fatigue—right vs. left? (calf, hip, and/or ankle control)
	Sagittal	Postural adaptations to lower BOS?
Undirected arabesque, each side	Posterior and Sagittal	ROM taken up at hip before spine? Lumbosacral dysfunction? Level of maximal spinal hyperextension? Spondylo step-off? Hip hike? Symmetry of and locus of rotation
		Stance limb COP; COG over BOS, maintenance of turnout? Cervical, thoracic spine; scapular/UE relationship, head alignment?
Gait	Sagittal and Coronal	Observation for planar dominances and asymmetries Comparisons/contrasts with normative kinematics

Abbreviations: COG, center of gravity; BOS, base of support; LE, lower extremity; STJ, subtalor joint; PSIS, posterior superior iliac spine; ROM, range of motion; COP, center of pressure; MTP, metatarsophalangeal.

Functional Testing in Dance

Functional control of the dancer is governed in part by strength, ability to rapidly adapt between mobility and stability demands, and cardiovascular power, but is also under voluntary stylistic control and perception of the dancer. The dancer's effort is affected not only by normal joint motion and baseline muscular strength, but also by recruitment sequencing, proprioceptive awareness, energetic and cognitive intent, concentration, relaxation, attention, motivation, and confidence.

According to Kirstein,[90] selection for professional status is based not on measures of time or distance, but on emotional and aesthetic attributes. Although dance can be a difficult activity to assess because of its qualitative components, some variables may be measured objectively by time, height, or distance gauges. Ergonomically, we can make some presumptions about the demands a dancer must be able to safely endure, and build a testing and training program accordingly.

Since dance is assessed primarily in techni-cal and interpretative terms that rely upon artistic judgment, some additional aspects of progression criteria should be considered. Tippett and Voight[186] suggest observing the performers' "control, confidence, and carriage" during functional progression protocols. This is a useful and elegant proposition. This type of observational assessment can be enhanced by asking the dancer for subjective feedback during rehabilitation tasks. Changes in physiologic and perceptual measures are expected in the clinic over time. Fitness training and mental anxiety both produce changes in heart rate.[187,188] However, one's perceived exertion of a task does not necessarily increase or decrease linearly with physical workload. Some measurement of perception is of value.[189] The scale developed by Borg can provide some information to the therapist about how his or her client is responding and adapting to a given task over time. Another subjective, psychological rating scale that has been validated in measuring fatigue among athletes and dancers is the Profile of Mood States.[190] This scale is a 50-item assessment, and is not practical for everyday, immediate feedback. Used on a weekly

TABLE 8-4 *Dynamic (technical) functional dance evaluation*

This is a continuation of Table 8-3, using dynamic ballet techniques in place of static positioning. Dynamic evaluation is usually carried out after the clinician is satisfied of the dancer's ability to maintain static postures. Clinicians may go directly to dynamic evaluation if they are familiar with the dancer's performance, rehearsal, training, and injury history.

DANCER POSITION/ACTION	CLINICIAN OBSERVATION	EVALUATION CRITERIA
Demi-plié, parallel	Posterior	Changes in: Navicular tuberosity position Calcaneal-crural alignment Iliac crest and above symmetry
	Sagittal	Symmetrical dorsiflexion? Primarily ankle or midtarsal? COP location Trunk alignment stable?
Grand-plié, turned-out	Sagittal and Anterior	Pre-movement: re-assessment for turned-out stance motion: Symmetrical flexion at MTPs, ankles, knees, hips? Lateral rotation maintained and aligned over first or second MT? Spine and pelvis neutral and stable? Muscular control eccentric and concentric? ROM taken up at demi- before grand-plié action? COP distribution and foot and ankle alignment throughout?
Plié to relevé (observe bi- and unilaterally)	Sagittal and Posterior	Postural integrity with weight shift? Initiation of movement? Control of movement?
Plie to relevé with port de bras	Sagittal and Posterior	Neutral postural stability? COP distribution? COG over BOS location?
Second position plié, weight shift into passé retire	Sagittal	Flexion at hip or lumbar spine? Spine and pelvis neutral? Posterior pelvic tilt? Lumbar flexion? COG over BOS? COP distribution? Sufficient hip abduction strength?
	Posterior	Femoral glide symmetrical[127]? Lateral shift of neutral pelvis? Hip hike or hip sink? Appropriate adaptation at ankle/foot?
Plié, fifth position to tendu fourth position, close fifth. Reverse to back. Reverse to other side.	Sagittal	Pelvis and spine neutral? Postural stability and weight shift on stance leg? Foot/ankle adaptation of stance foot? Full surface area of gesturing foot on floor? Full weight shift to front leg? Pelvic/spine adaptation (functional unilateral hip extension) Movement controlled? Abdominal activation? Maintenance of lateral thigh rotation? Square pelvis? Symmetry and location of distal lower extremity rotation?

(Continues)

TABLE 8-4 *(Continued)*

DANCER POSITION/ACTION	CLINICIAN OBSERVATION	EVALUATION CRITERIA
Sissone	Sagittal and Anterior	Check locus of landing force Appropriate muscular control of landing forces through kinetic chain? Proper overall alignment maintained?
Unilateral sautés with opposite foot in coup de pied position	Sagittal and Anterior	Depth and control (maintenance of lateral rotation without anterior pelvic tilt; hip sink; excessive or late pronation) of plié and subsequent height of jump Postural control Surface area of feet and COP distribution on take off and landing. Zero, single, or double heel strike on landing? Pronatory and supinatory control on take-off and landing? Control of lateral thigh rotation? Compensations at distal lower extremity? Time to onset of fatigue (recruitment of trunk musculature)

or monthly basis, however, the clinician might find it helpful in monitoring training.

Functional tests may include tasks like the number of successful single-leg jumps the dancer is able to accomplish without fatigue-induced technical adaptations; vertical jump height in sauté position, long jump distance for jeté from each leg (Fig. 8-17); limb position replication with eyes closed; Rhomberg time tests; length of time a dancer can hold single-leg plié-like wall-sit at varying angles; number of mistakes made in reaction time drills such as the ability to follow rapid commands to jump to a specified quadrant within a four-square box; and dancer's ability to sustain postural control while changing weight-bearing responsibility from limb to limb to trunk (Tables 8-6 and 8-7).

The traditional orthopaedic sports and dance medicine rehabilitation protocols utilize three phases: healing time, restoration of motion and basic strength, followed by retraining of supernormal strength and skill. In what is described as the fourth phase, below, metabolically specific overload conditioning and cognitive awareness coaching is also included.

Incorporating and building upon the three-stage, spectrum-based rehabilitation structure for dance injury rehabilitation described by Hamilton and Molnar,[191] a four-stage progressive reconditioning program is described below and encapsulated in Table 8-8. The progression is designed in such a way that the clinical goals coincide with progression back into dance motions and the formal dance setting.

Two general considerations are important when developing a functionally progressive program for injured dancers:

1. Dancers rarely, if ever, vary or augment their daily training with other conditioning modalities. Therefore, not only are they exposed to repetitive stresses, but they reinforce one set of motor patterns which creates imbalances.[168] One of the major factors in creating imbalances is that ballet does little to strengthen abdominals, UEs, or ankle dorsiflexors.

2. Although dancers are required to maintain very lean body masses, a 1-hour ballet class utilizes only 200 kcal in women and 300 kcal in men.[2]

Important components to every rehabilitation program include:

1. Design exercise regimens that will rebalance the underutilized movement ranges while resting the overused tissues.

2. Include an aerobic component that will increase energy expenditure and allow the dancer to improve nutritional intake. (Clinicians should keep an eye out for those dancers suspected of eating disorders. These

TABLE 8-5 *Functional evaluation: dance coordination/integration assessment tasks*

This table reviews selected evaluation of basic and advanced ballet functional tasks. These test movements can be used during the rehabilitation period, as long as the clinician has determined that the dancer is capable of performing these tasks, based upon evaluation of static and dynamic techniques (Table 8-3, 8-4).

TASK	COMMON TECHNICAL FAULT	MOVEMENT EVALUATION CRITERIA	POSSIBLE INJURY RISKS
Stance Task Lower limb task Have the dancer accomplish his/her maximal turnout for first position from an unloaded approach such as via low-friction, lazy-susan-type rotation discs or having the dancer press up with upper extremities on parallel bars, rotate hips while raised and then lower to stance, making no further lower extremity rotational adjustments. Compare this to the undirected turnout stance accomplished by the dancer as typically done in the studio.	Turnout accomplished other than by hip Cannot maintain proper lower extremity or spinal alignment relationships (poor line)	Angle differential—locus of compensation Screw home foot placement Excessive pronation Excessive tibial rotation Anterior pelvic tilt Hyperlordosis Overall postural assessment Patella center over second MT Level pelvis Neutral spine/square torso Hip ER and adduction strength Trunk muscle strength COG over BOS	Medial ankle tendinitis Cuboid subluxation Hallux valgus—capsular strains Neuromas Meniscal, MCL, and/or PFPS Closed chain ACL overloading Spondylolysis ITB/psoas contractures
Upper limb tasks Port de bras En bas to en haut (flexion) En bas to second (abduction)	Dropped or saggy arms (external rotation of the humerus). Suboptimal thoracic extension or scapular elevation	Scapula stabilization Scapula symmetry Neutral spine/square torso	Weak scapula stabilizers Weak rotator cuff muscles Insufficient cervical/thoracic stabilization
Weight Shift Task Piqué Turned out plié to relevé shifts: forward to backward (sagittal) step ups or side to side (coronal) step ups. Temps Lié Fifth position, slide and close or tendu, plié, and close to fifth on front leg. Reverse. Chassé Temps lié with jump to close.	Lack of postural stabilization Poor weight shift strategy (resulting in unsuccessful transfer and/or poor line) Dynamic position of foot/ankle Sickling (ankle and midtarsal plantar flexion and inversion with forefoot adduction) Winging (ankle and midtarsal plantar flexion and eversion with forefoot abduction)	Postural dys-automatization: loss of feedforward control or motor program for basic dance postures Poor kinesthetic reproducibility Weak trunk and/or lower extremity musculature Functional scoliosis Placement of foot Suboptimal movement strategy: Hip sinks on stance leg (Trendelenberg) Weak hip abductors Diminished medial femoral glide Anterior ankle impingement Hallux limitis or rigidis	

Task	Observable faults	Contributing factors	Potential injuries
Unilateral Stance/lower extremity gesture Task Arabesque balance while executing transverse plane, counterbalanced port de bras rotations. Passé Ronde de jambe Developpé	Poor ROM flow (take-up) Timing of muscle activation Loss of alignment in stance limb Loss of balance	Hip hikes on gesture leg Quadratus lumborum recruitment 2 degree hip flexor weakness and/or uncoupling of lower extremity pelvis Hamstring tightness Contributing factors Ligamentous laxity Intrinsic/extrinsic muscle weakness Capsular shift—fixed equinus Excessive and/or late pronation Genu valgum Genu recurvatum Pelvic/spinal adaptation Spinal flexion, lateral flexion or hyperextension before full movement range utilized in hip flexion, abduction and extension, respectively COG over BOS integrity Muscle fatigue onset Placement of gesture leg foot	Ankle sprains Spiral fractures Facet impingements Osteophytes Trochanteric bursitis MCL sprains Mechanical LBP Spondylolysis Ankle sprains and tendinitis
Jump Task Bilateral Sauté first position Entréchat quatre Cabriole Unilateral Sauté with contralateral foot in coup de pied posture Jeté	Labored appearance Hard landing	Dynamic LE malalignment Excessive trunk muscle recruitment (heaving with shoulder girdle and torso) Knee valgus Excessive and/or late pronation Suboptimal propulsion at first ray Heel contact Multiple None Ankle, knee and hip ROMs Impingement suspected Lacks eccentric plantar flexion and/or quadriceps/hamstring control	All of the above Shin splints Tibial and metatarsal stress fractures Calf strains
Turn Task Double pirouette en dehors beginning in fourth position, finishing in fifth position. Piqué Fouetté	Fall out of turn Lose verticality of square torso Imprecise landing Lose control over angular acceleration	Movement skills Inability to select movement patterns which require changing reference frames increased degrees of freedom leading to loss of optimal movement strategies trunk and/or LE strength Suboptimal kinesthetic awareness	Torsion stresses along spine Ankle sprains (anterolateral sprains often accompanies by fifth metatarsal and/or fibula fracture)

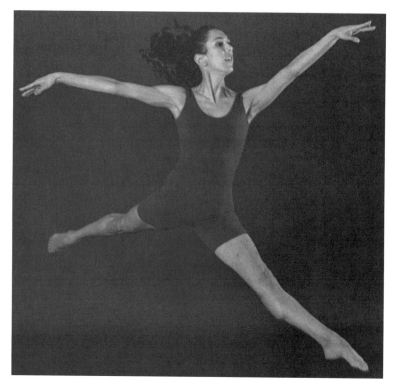

FIGURE 8-17 *Jeté or leap.*

dancers should be referred for professional medical evaluation and *not* be put on a fitness program that may serve as an incentive for further self-starvation and weight loss.)

Functional Progressions in Dance Injury Rehabilitation

DESIGN RATIONALE

Considering the lack of periodization and specificity of training issues, dancers should first recover and balance neutral function, develop a solid base of strength, stability, and endurance and then begin dance-specific motions, exercises, and skill training after injury. Skill patterning and overload training is dependent upon baseline fitness and balanced function as well as on psychological readiness.

Rehabilitation must begin immediately after injury and end when the dancer returns to full activity without limitations imposed by the injury and with full confidence in the stylistic demands of movements, stage sets, partners, and costumes. They must be fully educated about overall lifetime conditioning requirements for the prevention of reinjury.

Specificity of movement demands are important in the design of every program. Dance-specific exercises work best when they are reserved for the final stages of this reconditioning protocol where they may be incorporated into the context of an overall conditioning sequela.

Noyes believes that injuries are sport-specific and there are motions peculiar to each sport.[192] A functional progression for dancers must emphasize not only the typical agility, twist, squat, and vertical jump activities common to sports protocols today,[193] but also multiple and dynamic balances, jumps to and from one (and both) leg(s) in multiple directions, reacquisition of visual/somatic field in multiple lighting environments, and a recovered kinesthetic sense of side and back space. They must be non-

TABLE 8-6 *Functional skill tests for dance*

This table reviews the basic skills that are integrated in the performance of dance and dance techniques.

PARAMETER	EXAMPLE OF TASK	SCORE UNIT
Balance	Basic and dance-specific Rhomberg-type tests	Time
Agility	Direction oriented, dance-specific reaction time drills	Number of successful comprehension with time limitations imposed
Concentration	Movement task with changing instructions in chaotic environment	Number of successful comprehensions with sound and space distractions imposed
Proprioception	Above balance tests with changing surface and/or light environments	Time
	Vision restricted joint angle replication	Goniometric accuracy
Trunk strength and endurance	Pike sit-ups with mobile upper extremities	Number of repetitions without fatigue-induced movement errors
Trunk power	Transfer of lower extremity weight	Number of successful transfers utilizing translation strategy
	Efficiency of lower extremity placement following change in body level or directional facing	Number of successful foot placements with time-dependent level or direction changes
Lower extremity strength and endurance	Unilateral limb wall sits at varying angles	Time
Lower extremity power	Unilateral sauté jumps	Height and/or number of repetitions without fatigue-induced movement errors
	Unilateral jeté jumps	Distance

TABLE 8-7 *Functional training exercises*

This table reviews exercise and training techniques that can be used to rehabilitate deficiencies in the basic skills (noted in Table 8-6) of dance.

PARAMETER	EXAMPLE OF FUNCTIONAL TRAINING EXERCISE
Balance	Balance beam, trampoline weight shifts, Pro-Fitter in fourth position
Coordination	Standing bike with dowel rod
Agility	Four-square box changes with tendu releve and/or small jumps
Bilateral stance leg strength	Leg press with turned out plie, jumps
Unilateral stance leg strength	Airplane Rhomberg-variant
Gesture leg strength	AK resisted pulley on Universal system
Specific trunk strength	Pike sit ups, Swiss ball port de bras
Ankle strength	Closed chain press, backward treadmill walking
Concentration	Spontaneous recall and recitation of yesterday's activities while keeping precise movement and rhythm combination with unpredictable variations of floor surface, attempted conversations of others, light source changes
	Reversal exercises
Cardiovascular endurance	
aerobic	Aquatrex running and leaping, Nordic track, bike, Stairmaster, Treadmill
specific anaerobic	Jump rope with mixed foot patterns

TABLE 8-8 *Spectrum-based clinic-studio progression goals*

This table provides an example of a phased rehabilitation program for a FHL injury (see text). Note that the dancer's rehab program requires simultaneous clinical and movement training. Generally, techniques are cleared in the clinic prior to performance in the studio, although some overlap may occur, depending upon the severity of the injury and performance demands of the dancer.

PHASE	CLINICAL GOAL IN THERAPEUTIC SETTING	MOVEMENT GOAL IN STUDIO SETTING
Restricted Phase[187]	Reduce swelling and pain Active rest—maintain or build fitness level "around" the injury Evaluate kinetic chain for dysfunction Aerobic conditioning	Assume inability to dance safely Restrict tissue loading Develop motor control via Alternate non-weight bearing classes (floor barre, underwater barre, Feldenkrais, Alexander, yoga) Cognitive activities (mental practice, sympathetic overflow, observation of dancing classmates for knowledge of performance error learning[213])

Restoration Phase[187]	Restore ROM and baseline strength
	Pedal intrinsics and proximal PREs
	Open and closed chain therapy exercises
	Continue aerobic conditioning limiting planes of motion to 1 or 2 stationery bike, Nordic track, stairclimbers as appropriate
	Introduce functional weight-bearing work utilizing following concepts:
	  Parallel before turned-out
	  Wide base before narrow base
	  Slow tempos before fast tempos
	  Eyes open before eyes closed
	  Bilateral before unilateral
	  Uninjured before injured weight-bearing side
	  Linear before angular jumps
	  Progress from bi- to unilateral, supported functional tasks as tolerated
	Stance:
	  Pliés
	  Relevés
	  Rhomberg tasks (change surfaces)
	  Incorporate port de bras
	Turns:
	  Start 1/4 turn rotations from fourth position and progress as tolerated for greater angular displacement and velocities. Decrease lever arm by progressing from fourth to fifth—this requires greater force generation and loading of tissues.
		Restrict tissue loading exposure of injured tissues
		Tape, pad, shoe, or brace as indicated
		Restrict time in stance activities
		Allow maximal movement/training of non-injured areas
		Maximize functional strength building
		Barefoot work if teacher permits for optimal pedal intrinsic work and for enhanced proprioception (may need shoe support)
		Concentrate primarily on alignment and stability
		Return to standing barre with following limitations:
		Beginner's level class for slower pacing and more attention to baseline postural principles and fundamental foot placements.
		Focus on deconstructed technical skills.
		No jumps
		Elemental turns only
		Build from 1/4 turn rotations
		No opposition/épaulement
		Demi-relevé only
		No fourth and fifth position unless done with modified turn out.
		Continue adjunctive somatics classes

296

Chaines
Pirouette from fourth
Pirouette from second
Prelude to jumps:
Lunges in all directions
Plyometrics-leg press to boxes
Prances
Jump rope
Echappé

Reacquisition phase[187]

Progress overall strength and conditioning program to now include multi-planar WB activities: skate-gliding, treadmill tasks, obstacle courses
Progress bi- to unilateral supported work
Stance
  Women begin pointe strength and alignment retraining
Turns
  Pirouette from fifth
  Pique
  Fouette
  Turns with embellished posture
Jumps
  Bi- to unilateral sautés
  Linear:
    Assemblé
    Pas de chat
    Entréchat quatré
    Sissone
    Jeté
  Angular:
    Tour jeté
    Grand jeté en tournant
    Tour en l'air

Return to appropriate level class. Progress gradually from one class per day to number of classes taken during pre-injured status as fitness/fatigue level indicates and as other outside activity warrants
Limit number of jumps per class to one repetition cycle only
Begin repertory rehearsals of moderate technical and cardiovascular difficulty
Limit rehearsal exposure to approximately 2–3 hours
Soft leather or canvas shoes. Women may begin to wear their pointe shoes around the home to reacquire feel and calluses

Refinement phase

Build confidence, carriage, and control
Complicate skills training environment
Progress intensity, duration, and frequency of cross-training C-V drills
Introduce anaerobic bursts into C-V work
Progress port de bras, port de corps, opposition and épaulement into movement tasks
Increase speed and repetitions of specific skill tasks as appropriate
Progress cognitive integration with reversal, concentration and self-reports
Progress ROM expansion in dynamic balance work

Unrestricted dance movement and rehearsal exposure with clear understanding of issues surrounding fatigue, repetitive stress, muscle imbalance, and proper nutrition
Prescribed warm-up program
Discharge maintenance plan scheduled

verbally able to anticipate other movers in the same space, through peripheral vision and heightened attention to surroundings.

Specificity is emphasized with a concept of individually tailored and epigenetically governed overall program goals. That means that each dancer is assumed to have a unique body structure, injury mechanism, history of training experiences, level of personal development, and maturation (physically and cognitively) that will affect their psychomotor skill level and perception of personal responsibility. A dancer has learned body control through an integrated process of attention and concentration, which leads to cognitive-somatic awareness. That awareness must be used in successful relearning of motor tasks through practice with manual/verbal feedback from the clinician. Each dancer will have different levels of fitness, fatigue, depression, or language association. All of these variables (and more) affect re-education in the clinic and successful healing.

As in all sports, dance is dependent upon all of the neuromusculoskeletal components operating at peak efficiency when performance demands are high. This means adequate strength, cardiovascular endurance, somatic and kinesthetic control, and environmental awareness must be restored following an injury. For everyone, bilateral tasks precede unilateral tasks; supported tasks precede unsupported tasks; and linear motion precedes angular motion. Coordination of the rehabilitation stage with return to technique class (Table 8-8) provides important motivation to the dancer. Generalized restrictions are provided but should be modified for specific diagnoses, individual kinetic chain problems, or technique requirements (Table 8-9).

Balance is re-educated with changing visual, auditory, and stability stimuli. Begin static bal-

TABLE 8-9 *Functional Progressions for Dance*

This table gives examples of basic and advanced levels of movement requirements for dancers. Each dancer's training and rehabilitation regimen should include as many of these elements as possible. Exact progressions from basic to advanced will depend upon available equipment, dance background and requirements, and nature of current injury(ies).

PARAMETER	BASIC LEVEL	ADVANCED LEVEL
Movement Patterns	Pedestrian stance and gait	Ballet stances and skills
C-V	20–40 minutes, QIW, target HR	40 mins QD, alternate aerobic metabolism BIW with anaerobic bouts of ratio 2 minute max HR:5 minute rest
Strength	Wide, parallel base with proximal resistance keeping trunk in sagittal plane	Sagitally restricted base, i.e., "turned-out" with distal resistance; moving trunk, UEs, head and eye focus throughout frontal and transverse planes
Exercise Tempos	Slower	Faster
Mechanical Loads	Lighter	Heavier
Balance	Two legs	Single leg
	Grounded base of support (e.g., plié)	Narrow base of support (e.g., relevé)
Surface	Stable floor	Trampoline, sand, mattress, moving treadmill
Vision	Eyes open	Eyes closed
	Comfortable light level	Dim or very bright light level
Jumping	Low height, low repetitions	High height, moderate repetitions
	Two feet	One foot
Concentration surface	Perform simple verbal recall while performing balance task on stable floor surface	Perform complex verbal recall while executing unstable balance tasks, intermittently assessing HR
		Reverse exercises

ance training once the dancer can safely bear weight. Progression is recommended from bi- to unilateral,[139] from activities performed with eyes open to eyes closed, and from activities performed on a stable to an unstable surface, and ultimately to balancing while distracted from the concentration of balance (catching or throwing a ball, or reciting what was had for dinner the night before while lifting small dumbbells through a port de bras pattern). With regard to dynamic balance, the recommendations are to move from slow to fast speed, from low to high force activities, and from controlled to uncontrolled activities that are acceleration- and deceleration-specific.

Challenge the dancer with textural surface changes such as sand pits, mattresses, beams, and trampolines (Fig. 8-18); impose visual limitations; ask for progressive pliometric jumps from the leg press and then from boxes of variable heights. Progress them to backward and reversal exercises, high-load, high-level dance skills such as multiple turns; "partnering" with weights, then rolls, then skilled partners; bilateral to unilateral and multiple leaping sequences that may be first practiced in a pool or underwater tank or in a deconstructed pattern—gradually accumulating length, difficulty, complexity, and angularity.

The dancer can use the Pro-Fitter ski simulator in conventional and dance-specific ways. Have the dancer stand sideways on it in turned-out fourth position stance and work it anterior-posteriorly. Slide boards are also useful in helping the dancer learn how to control deceleration and coordinate overall timing when re-educating turn skills. For safety reasons, the dancer should always be spotted during such tasks.

ADDITIONAL DANCE-SPECIFIC CONSIDERATIONS

The abdominals in dance, especially ballet, primarily function as isometric stabilizers and as eccentric controllers. In rehabilitation, therefore, the clinician should choose strengthening that not only dynamically strengthens this muscle group to make up for the undertraining inherent in a dance education, but that also mimics

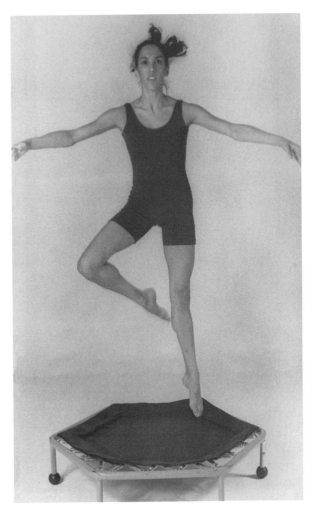

FIGURE 8-18 *Petit allegro jumps on a trampoline.*

motions needed by the dancer for performance. By and large, this means lifting the leg or legs up against gravity on a fixed pelvis and erect torso. Universal gym systems are useful for this (Fig. 8-19). In this case, there is cocontraction of the erector spinae and abdominals for torso and pelvis stabilization while the hips flex. Keeping the hips at less than 70 degrees will use the psoas and rectus femoris more than abdominals. Erect and supine work should emphasize a starting point of at least 70 degrees of hip flexion.

Abdominal exercises designed to be dance-shape specific and multisegmental, both on the

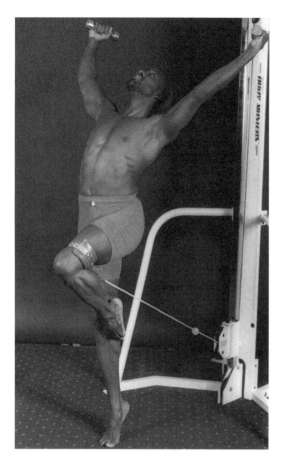

FIGURE 8-19 *Dance-specific movement with cable resistance.*

floor and standing, can be very challenging for the dancer. Have the dancer sit with the desired hip flexion angle accompanied by knee flexion so that the dancer's feet can rest on the floor or plinth and ask them to roll through a flexed spine down to a flat position for an eccentric component to overall abdominal training.

The overall coordination of the limbs, torso, and head in dance is complex and exacting. They must be specifically considered in the reconditioning of the dancer following injury. For example, ask the dancer to assume a tightly held pike position and perform a controlled separation of legs and torso to 70–90 degrees, while performing a port de bras with hand weights (Fig. 8-7). Progress to alternating leg action and add spinal rotation and shifting visual focus direction. This

will also incorporate the obliques and accomplish both exercise and functional progression.

The popular spinal stabilization (Swiss ball) protocols that have been introduced over the past few years are invaluable in the dance population. They are an excellent way to start the dancer off on a strength training program while they cannot aggressively weight-bear.

Other stabilization exercises can be specifically and functionally designed, when weight-bearing is tolerated, by attaching a weight resisted pulley to either the dancer's lower or upper extremity. A proximal placement is used initially. Movement phrases can incorporate spatial and rhythmic patterns for the UE/LE, with spinal flexion or extension and varying port de bras for broader coordination and phrasing. This can be initiated in parallel positions and progressed to turned-out postures. Progression also includes two- to one-leg stances, spinal rotation, changing eye focuses and light levels, and relevé for decreased base of support.

Dancers are accustomed to learning movement through imagery and respond very well to somatic techniques such as ideokinesis. Developed by Sweigard,[52] ideokinesis is a means of using the declarative memory system to "mentally visualize imagery which will facilitate improved neuromuscular coordination"[196] by creating moving images with directed, energetic, intentional lines of movement through specific anatomic sites within the body. Dancers are called upon to actively participate in the reintegration process of their injury by enhancing their sensorimotor awareness.

Interaction with the clinician, other patients, and other dancers is vitally important for the dancer to fill the socialization void they will encounter when removed from their regular daily setting and schedule. Feelings of connectedness or association with other people, groups, or activities will enhance wellness. It is important to monitor how information is conveyed to and interpreted by dancers. It is useful to have them execute introspective tasks, such as reporting on how they are feeling, what thoughts or images are coming up during their exercises, how many respirations or heart beats they are having per minute, how it changes with different workloads or exercises, and how it affects their mood. Demand that they pay full concentrated attention to given tasks. Vary and complicate their routines often to promote attention vigilance. Have them execute maximal effort in some exercises so they begin to comprehend what optimal effort is by comparison. These effort exercises should be repeated in many different forms, many times. By contrast, independent activities are built into every session, so that they develop a feeling of autonomy, achievement, and gratification. It may be appropriate to ask them to keep a log of their food intake and other activity and have them perform an analysis of how that affected their physical performance and their mood. Each of the integral parts plays a role toward greater development of kinesthetic awareness and body control.

One potential problem is that dancers become so accustomed to internal judgment and feedback that they assess themselves based on past experiences of success and familiarity. This type of "muscle memory" can be a help if the dancer is encouraged to retain the sense of their past movement experience for the valuable awareness it provides in knowing optimal levels of effort for a given task. Remind them that the only way to attain that level of finesse again is by setting future goals, accomplished only by fully concentrating on the present task phase.

Therapeutic and home exercises should always include linked and closed chain approaches since somatosensory integrity and environmental adaptability is critical and since injury to the musculoskeletal system will always have an impact on structures proximal and distal to the site of injury.

Dancers may often perform well in the clinic and then leave your setting resuming many previous postural habits that degrade their therapeutic gains. It is not unusual for young dancers to affect a toed-out gait during ADLs or habitually carry heavy bags over one shoulder. They will benefit by being reminded that what they do outside of your clinic and the studio is very important to their progression as well as their formal training. Coach the dancer that correct use of their posture and gait outside the studio and clinic, as well as appropriate rest, conditioning, and eating habits is helpful in affecting their therapeutic outcomes.

Example: Protocol for Grade I Flexor Hallucis Longus Tendinitis

Flexor hallucis longus (FHL) tendinitis is an injury that is fairly unique to and common within dance. The postural adaptations, numerous exposures to extreme plantar flexion, as well as excessive weight-bearing and unilateral loading, on turned-out and pronated LEs, contribute to this condition.

A thorough personal history, training history (current or recent and past as well as short and long term future goals) and family history from the dancer is important. If one is unfamiliar with the style or teacher the dancer is working with, try to find out more about it through interview or observation of a performance, rehearsal, or class video.

As in all orthopaedic injuries, it is essential that offending postures and movement patterns be identified and modified; that tissue swelling be reduced; motion restored; and functional strength, endurance, and technical skill be achieved. With regard to FHL injury, often the culprit is the diminished range of dorsiflexion at the talocrural joint that was discussed earlier. In essence, the trained and adapted excessive plantar flexion at this joint can offset available dorsiflexion. The midtarsal joints subsequently accommodate for dorsiflexion, throwing off the moments of pronation and propulsion.

Traditional orthopaedic measures for ROM and strength are measured. With dancers, it is recommended that these measures always include assessments of the hallux, foot/ankle (talocrural, subtalar, midtarsal, tarsal phalangeal), knee, thigh, hip, pelvis, and full spine. The dancer should be observed in simple stance and pedestrian tasks as well as in dance skills (Table 8–3, 8–4, 8–5), where one can observe alignment, movement style, and energetic approaches to the movement. ADL motions should be evaluated for symmetry, endurance, and strength before advanced skills are inspected. Reflexes and proprioceptive functions are assessed.

Neutral anatomic ROMs should be noted and judiciously restored. Most importantly, basic stance, gait, and movement patterns in neutral and fundamental dance postures should be re-educated so that an appropriate engram is established and potentially destructive patterns discouraged before the skill is imposed.

Electric stimulation (ES) for muscle re-education can be useful in the functional rehabilitation of dancers in all of the ways it is used for athletes and other orthopaedic patients. Its use in conjunction with movement specific postures and weight borne movements as part of pattern re-education arena is beneficial. One particularly interesting clinical application of ES for dancers with FHL tendinitis is over the abductor hallucis muscle in the foot, in order to promote kinesthetic awareness of pronatory control of the foot and to begin to recover subtalar neutral. The purpose of learning subtalar neutral is primarily so that they will understand the *sensation* of pronation in order to reduce their inefficiency in shock absorption at heel strike as well as the tensile loading in turned-out stance. Actively contracting their great-toe abductor muscles simultaneously with the on-cycles aids in this goal.

The pedal muscles are often extremely weak in ballet dancers, due to pointe shoe constriction and repetitive trauma. A battery of intrinsic foot exercises, such as doming (Fig. 8-20) should be initiated. Emphasize that the dancer should work in a pain-free manner.

Dancers have to initiate strong muscle contractions from maximally stretched positions and execute isometrically controlled balances and multisegmental shapes. These postures can be mimicked in ankle strengthening exercises (Fig. 8-21). Remember that choreographic de-

mands vary in terms of speed of motion and load. In general, the dancer must possess both isometric and isotonic trunk and extremity strength in order to control their movement. The dancer is put on a program of proximal thigh, functional abdominal, and cardiovascular fitness exercises as warranted. Style and modality of exercise is determined on a case-by-case basis depending on preinjury status, and stage of healing with regard to weight-bearing. For example, aerobic conditioning may progress from underwater treadmill, to bike, Nordic track, slide board, stairmaster or treadmill, jump rope, and dance-specific obstacle course. Treadmill walking is an extremely useful tool for recoordinating lumbo-pelvic rhythm and, with retro-walking, for reacquisition of back space awareness as well as for eccentric plantar flexion strength training. If performed barefooted, proprioceptive and sensory tasks can also be implemented. Once tissue healing has sufficiently occurred and resistance work is tolerated, the dancer is placed on a program of active dorsiflexion exercises with theraband and gravity resisted tasks, which have been shown to decrease navicular tuberosity deviation,[195] and extensive overall strength training.

Shoewear, both dance and street shoes, should be checked for wear patterns and construction. Encourage them to wear shock-absorbing shoes out of the studio. Their shoes should be checked for true fit. All shoes should have a flex point aligned with the first MTP joint and enough room to allow for shear absorption and decompression of the toenails and plantar nerves. In FHL cases where overuse versus pathomechanics is determined, a simple $\frac{1}{8}$ to $\frac{1}{2}$ inch soft medial arch support may help alleviate the otherwise normal pronatory forces from excessive repetitive loading on the tendon at the medial aspect of the ankle. The pad can be taped right on to the foot with a medially directed elastic tape for security without restriction. One should compare the injured to noninjured limb in all motions and both sides of the spine and re-educate them about safe ROMs within which to work.

Dancers are a satisfying population to work with. Their movement demands and accomplishments are fascinating, and they are, generally speaking, an extremely motivated popula-

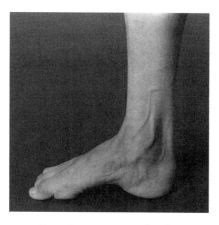

FIGURE 8-20 *Doming exercises for foot intrinsics.*

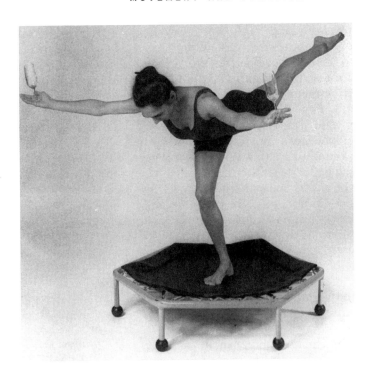

FIGURE 8-21 *Balancing on an unstable surface.*

tion, eager to learn and to excel. Transference of personal education will go a long way in promoting a healthier dancer and art form and in providing gratification to the practitioner for creative application of clinical skills.

Special thanks to Marni Larkin, PT for her critical review of this chapter and to the editors, Shaw Bronner and Bruce Brownstein, for their direction.

Glossary of Terms

Arabesque: A unilateral leg gesture to the back of the dancer's body which requires hip and spine hyperextension, knee extension, and ankle and foot plantar flexion

Battement: A unilateral leg raise that begins and ends with a knee-extended position

Cabriole: A jump where one leg is kicked up into the air and the other leg is brought up to meet it[214]

Chaînés: A series of small turning steps performed continuously in rapid succession[196]

Chassé: A "chasing step" where one foot and leg slides out from a stance position and is then followed by the other limb. When the second foot meets the first foot in space, a small sauté ends the action

Cloche: A unilateral, sagittal plane swinging action of the LE

Coup-de-pied: A unilateral standing posture where the gesturing foot is held in "the neck of the opposite foot",[196] just anteromedial of the medial malleolus

Developpé: A unilateral leg action where the gesturing limb begins from a knee-flexed position (passé) and ends in a knee-extended position

En bas: A lowered position of the arms[196]

En croix: Unilateral leg gestures carried out in three directions relative to the dancer's front, side and back space, making the shape of a cross.

En haut: A high position of the arms[196]

Entréchat quatré: A jump where the dancer beats the legs in the air, changing the foot positions[196]

Envelopé: A unilateral leg "kicking" activity where the gesturing limb begins in a knee extended position and "folds" back into the body to end in a knee-flexed position

Épaulement: A rotary movement of the shoulders made in sympathy with a simultaneous movement of the arms and/or legs[13]

Fouetté: A "whipping[196]" turn requiring coordinated hip and leg extension, adbuction, and flexion of one gesturing lower limb with opening and closing arm action to create spin on the opposite stance limb

Grand ronde de jambe en l'air: A unilateral, circumducted hip action where the gesturing limb describes a semi-circle in space at ≥90 degrees of hip flexion

Jeté: A "throwing step"[196] where a leaping jump is executed from one foot to the other

Passé: Similar in shape to the retiré, "the [spatial] point of the working foot as it passes the supporting knee on its way to another position."[196]

Piqué: A step in which the body shoots sharply onto the pointe or demi-pointe of the opposite foot.[196] This action can be immediately followed by a turning motion, known as a piqué turn

Pirouetté: A "whirl"[196] turn such that the body is supported by one leg while it rotates around its vertical axis

Plié: There are two types of pliés: demi- and grand. Both represent a bend of the knees while the torso is held upright. The action relies on varied degrees of hip and knee flexion, with ankle and MTP dorsiflexion

Port-de-bras: Carriage of the arms[196]

Port-de-corps: Carriage of the body. Basically, port-de-bras action supplemented with flexion, lateral flexion, or hyperextension movement of the spine

Relevé: A toe raise of varying height where the hip is neutral, the knee is extended, the ankle is plantar flexed and the MTPs are dorsiflexed. In full relevé, or pointe, the MTPs would be plantar flexed

Retiré: A static position in which the thigh of the gesturing leg is flexed, laterally rotated and abducted. The knee is flexed and held so that the toes of the gesture leg point into the knee of the stance leg[196]

Ronde de jambe: A unilateral leg action where the gesturing leg is circled from front to back of the dancer's body, or vice versa

Sauté: A simple jump in the vertical direction

Sissone: A jump from two feet onto one foot in various directions[196]

Temps Lié: A smooth transfer of weight from one stance posture to another[196]

Tendu: A "stretched[196]" action of the unilateral gesturing limb from a stance position

Tour en l'air: A sauté (see above definition) which incorporates airborne rotations

Tour jeté: A jeté (see above definition) which incorporates an angular rotation

References

1. Cohen JL, Gupta PK, Lichstein E et al: The heart of a dancer: non-invasive cardiac evaluation of professional ballet dancers. Am J Cardiol 45: 959–65, 1980

2. Cohen J, Segal KR, McArdle WD: Heart rate response to ballet stage performance. Phys Sports Med 10:120–33, 1982a

3. Liederbach M, Gleim G, Nicholas, J: Monitoring training status in professional ballet dancers. J Sports Med Phys Fitness 32:187–95, 1992

4. Hamilton L, Hamilton W, Meltzer J et al: Personality, stress, and injuries in professional ballet dancers. Am J Sports Med 17:263–7, 1989

5. Sheskier S, Rose D: Differences in injury patterns between ballet and modern dancers in a hospital-based orthopaedic clinic. Proceedings of the Third Annual Conference of the International Association for Dance Medicine and Science, New York, June 1993

6. Nicholas J, Grossman R, Hershman E: The importance of a simplified classification of motion in sports in relation to performance. Orthop Clin North Am 8:499–532, 1977

7. Gray M, Skrinar M: Base support used in two dance idioms. Res Q 55:184–7, 1984

8. Ryman R, Ranney D: A preliminary investigation of skeletal and muscular action in the grande battement devant. Dance Res J 11:1–2, 1979

9. Gentile AM: skill acquisition: action, movement and neuromotor processes. p. 93. In Carr JH, Shepherd RB (eds): Movement Science: Foundations for Physical Therapy in Rehabilitation. Aspen Publishers, Rockville, MD, 1987

10. Ranney D: Biomechanics of dance. p. 125. In Clarkson P, Skrinar M (eds): Science of Dance Training. Human Kinetics Publishers, Champaign, IL, 1988

11. Laws K: The physics of dance. Physics Today, 37:24–31, 1985

12. Galea V, Norman R: Bone on bone forces at the ankle joint during a rapid dynamic movement. p. 71. In Winter D (ed): Biomechanics IX A. Human Kinetics Publishers, Champaign, IL, 1985

13. Lawson J. The Principles of Classical Dance. Knopf, New York, 1980

14. Lopez-Ortiz C: Kinematic trend of piroutte performances as a function of skill level. Master's Thesis, SUNY, Brockport, 1994

15. Clarkson P, Kennedy T, Flanagan J: A study of three movements in classical ballet. Research Quarterly 55:175–9, 1984

16. Mouchnino L, Aurenty R, Massion J, et al: Coordination between equilibrium and head-trunk orientation during leg movement: a new strategy built up by training. J Neurophysiol 67: 1587–1598, 1992

17. Allen B: Teaching training and discipline-based dance education. J Phys Ed Rec Dance 59:65–9, 1988

18. Puretz S: Psychomotor research and the dance teacher, p. 279. In Clarkson P, Skrinar M (eds): Science of Dance Training. Human Kinetics Publishers, Champaign, IL, 1988

19. Puretz S: Bilateral transfer: the effects of practice on the transfer of complex dance movement patterns. Res Q 54:48–54, 1983

20. Gruen A: The relation of dancing experience and personality to perception. Psych Monogr 69: 1–16, 1955

21. Shea J, Hunt J: Motor control. Clins Sports Med 3:171–183, 1984

22. Skrinar M: Motor learning may help the dancer. p. 187. In Shell (ed): The Dancer as Athlete. Human Kinetics Publishers, Champaign, IL, 1986

22a.Bowman B: Learning experiences in selected aspects of a dance movement sequence. Unpublished doctoral dissertation. University of Michigan, Ann Arbor, MI, 1971

22b.Corsi-Cabrera M, Gutierrez L: Spatial ability in classical dancers and their perceptual style. Percep Motor Skills 72:399–402, 1991

22c.Barrell G, Trippe H: Field dependence and physical ability. Percept Motor Skils 41:216–218, 1975

22d.Soechting J, Flanders M: Moving in three-dimensional space: frames of reference, vectors, and corrdinate systems. Ann Rev Neurosci 15: 167–191, 1992

22e.Stein J, Glickstein M: Role of the cerebellum in visual guidance of movement. Physiol Rev 72(4): 967–1017, 1992

22f.Rieser JJ, Pick HL, Ashmead DH, Garing AE: Calibration of human locomotion and models of perceptual motor organization. J Exp Psych 21(3):480–497, 1995

22g.Hamilton W: Stenosing tenosynovitis of the flexor hallucis longus tendon and posterior impingement upon the os trigonum in ballet dancers. Foot and Ankle 3:74.

23. Higgins S: Motor skill acquisition. Ann Rev Psych 71:123–39, 1991

24. Schmidt RA: A schema theory of discrete motor skill learning. Ann Rev Psych 42:225–60, 1991

25. Ryman R: A kinematic analysis of selected grand allegro jumps. CORD Dance Research Annual 9: 231–242, 1978

26. Hinson M, Buckman S, Tate J et al: The grande jeté en tournant entrelace: an analysis through motion photography. Dance Res J 10:9–13, 1978

27. Laws K: An analysis of turns in dance. Dance Res J 11:12–19, 1979

28. Winter D, Patla A, Frank J: Assessment of balance control in humans. Med Progress Technol 16:31–51, 1990

29. Kogler A: Yoga for Every Athlete. Llewellyn Publications, St. Paul, MN, 1995

30. McDermott KB, Roediger HL: Effects of imagery on perceptual implicit memory tests. J Exp Psych 20:1379–1390, 1994

31. Posner MI, Petersen SE: The attention system of the human brain. Ann Rev Neurosci 13:25–42, 1990

32. Gelabert R: Posture. Dance-magazine 10:85–7, 1977

33. von Laban R, Lawrence FC: Effort: Economy in Human Movement. 2nd Ed. Plays, Boston, 1974

34. Shick J, Stoner L, Jette N: Relationship between modern dance experience and balancing performance. Res Q 54:79–82, 1983

35. Bushey S: Relationship of modern dance performance to agility, balance, flexibility, power and strength. Res Q 37:313–316, 1966

36. Crotts D, Thompson B, Nahom M et al: Balance abilities of professional dancers on select balance tests. J Orthop Sports Phys Ther 23:12–17, 1996

37. Byl, N: Spatial orientation to gravity and implications for balance training. Orthop Phys Ther Clin North Am 1:207–236, 1992

38. DeWitt G: Optic versus vestibular and proprioceptive impulses measured by posturometry. Aggressologie 13b:75–9, 1972

39. Irrgang J, Whitney S, Cox E: Balance and proprioceptive training for rehabilitation of the lower extremity. J Sport Rehab 3:68–83, 1994

40. Haines R: Effect of bed rest and exercise on body balance. J Appl Physiol 36:323–7, 1974

41. Lentell G, Katzman L, Walters M: The relationship between muscle function and ankle stability. J Orthop Sports Phys Ther 11:605–616, 1990

42. Hughson B: Balance training for the dancer using the B.A.P.S. Master's Thesis, SUNY Brockport, 1991

43. Woodhull-McNeal A, Clarkson P, James R et al: How linear is dancers' posture? Med Probs Perf Artists 5:151–4, 1990

44. Hamilton WG: Tendinitis about the ankle joint in classical ballet dancers. Am J Sports Med 5: 84, 1977

45. Horak F, Nashner L, Diener H: Postural strategies associated with somatosensory and vestibular loss. Exp Brain Res 82:167–77, 1990

46. Werner L: An electromyographic analysis of balance control in dancers: on relevé, with and without hyperextended knees. Master's Thesis, University of Oregon, 1987

47. Smeets JB, Brenner E: Perception and action are based on the same visual information: distinction between position and velocity. J Exp Psych 21:19–31, 1995

48. Wolpaw J: Acquisition and maintenance of the simplest motor skill: investigation of central nervous system mechanisms. Med Sci Sports Exerc 26:1475–9, 1994

49. Bartenieff I, Lewis D: Body Movement: Coping with the Environment. Gordon and Breach Science Publishers, New York, 1980

50. Marr SJ: The ballet foot. J Am Pod Assoc 73: 124–132, 1983

51. Deutsch JA, Deutsch D: Attention: some theoretical considerations. Psyc Rev 70:80–90, 1963

52. Sweigard L: Human Movement Potential: its Ideokinetic Facilitation. Harper & Row, New York, 1974

53. Sparger C: Ballet Physique. Macmillan, New York, 1958

54. Todd M: The Thinking Body. Dance Horizons, Brooklyn, NY, 1937

55. Gardner E: The neuromuscular base of human movement: feedback mechanisms. J Health Phys Ed Rec 36:61, 1965

56. Goode D, Van Hoven J: Loss of patellar and achilles tendon reflexes in classical ballet dancers. Arch Neurol 39:323, 1982

57. Koceja D, Burke J, Kamen G: Organization of segmental reflexes in trained dancers. Int J Sports Med 12:285–289, 1991

58. Nielsen J, Crone C, Hultborn H: H-reflexes are smaller in dancers from The Royal Danish Ballet than in well-trained athletes. Eur J Applied Physiol 66:116–21, 1993

59. Rochcongar P, Dassonville J, LeBars R: Modification of the Hoffmann reflex in function of athletic training. Eur J Appl Physiol 40:165–70, 1979

60. Heckman CJ: Alterations in synaptic input to motoneurons during partial spinal cord injury. Med Sci Sports Exerc 26:1480–91, 1994

61. Dahlstrom M, Esbjornsson M, Jansson E et al: Muscle fiber characteristics in female dancers during an active and an inactive period. Int J Sports Med 8:84–7, 1987

62. McComas AJ: Human neuromuscular adaptations that accompany changes in activity. Med Sci Sports Exerc 26:1498–1509, 1994

63. Glenncross D, Thornton E: Position sense following joint injury. J Sports Med 21:23–27, 1981

64. Marteniuk R, Roy E: The codability of kinesthetic location and distance information. Acta Psychologica 36:471–9, 1972

65. Mountcastle VB, Poggio GR, Werner G: The relation of thalamic cell response to peripheral stimuli varied over an intensive continuum. J Neuroph 26:807–34, 1963

66. Barrack R, Skinner H, Brunet M et al: Joint laxity and proprioception in the knee. Phys Sportsmed 11:130–135, 1983

67. Barrack RL, Skinner HB, Brunet ME et al: Joint kinesthesia in the highly trained knee. J Sports Med 24:18–20, 1984

68. Armstrong T: Seven Kinds of Smart. Penguin Books, New York, 1993

69. Gardner H: Frames of Mind: The Theory of Multiple Intelligences. Basic Books, New York, 1992

70. Nicholas J: Risk factors, sports medicine and the orthopedic system: an overview. J Sports Med 3: 243–258, 1975

71. Liederbach M: Profiling data on the Joffrey Ballet. Proceedings from The Arts and Technology Conference, Connecticut College, New London, CT, April 12, 1986

72. Chmelar R, Schultz B, Ruhling R et al: A physiological profile comparing levels and styles of female dancers. Phys Sports Med 16:87–96, 1988

73. Schantz P, Astrand P: Physiologic characteristics

of classical ballet. Med Sci Sports Exerc 16: 472–6, 1984

74. Cohen J, Segal D, Witriol I et al: Cardiorespiratory responses to ballet exercise and the VO₂ max of elite ballet dancers. Med Sci Sports Exerc 14: 212–17, 1982

75. Dahlstrom M, Jansson E, Nordevang E et al: Discrepancy between estimated energy intake and requirement in female dancers. Clin Psysiol 10: 11–25, 1990

76. Gleim G, Small C, Liederbach M et al: Anaerobic power of professional ballet dancers. Med Sci Sport Exerc 16:193–194, 1984

77. Nisonson B, Liederbach M, Nicholas JA et al: Normative Cybex data on elite ballet dancers. Proceedings of the Sixth Annual Conference of the Medical Problems of Musicians and Dancers, Aspen, CO, July 1989

78. Nisonson B, Liederbach M, Nicholas JA: Comparison of ankle strength ratios between ballet dancers, soccer players and football players. Proceedings of the Sixth Annual Conference of the Medical Problems of Musicians and Dancers, Aspen, CO, July 1988

79. Kirkendall D, Bergfeld J, Calabrese L et al: Isokinetic characteristics of ballet dancers and the response to a season of ballet training. J Orthop Sports Phys Ther 5:207–11, 1984

80. Westblad P, Fellander LT, Johansson C: Eccentric and concentric knee extensor muscle performance in professional ballet dancers. Clin J Sports Med 5:48, 1995

81. Micheli L, Gillespie W, Wasaszek A: Physiologic profiles of female professional ballerinas. Clin Sports Med 3:199, 1984

82. Hamilton W, Hamilton L, Marshall P et al: A profile of the musculoskeletal characteristics of elite professional ballet dancers. Am J Sports Med 20: 267–73, 1992

83. Clippenger-Robertson K: Flexibility among different levels of ballet dancers. Proceedings of the Fourth Annual Conference of the International Association for Dance Medicine and Science, San Francisco, CA, June 12, 1994

84. Freedson P: Body composition characteristics of female ballet dancers, p. 109. In Clarkson P, Skrinar M (eds): Science of Dance Training. Human Kinetics Publishers, Champaign, IL, 1988

85. Jensen RK: Human morphology: its role in the mechanics of movement. J Biomech 26:81–94, 1993

86. Gleim GW: The profiling of professional football players. Clins Sports Med 3:185–9, 1984

87. Hamilton WG: Physical prerequisites for ballet

dancers. J Musculoskeletal Medicine 3:61–6, 1986

88. Hellerman A, Skrinar M: Relationship of technical skill rank to age, gender, and number of years in dance training. Res Q 55:188–90, 1984

89. Gelabert R: Classic lines: the ballet dancer's physique. Sportcare & Fitness 2:46–50, 1989

90. Kirstein L, Stuart M, Dyer C: The Classic Ballet: Basic Technique and Terminology. Alfred A. Knopf, New York, 1952

91. Cohen SJ: The Modern Dance: Seven Statements of Belief. Wesleyan University Press. Middletown, CT, 1965

92. Dunning J: But First a School: The First Fifty Years of the School of American Ballet. Viking Press, New York, 1985

93. McLean D: Artistic development in the dancer. Clin Sports Med 2:563–570, 1983

94. Brooks-Gunn J, Warren M, Hamilton L: The relation of eating problems and amenorrhea in ballet dancers. Med Sci Sports Exerc 19:41–4, 1987

95. DeCherney A: Physiologic and pharmacologic effects of estrogen and progestins on bone. J Reprod Med 38:1007–1014, 1993

96. Warren M, Brooks-Gunn J, Fox R et al: Lack of bone accretion and amenorrhea: evidence for a relative osteopenia in weight bearing bones. J Clin Endocr Metab 72:847–53, 1991

97. Karlsson M, Johnell O, Obrant K: Bone mineral density in professional ballet dancers. Bone and Mineral 21:163–69, 1993

98. Young N, Formica C, Szmukler G et al: Bone density at weight-bearing and nonweight-bearing sites in ballet dancers: the effects of exercise, hypogonadism and body weight. J Clin Endocr Metab 78:449–54, 1994

99. Garner D, Garfinkel P: Sociocultural factors in anorexia nervosa. Lancet 2:674, 1978

100. Garner D, Garfindel P: Socio cultural factors in the development of anorexia nervosa. Psychol Med 9:273–9, 1980

101. Druss R: Body image and perfection of ballerinas: comparison and contrast with anorexia nervosa. Gen Hosp Psychiatr 2:115–21, 1979

102. Yeager KK, Agostini R, Nattiv A et al: The female athletic triad: disordered eating, amenorrhea, osteoporosis. Med Sci Sports Exer 25:775–777, 1993

103. Calabrese L, Kirkendall D, Floyd M et al: Menstrual abnormalities, nutritional patterns and body composition in female classical ballet dancers. Phys Sports Med 11:86–98, 1983

104. Dolgener F, Spasoff T, St. John W: Body build

and body composition of high ability female dancers. Res Q 51:599–607, 1980

105. Benson J, Gillien D, Bourdet K et al: Inadequate nutrition and chronic calorie restriction in adolescent ballerinas. Phys Sportsmed 13:79–90, 1985

106. Hamilton L, Brooks-Gunn J, Warren M: Nutritional intake of female dancers: a reflection of eating problems. Int J Eating Dis 5:109–118, 1986

107. Hamilton L, Brooks-Gunn J, Warren M et al: The impact of thinness and dieting on the professional ballet dancer. Med Probl Perf Artists 2: 117–22, 1987

108. Lowenkopf E, Vincent L: The student ballet dancer and anorexia. Hillside J Clin Psychiat 4: 53–64, 1982

109. Schnitt J, Schnitt D, Del A'une W: Anorexia nervosa or thinness in modern dance students: comparisons with ballerinas. Ann Sports Med 3: 9–13, 1986

110. Van Dijk CN, Lim LS, Poortman A et al: Degenerative joint disease in female ballet dancers. Am J Sports Med 23:295–300, 1995

111. Micklesfield LK, Lambert EV, Fataar AB et al: Bone mineral density in mature, premenopausal ultramarathon runners. Med Sci Sport Exerc 27: 688–96, 1995

112. Claessens A, Beunen G, Nuyts M et al: Body structure, somatotype, maturation and motor performance of girls in ballet schooling. J Sports Med 27:310–14, 1987

113. Clarkson P, Freedson P, Keller B et al: Maximal oxygen uptake, nutritional patterns, and body composition of adolescent female ballet dancers. Res Q 56:180–4, 1985

114. Eisenman P, Mikat R, Hamblin B: Relationship of body composition and performance ratings of pre-professional female collegiate ballet dancers. Proceedings of the Third Symposium of Science and Somatics of Dance, University of Utah, Salt Lake City, Utah, Feb 10–12, 1995

115. Bonbright J: Developing screeing and education programs at the subclinical level in dancers. Impulse 3:303–311, 1995

116. Liederbach M: Anthropometric and perceptual determinants of performance capability in elite, classically trained dancers. (In press)

117. Hamilton WG: A dancer (like a fine racehorse) doesn't know when to stop. Orthopaedics Today 1:25–7, 1981

118. Nilsson C, Wykman A, Leanderson J: Spinal sagittal mobility and joint laxity in young ballet dancers. Arthroscopy 15:206–81, 1993

119. Warren M, Brooks-Gunn J, Hamilton L et al: Scoliosis and fractures in young ballet dancers: relation to delayed menarche and secondary amenorrhea. N Engl J Med 314:1348–1353, 1986

120. Molnar M: Personal communication. Third Annual Conference of the International Association for Dance Medicine and Science, Baltimore, MD, June 1993

121. Morais T, Bernier M, Turcotte F: Age and sex specific prevalence of scoliosis and the value of school screening programs. Am J Pub Health 75: 1377–1380, 1985

122. Bylund P, Jansson E, Dahlberg E et al: Muscle fiber types in thoracic erector spinae muscles: fiber types in idiopathic and other forms of scoliosis. Clin Orthop Rel Res 214:222–8, 1987

123. Fidler M, Jowett R. Muscle imbalance in the etiology of scoliosis. J Bone Joint Surg 10:200–1, 1976

124. Ford D, Bagnall K, McFadden D et al: Paraspinal muscle imbalance in adolescent idiopathic scoliosis. Spine 9:373–6, 1984

125. Spencer G, Eccles M: Spinal muscle in scoliosis. J Neuro Sci 30:143–54, 1976

126. Rosenberg C, Derman G: Letter to the editor. N Engl J Med 315:1417–1418, 1986

127. Keller K, West JC: Functional movement impairment in dancers: an assessment and treatment approach utilizing the Biomechanical Asymmetry Corrector (BAC) to restore normal mechanics of the spine and pelvis. J Back Musculoskeletal Rehab 5:219–233, 1995

128. Teitz CC: Sports medicine concerns in dance and gymnastics. Clin Sports Med 2:571, 1983

129. Nicholas J, Strizak A, Veras G: A study of thigh muscle weakness in different pathological states of the lower extremity. Sports Med 4:241–8, 1976

130. Bullock-Saxton J, Janda V, Bullock M: The influence of ankle sprain injury on muscle activation during hip extension. Int J Sports Med 15: 330–334, 1994

131. Marshall P: Management adaptations for sacroiliac joint dysfunction in classical dancers. J Back Musculoskeletal Rehab 5:235–246, 1995

132. Staheli L, Wyss C et al: Lower extremity rotational problems in children: normal values to guide management. J Bone Joint Surg 67A: 39–47, 1985

133. Watkins A, Woodhumm-McNeal A, Clarkson P et al: Lower extremity alignment and injury in young, preprofessional, college and professional ballet dancers. J Med Probl Perf Artists 4: 148–153, 1989

134. Sammarco G: The dancer's hip. Clin Sports Med 2:485, 1983

135. Thomassen E: Diseases and injuries of ballet dancers. Universitetsforlaget I Arhus, Denmark, 1982

136. Renstrom P: Tendon and muscle injuries in the groin area. Clin Sports Med 11:815–831, 1992

137. Lee D. The Pelvic Girdle. Churchill Livingstone, New York, 1989

138. Kushner S, Saboe L, Reid D et al: Relationship of turnout to hip abduction in professional ballet dancers. Am J Sports Med 18:286, 1990

139. DeMeo D: An investigation of trunk-pelvic flexibility and strength of female ballet dancers. Master's Thesis, Long Island University, 1995

140. Parnianpour M, Davoodi M, Forman M et al: The normative database for the quantitative trunk performance of female dancers: isometric and dynamic trunk strength and endurance. Med Prob Perf Artists 9:50–7, 1994

141. Ellison J, Rose S, Sahrmann S: Patterns of hip rotation range of motion: a comparison between healthy subjects and patients with low back pain. Phys Ther 70:537–541, 1990

142. Bauman P, Singson R, Hamilton W: Femoral neck anteversion in ballerinas. Clin Orthop Rel Res 302:57–63, 1994

143. Calliet R: Foot and Ankle Pain. FA Davis Co, New York, NY, 1983

144. Hoppenfeld S: Physical Examination of the Spine and Extremities. Appleton-Century-Crofts, East Norwalk, CT, 1976

145. Hardaker W, Myers M: The pathogenesis of dance injury. p. 31. In Shell C (ed): The Dancer as Athlete. Human Kinetics Publisher, Champaign, IL, 1986

146. Garrick J, Requa R: Turnout and training in ballet. Med Prob Perf Artists 9:43–49, 1994

147. Fung L: A comparison of Chinese and American female artistic dancers on selected physical fitness measures. Paper presented at The 24th World Congress on Health, Physical Education and Recreation. Manila, Philippines, July 21–25, 1981

148. Tombeur S, Heyters C: L'attitude et la statique de la danseuse académique comparées à celles d'une population témoin. Sport (Adeps) 24: 130–43, 1981

149. Solomon R, Micheli LJ, Solomon J: The "cost" of injuries in a professional ballet company: Med Prob Perform Artists 10:3–10, 1995

150. Garrick JG. Ballet Injuries. Med Prob Perform Art 1:123–130, 1986

151. Sammarco GJ: Dance injuries. p. 1406. In Nicho-las J, Hershman E (eds): The Lower Extremity and Spine in Sports Medicine. CV Mosby, St. Louis, 1986

152. Hamilton W: Foot and ankle injuries in ballet dancers. Clin Sports Med 7:143–150, 1988

153. Howse AJ: Disorders of the great toe in dancers. Clin Sports Med 2:499–506, 1983

154. Schon LC, Biddinger KR, Greenwood P: Dance screen programs and development of dance clinics. Clin Sports Med 13:865, 1994

155. Trepman E, Gellman R, Solomon R et al: Electromyographic analysis of standing posture and demi-plie in ballet and modern dancers. Med Sci Sports Exerc 26:771–82, 1994

156. Marshall P: The rehabilitation of overuse foot injuries in athletes and dancers. Clin Pod Med Surg 6:639–655, 1989

157. Novella T: An easy way to quantify plantar flexion in the ankle. J Back Musculoskel Rehab 5: 191–99, 1995

158. Michaud TC: Foot Orthoses and Other Forms of Conservative Foot Care. Williams & Wilkins, Baltimore, 1993

159. Marshall P: The rehabilitation of overuse foot injuries in athletes and dancers. Clin Sports Med 7:175, 1988

160. Sammarco G, Miller E: Forefoot conditions in dancers, part 2. Foot and Ankle 3:93–98, 1982

161. Schneider H, King A, Bronson J: Stress injuries and developmental changes of the lower extremities in ballet dancers. Radiology 113:627–32, 1974

162. Kravitz S, Huber S, Murgia C et al: Biomechanical study of bunion deformity and stress produced in classical ballet. J Am Pod Med Assoc 75:338–45, 1985

163. Stacey J: The relationship between the activity of the lower leg muscles and the foot impulse patterns in a balletic vertical jump. UMI Dissertation Services, Ann Arbor, MI, 1994

164. Ambre T, Nilsson BE: Degenerative changes in the first metatarsophalangeal joint of ballet dancers. Acta Orthop Scand 49:317–9, 1978

165. Einarsdóttir H, Troell S, Wykman A: Hallux valgus in ballet dancers: a myth? Foot and Ankle Int 16:92–4, 1995

166. Hagins M: The relationship between weight-bearing and non-weight-bearing measurements of ankle dorsiflexion in dancers. Impulse 2: 165–175, 1994

167. Marshall P, Hamilton WG: Cuboid subluxation in ballet dancers. Am J Sports Med 20:169–175, 1992

168. Myers M: Is the grande plié obsolete? Dance Magazine June: 78–80, 1982. Liederbach M,

Gleim G, Nicholas J: Physiologic and psychological measurements of performance stess and onset of injuries in professional ballet dancers. Med Prob Perform Artists 9:10–14, 1994

169. Reber L, Perry J, Pink M: Muscular control of the ankle in running. Am J Sports Med 21:805–810, 1993

170. Garth W: Flexor hallucis tendinitis in a ballet dancer: a case report. J Bone Joint Surg 63A: 1489, 1982

171. Tudisco C, Puddu G: Stenosing tenosynovitis of the flexor hallucis longus tendon in a classical ballet dancer: a case report. Am J Sports Med 12: 403, 1984

172. Gans A: The relationship of heel contact in ascent and descent from jumps to the incidence of shin splints in ballet dancers. Phys Ther 65: 1192–6, 1985

173. Lycholat T: Lifting technique in dance. Dancing Times 73:123, 203–204, 287–288, 381, 383, 1982

174. Kerr G, Krasnow D, Mainwaring L: The nature of dance injuries. Med Prob Perform Artists 9: 7–9, 1994

175. Monad H: Contractility of muscles during prolonged static and repetitive dynamic activity. Ergonomics 28:81–89, 1985

176. Landry M, Zebas C: Biomechanical principals in common running injuries. J Am Podiatr Med Assoc 74:48–52, 1985

177. Clement D: Tibial stress syndrome in athletes. J Sports Med 2:81–85, 1974

178. Tauton JE, Clement DB, Webber D: Lower extremity stress fractures in athletes. Physician Sports Med 9(10):77–86, 1981

179. Kadel N, Teitz C, Kronmal R: Stress fracture in ballet dancers. Am J Sports Med 20:445–449, 1992

180. Burrows H: Fatigue infarction of the middle tibia in ballet dancer. J Bone Joint Surg 38B:83–94, 1956

181. Hamilton W: Sprained ankles in ballet dancers. Foot and Ankle 3:99–101, 1982b

182. Burton E, Amaker B: Stress fracture of the great toe sesamoid in a ballerina: MRI appearance. Pediatr Radiol 24:37–8, 1994

183. Micheli L, Sohn R, Solomon R: Stress fractures of the second metatarsal involving Lisfranc's joint in ballet dancers. J Bone Joint Surg 67A: 1372–5, 1985

184. Noonan T, Best T, Seaber A et al: Identification of a threshold for skeletal muscle injury. Am J Sports Med 22:257–261, 1994

185. Steffen R: The effects of fatigue on the performance vertical jump in dance. Master's Thesis, SUNY Brockport, 1986

186. Tippett SR, Voight ML: Functional Progressions for Sport Rehabilitation. Human Kinetics, Champaign, IL, 1995

187. Anderson EA, Wallin BG, Mark AL: Dissociation of sympathetic nerve activity in arm and leg muscle, during mental stress. Hypertension 9: 114–19, 1987

188. Saito M, Mano T, Abe H, et al: Responses in muscle sympathetic nerve activity to sustained handgrips of different tensions in humans. Eur J App Physiol 55:493–8, 1986

189. Borg G: Perceived exertion as an indicator of somatic stress. Scand J Rehab Med 2:92–8, 1970

190. McNair DM, Lorr M, Droppelman LF: Profile of Mood States Manual. Educational and Industrial Testing Service, San Diego, 1980

191. Hamilton WG, Molnar M: Back to dancing after injury. Dance Magazine 4:88–90, 1983

192. Noyes F, Lindenfeld T, Marshall M: What determines an athletic injury (definition)? Who determines an injury (occurence)? Am J Sports Med 16(suppl):S65–8, 1988

193. Tegner Y, Lysholm J, Lysholm M et al: A performance test to monitor rehabilitation and evaluate anterior cruciate ligament injuries. Am J Sports Med 14:156–9, 1986

194. Batson G: The role of somatic education in dance medicine and rehabilitation. North Carolina Med J 54:74–78, 1993

195. Liederbach M: The effect of a dorsiflexor strengthening program on the amount of foot pronation and the symptomatic relief of the shin splint syndrome in female classical dancers. Master's Thesis, Virginia Commonwealth University, Richmond, VA, 1981

196. Mara T: The Language of Ballet: A Dictionary. Princeton Book Company, Princeton, NJ, 1966

197. Quirk R: Injuries in classical ballet. Austr Fam Physician 13:802–4, 1984

198. Liederbach M: Performance demands of ballet: a general overview. Kines and Med for Dance 8: 6–9, 1985

199. Solomon R, Micheli L: Technique as a consideration in modern dance injuries. Phy Sports Med 14:83–90, 1986

200. Garrick J, Requa R: Ballet injuries: an analysis of epidemiology and financial outcome. Am J Sports Med 21:586–90, 1993

9

Function in Older Individuals—Orthopaedic Geriatrics

RAY PLONA

BRUCE BROWNSTEIN

Treatment of the aging or older adult contains many challenges and potential rewards. In a certain sense, the older adult as a patient is not unlike the sports medicine patient. Both populations represent a group of people with activity demands, lifestyles, physical capabilities, and responses to injury and the rehabilitation process that are different from the "average." As physical therapists, we are obligated to master the body of knowledge that has been amassed regarding the science of treating the geriatric orthopaedic patient. As in the sports medicine patient, injury causes significant changes in the ability of the older adult to live in the manner in which they would like. In this instance, however, the functional loss is not a missed season of skiing, it is the capability of walking to the grocery store, caring for oneself, maintaining quality of life.

We are concerned with movement in a more basic sense when the patient is an older individual. Diminished physical capacity as a result of disuse, previous and current injuries, possible disease process, reduced sensory and somatosensory functions, and physiologic changes results in a more precarious functional level. The overlapping role of multiple systems that could accommodate for injury are no longer able to exert the compensatory role of a younger adult. The range of movement skills that allowed for exploration of the environment as a child and mastery as a younger adult are waning in the older adult. An understanding of this process is essential to working with the older population. As is often the case, physical therapists occupy a unique position at the crossroads between injury and recovery of function.

Approximately 15 percent of the U.S. population is over the age of 65.[1] This percentage will grow to almost 20 percent in the next 25 years. The U.S. Census Bureau expects that the number of people older than 45 will increase from 82,000,000 to 124,000,000 between 1990 and 2010.[2] Approximately 25 percent of elderly people cannot walk half a mile or lift 10 lbs.[3] Fifteen percent are unable to climb stairs.[4] Additionally, there are 2.5 million injuries per year in the elderly. Between the years of 1984 and 1987, there were almost 800,000 hip fractures reported by Medicare in the United States.[5] The cost of these fractures was more than $7 billion.[4] Most of these fractures occurred during or as a result of a fall.

This chapter on the aging adult explores the issues in treating this population. Reductions in reimbursement and available treatment time compel therapists to be aware of the range of functional challenges facing the older adult. We must tailor our treatment efforts toward a multi-dimensional treatment approach that addresses the overall needs of the patient, not just recovery from the immediate orthopaedic incident. Training in movement skills, increasing awareness of the environment, encouraging continued exercise and conditioning, and educating the patient regarding their body's physical capabilities should be part of a comprehensive program.

Physical Changes with Aging

With advancing age, changes may be seen in the cardiovascular, respiratory, musculoskeletal, and somatosensory systems. All of these changes affect the quality of life that is possible to the older adult. These changes can obscure or magnify symptoms that accompany orthopaedic pathology. From an orthopaedic standpoint, we are most concerned with changes in tissue strength, muscular capability, and sensorimotor control.

CARDIOVASCULAR RESPIRATORY CHANGES

Maximal VO_2 (cardiac function) is the best indicator of a person's ability to deliver oxygen throughout the body. VO_2 maximum declines with age in both men and women.[6] Older people who participate in regular activity have a higher capacity, but the rate of decline is unchanged[6,7] (Fig. 9-1). Cardiovascular disease and physical frailty can hasten the decline in VO_2 maximum. Eventually, some individuals lose the physical work capacity to perform activities of daily living independently. The reduction in VO_2 max is associated with a decrease in maximal heart rate, stroke volume, and cardiac regulation.[1] Pendergast et al.[1] contends that the loss of cardiac function is due to a reduction of the ability of cardiac muscle to generate force, paralleling the process that occurs in skeletal muscle.

VO_2 maximum can be improved in the elderly with an appropriate training program.[8-10] It should be noted that the effects of training in older individuals take longer and are less effective than in younger subjects. Subjects have improved with both high and low intensity exercise. Seals et al.[9] reported that orthopaedic injuries as a result of exercise were more common and of greater severity in the high intensity exercise group. It is suggested that low level activities, such as walking, are more beneficial in the elderly than high intensity exercise, since low intensity training can result in equal cardiovascular benefit, while minimizing the risk of musculoskeletal or cardiovascular injury.[11-13]

Similar changes occur in pulmonary function. Pulmonary capacity, air volume, and the elasticity of lung tissue decreases with age, resulting in diminished vital capacity. Postural changes resulting from increased kyphosis, decreased thoracic flexibility, and strength also contribute to less efficient respiratory function.[14]

MUSCULOSKELETAL CHANGES

Diminished musculoskeletal capability, along with cardiovascular disease, represents the major cause of functional loss in the elderly. Changes in the mechanical properties of bone,[15] articular cartilage,[16] and muscle,[17] combined with altered neural control,[18] act to reduce the effectiveness of our body to move efficiently. Reduced joint mobility, increased frailty, diminished sensory perception, and generally decreased motor output prevent the elderly from accomplishing daily tasks to which younger adults are accustomed.

Despite increasing knowledge regarding the age-related changes that occur to the various tissues of the musculoskeletal system, there is no method to predict which individuals will become impaired. Age-related changes in articular cartilage do not always result in osteoarthritis and functional loss. Not all people who demonstrate decreased bone mass suffer hip fracture, and only a small percentage of elderly persons rupture the rotator cuff or Achilles tendon. A conflu-

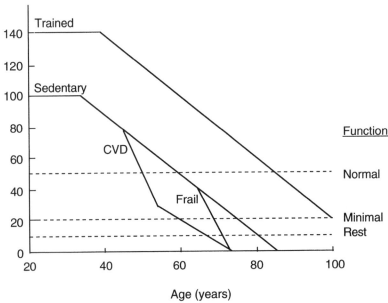

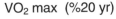

FIGURE 9-1 *Cardiovascular function (expressed by VO_2 maximum) in aging individuals. Patients with disease and frailty have sharp declines in CV capacity, which limits overall function. (From Pendergast DR, et al with permission.)*

ence of variables including anatomic, environmental, and metabolic factors cause the natural reduction in physical capability to become pathologic and disabling.

Bone

Fractures represent one of the major causes of morbidity in the elderly. Fractures are rarely fatal, although the mortality rate of older persons within a year after hip fracture ranges from 14–36 percent.[19] Approximately 25 percent of persons who fracture their hip lose their independence in walking and approximately 60 percent do not regain their pre-injury level of ambulation, regardless of the definition of functional or ambulatory level.[19,20] Other fractures cause functional problems in the elderly. Colle's fracture can be significant when an individual already has decreased grip strength and precision grip,[21] as well as limited ROM (range of motion)

in the shoulder complex.[22] Fracture of the lumbar vertebrae is seen frequently as a consequence of osteoporosis and can have a significant impact on ADL (activities of daily living).

Bone resorption is a natural consequence of aging.[23] Humans are capable of increasing their bone mass until the age of 40.[24] Generally, age-related bone loss begins between the ages of 30 and 40. Bone mineral density, which is correlated with bone strength,[25] decreases by approximately one percent after the age of 50.[26] McCalden et al.[15] states that bone density is a function of the amount of bone and the degree of mineralization. They contend that the volume of bone decreases with age; the degree of mineralization is unaffected by aging. Bone microstructure and architecture are affected by aging. Trabecular width decreases and spacing increases, reducing resistance to both tensile and compressive forces.[27,28] Nash and Spieholz[29] suggest that trabecular disintegration explains the skeletal degeneration that occurs out of proportion to mineral loss itself.

From a functional standpoint, bone resorption and loss is related to the overall impact of reduced activity levels, which results in reduced physical capability and fosters a further cycle of inactivity. Bone density, mineral content, and strength are higher in physically active people. Nilsson and Weslin[30] studied age-matched controls and concluded that male athletes have higher bone density of the distal femur than sedentary men. Similar findings were found in the bone density of middle-aged runners[31] and spinal bone density of women over 50.[32]

Regional changes in bone density can occur with exercise programs. Dalsky et al.[33] found that nonweight-bearing exercise can increase spinal bone density in postmenopausal women. Ayalon et al.[34] found an increase in radial bone density in osteoporotic women following a 5-month program of specific wrist and forearm exercises. Krolner et al.[35] found that lumbar spine density, but not radial density, were increased following a program of calisthenics and low level aerobics over a long period. Unfortunately, increased bone density as a result of exercise is not permanent; bone loss occurs as a result of deconditioning if the exercise regimen is discontinued.[33] It appears that exercise programs that incorporate specific muscle-oriented routines are more effective in increasing bone mass. Cavanaugh and Cann[36] found that postmenopausal women who participated in a brisk walking program actually lost bone mass. This is probably due to the nature of the loading that occurs with strength training versus impact loading. Bone can increase or decrease its mass in response to the type of stress placed upon it.[37] Care must be taken to account for the initial level of potential bone deterioration when designing exercises programs for people to increase their bone density.

Tendons and Ligaments

Degenerative changes in dense fibrous tissues also occur as a result of the aging process. These changes occur at the cellular and morpho-logic level with corresponding decreases in biomechanical capacity. Anatomic factors such as vascularity, patterns of use with regard to microtrauma and overuse, and underlying medical conditions such as diabetes, all play a role in the response of collagenous tissue to aging.[38] Although the cost of treatment of soft tissue injuries in the older adult does not match the cost of arthritis or osteoporosis, the rising number of older adults almost guarantees that this area will begin to become more costly. Laurencin and Gelberman[38] cite statistics that include the following:

- 72 percent of work-related injury health costs can be attributed to persons over 45.
- In 1988, 115,000 injuries related to soft tissue trauma at work were reported.
- Repetitive trauma-related injuries increased from 23 to 45 percent of occupational illnesses between 1983 and 1988.
- Surgery for repair of soft tissues (rotator cuff, Achilles tendon, etc.) rank in the top 20 most frequent musculoskeletal procedures performed.

Clearly, there is reason to believe that soft tissue injuries will increase as the population and workforce age.

The collagenous tissues include tendon, ligament, and joint capsule. Degradation of the biomechanical characteristics of these tissues may predispose an individual to injury, either spontaneous rupture or sprain at force levels far below the energy required to tear these tissues in younger adults.[2] Tendon and ligament age-related changes have not received as much attention from researchers as bone changes. Even less is known about the joint capsule. These tissues play a direct role in impairment in the elderly, as well as an indirect one as a secondary consequence of arthritis.

Butler[39] reviewed the age-related changes of the anterior cruciate ligament (ACL). He noted that older ACLs have much lower (approximately 40 percent of normal) failure strengths, elastic modulus, and strain energy to failure than younger ACLs.[40,41] No literature exists regarding the direct forces on the ACL with respect to age-related changes. Animal studies on the medial collateral ligament (MCL) of the knee have shown similar declines in mechanical properties, but not to the extent of the ACL.[42,43]

One would expect similar changes in the strength of tendons as a result of aging. Kannus and Józsa[44] examined biopsies of spontaneously ruptured tendons, including Achilles tendons, biceps brachii, extensors pollicis longus, quadriceps tendons, patellar ligaments, and various other tendons. They compared the histology of these specimens to fresh samples from age- and sex-matched cadavers. All of the samples from ruptured tendons were abnormal (showing signs of degenerative changes) as well as 35 percent of the control group. The results suggest that degenerative changes in tendon tissue are very common after 35 years of age. There is some evidence that biochemical changes also occur with aging, but this information remains limited in scope.[45] It is possible that age affects the attachment site of the capsular structure.[46]

The sensory role of ligaments, tendons, and capsular structures is also affected by aging. The ability to detect isolated movement of the knee joint decreases with age.[47,48] Skinner et al.[47] suggests that proprioception testing may serve to identify subclinical osteoarthritis. The role of neurogenic pathology in the origin of arthritis cannot be ignored. O'Connor et al.[49] identified accelerated osteoarthritic changes in a canine model in the presence of neurogenic influences. Finsterbush and Friedman[50] found similar results in the rabbit model. Barret et al.[48] noted that an elastic bandage improved detection of joint motion. It remains to be seen what information develops along the lines of proprioception training as a method to reduce injury and disability in the elderly.[51-53]

Articular Cartilage

Osteoarthritis (OA) is the end stage of degeneration of articular cartilage and subchondral bone. In 1988, OA accounted for 43 percent of the cost of musculoskeletal conditions in the United States, or $54.6 billion.[54] Each year, about 400,000 joint arthroplasties are performed at the knee and hip; OA is the cause of 85 percent of the knee procedures and 55 percent of the hip procedures.[55]

Development of OA is a combination of factors that include aging, trauma, and genetics. Risk factors include age, sex, race, obesity, use and abuse of joints, and joint geometry.[54] Participation in sports may not predispose an individual to OA, but injury as a result of sports (i.e. menisectomy) can lead to radiologic changes, if not symptomatic OA decades after the original injury. Dahlberg et al.[56] noted that patients diagnosed with a meniscal tear after the age of 30 often have radiologic changes consistent with OA within five years, while patients under the age of 30 at the time of injury do not show these changes for 20–25 years.

It is unclear why age is such a strong factor in the development of OA. Age-related changes include altered proteoglycan structure,[16] possible decreased chondroitin sulfate content,[57-59] and decreased water content, probably as a result of the proteoglycan changes.[60] Osteoarthritic articular cartilage demonstrates a different profile than normally aged cartilage Table 9-1 contrasts the two tissues. It may be that the changes in aged articular cartilage are precursors to osteoarthritic cartilage, given the appropriate environment. Radin et al.[61] found that the subchondral bone is stiffer than normal in patients with early OA changes. Perhaps altered bone stock, combined with neurogenic changes, previous trauma, and genetic factors can lead articular cartilage from normally aged tissue to diseased tissue.

Regardless of the exact mechanism, OA can lead to severe disablement. More than 60 million people in the United States probably have OA to some degree.[62] Arthritis is described as the second leading cause of limitation by men of middle age and older; it is the leading cause of limitation in women of the same age group.[63] People with arthritis (both OA and rheumatoid) report more disability in daily life than those without.[64,65] The impact of knee OA on physical function is greater than any other disease.[62,66]

TABLE 9-1 *Comparison of changes between normal aged and osteoarthritic articular cartilage*

MEASUREMENT	AGEING	OSTEOARTHRITIC
Tissue water content	Decreased	Increased
Glycosaminoglycans		
Chondroitin sulphate content	Normal or slightly decreased	Progressively decreased
Chondroitin sulphate chain length	Decreased	Increased early; decreased with progression of disease
Ratio of chondroitin 4-sulphate: chondroitin 6-sulphate	Decreased	Increased
Keratan sulphate content	Increased	Decreased
Hyaluronic acid content	Increased	Decreased
Proteoglycans		
Extractability	Decreased	Increased
Aggregation	Normal	Diminished
Size of monomers	Decreased	Decreased
Rate of maturation of hyaluronate-binding region	Decreased	Increased
Tissue content of free hyaluronate-binding region	Increased	Unknown
Link protein	Fragmented	Normal
Degradative enzyme activity		
Neutral proteoglycanase	Normal	Increased
Acid protease	Normal	Increased
Collagenase	Normal	Increased

(From Brandt KD and Fife RS,[60] with permission.)

Men and women with arthritis have lower work participation rates.[67] The disabling effects of arthritis have an impact on almost every aspect of life, from the social level to the cellular.

Intervertebral Disk

Complaints of neck and low back pain and stiffness are common complaints of middle-aged and older people.[55] Although radiographic evidence of disk degeneration does not correlate with pain symptoms, the widespread changes that occur in the intervertebral disk with aging place it in the same category as tissues already discussed. Age-related changes alter the function of the intervertebral disk and predispose it to pathology that results in pain, loss of mobility, and functional loss. Several investigators have noted that degenerative changes in disk complexes in the lumbar spine occur in almost every person.[68–70]

Factors influencing disk deterioration include physical labor,[71] previous injury,[72] and spinal deformities (such as scoliosis, spondylolisthesis).[73] Age-related changes are decreased proteoglycan and water concentration,[74] declining cell nutrition,[75] and reduced average failure torque.[76] Other changes associated with aging that may accompany degeneration of the intervertebral disk are disk herniation, spinal stenosis, and facet joint degeneration.

Skeletal Muscle

Perhaps the most obvious age-related effects are on skeletal muscle. Skeletal muscle mass begins declining at the rate of four percent per decade between the ages of 25 and 50 years old.[2] The rate of decline increases to ten percent per decade after age 50. Reduced skeletal muscle mass has a corresponding decrease in absolute strength of the major muscle groups in the body. Once again, the underlying reasons for strength loss are several, resulting in a spiral of reduced activity leading to reduced strength and functional capacity, which fosters reduced activity and further atrophy. The primary age-related changes in skeletal muscle are loss of muscle mass,[77] loss of type II muscle fibers,[77,78] reduced number of fibers,[77] and progressive denervation.

Several investigators have found that age-related strength loss can be reduced or reversed with appropriate exercise interventions. Strength training in older adults has the same benefits as in younger adults—increased muscle mass, cross-sectional area, motor unit recruitment, contractile proteins, and oxidative capacity.[79–84] There are some limitations to exercise in the elderly, particularly increased incidence of injury. Brown[85] compared the effects of low (flexibility and strengthening) and moderate (walk/jog/bike at 60 percent + VO_2 maximum) intensity exercise programs on the elderly. In the low intensity exercise program, 27 percent of the participants experienced painful episodes that required exercise modification (rest, ice, external support). Almost 65 percent of the participants in the moderate exercise group had a painful episode. In both groups, the knee was the joint with the greatest number of complaints.

Most of the age-related changes in skeletal muscle are linked to disuse atrophy, which has many underlying causes. Exercise can be beneficial in modifying these effects, resulting in higher potential functional levels.

INFORMATION PROCESSING—NEURAL ELEMENT CHANGES

One of the more important factors in function is the correct detection and processing of sensory information into appropriate movement responses and strategies. The major sensory providers—visual, vestibular, and somatosensory—can all be affected by aging and age-related pathology. It is more difficult to determine whether processing changes occur as well, not to mention selection of suitable musculoskeletal responses following the processing stage.

As mentioned earlier, joint position sense and movement detection of the knee are affected by age.[47,48] Total knee replacement (TKR) does not worsen position sense of the knee.[86] One study found that TKR slightly improved "propri-

oception."[48] The failure of TKR, regardless of prosthesis design, to restore normal joint position sense, indicates that the loss of this type of sensory detection is a result of age-related changes in the sensory systems that subserve detection of movement. Skinner et al.[86] noted that abnormal gait parameters persisted following TKR and attributed some of this to permanent loss of joint proprioceptive function. Corresponding loss of muscle function must also be included as a contributor to changes in gait following joint replacement.[87] Age-related changes in detection of movement in other joints may or may not mimic the changes that occur at the knee.[21]

Visual system changes also accompany aging. Cataracts and macular degeneration are two of the diseases of the eye that can reduce visual acuity. Retinal function also declines, causing loss of visual sensitivity, particularly in contrast, contour, and depth perception, and detection of movement.[88] These changes are important in determining the orientation of the body in its environment, particularly when the environment is changing, and avoiding obstacles is required.

Age-related changes in the vestibular system include loss of thick nerve fibers[89] and vestibular hair and nerve cells.[90] Nonetheless, severe vestibular deficits alone do not result in loss of balance control in the presence of intact visual and somatosensory systems, even though postural sway may be increased.[18,91] The loss of multiple sensory systems is termed "multisensory deficit"[92] and refers to the loss of several sensory systems with the inability of alternative systems to compensate for severe losses in any one system.[93]

The final mechanism of movement is the processing of information in the central nervous system (CNS) and the voluntary movement that occurs afterward. Light[94] reviewed information processing as it pertains to motor performance in older adults. Difficulty may occur at any of the steps between stimulus detection and movement output (see Fig. 9-2). Controversy exists as to which step of the processing paradigm is most affected by age. Hines et al.[95] stated that sensory

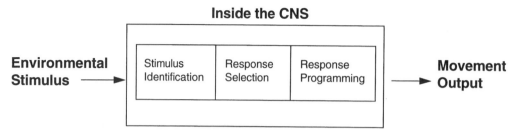

FIGURE 9-2 *Steps involved in processing outside information into a functional movement. Decrease in function can occur after alteration at any step. (From Light KE,[94] with permission.)*

encoding was the limiting factor in CNS processing. Botwinick[96] found that intensity of the stimulus could be related to CNS processing. Both of these studies place the greatest emphasis on stimulus identification. Stelmach and Wortingham[97] noted evidence of slower encoding, slower processing, and delayed response initiation in a normal elderly population.

Age also affects the second stage of processing. Rabbitt,[98] Rabbitt and Vyas,[99] and Salthouse and Somberg[100] all found that the choice of response was affected by aging. This may be related to problems with anticipation and expectancy under changing conditions.[94] A study by Goggin and Meeuwsen[101] related the increase in movement time to an index of difficulty that related the complexity and type of movement required to the response of the subject. They found that older subjects (average age, 78.8 years) had slower movements than younger subjects at all levels of complexity. They also found that older adults made fewer errors in their movements, indicating that they emphasize accuracy over speed in spatial aiming movements of the upper extremity. This effect may also carry over to the lower extremity and should be considered during studies of gait, obstacle avoidance, and falling.

Light and Spirduso[102] found that the complexity movement and the stage of response programming are related. Older people are more sensitive to movement complexity than younger subjects. This affects their ability to plan and execute appropriate responses even after the CNS has selected a response path.

In general, the speed of response to external stimuli is reduced in the elderly as a result of multiple peripheral and central factors. Older adults are capable of improving their motor performance with practice[94] combined with physical conditioning.[103] People who had been physically active during their lives had better response times than generally sedentary individuals. Subjects who undertook a training program also improved their processing capacity as measured by motor response times.[103]

Functional Limitations in the Elderly

Primary concern lies in the ability of individuals to function in their everyday lives at home and in society. It is useful to understand the nature of the age-related changes in the major tissues; however, age-related changes do not necessarily imply age-related loss of function. Functional loss of a joint or limb is a combination of the failure of many tissues, often overlaid by environmental factors, history of previous injury, and the social support that surrounds the individual. This section reviews the major functional areas affected in aging that provide clues as to how exercise programs should be directed to maximize function.

JOINT MOBILITY

As previously noted, normal aging results in changes in the biomechanical nature of all of the tissues of the synovial joints. Articular cartilage degenerates, resulting in less efficient lubrication and changes in the congruency of the joint surfaces. Muscle tissue is lost, with the end result being a potential inability to support the weight of a limb that is being moved. Capsular structures become stiffer. All in all, the synovial joint becomes more difficult to move.

These changes result in reduced range of motion in the joints. Reduced joint mobility affects both men and women, with similar functional results. Netzer and Payne,[104] using two-dimensional video analysis, found that neck rotation, total neck and back rotation, and side-bending (total motion referring to combined spinal motion) were significantly reduced in older adults. Older adults were represented by the age group of 60–80 versus all other groups (6–8, 12–15, 20–30, and 40–50 years old). The results of Netzer and Payne echoed Einkauf et al's.[105] findings of reduced spinal motion in older women. Netzer and Payne believed that declining physical activity may be a major contributing factor to loss of mobility. Loss of spinal motion can affect functional performance in simple daily tasks such as picking objects up from the floor, looking over one's shoulder, or dressing.

Chakravarty and Webley[106] studied the relationship between shoulder ROM and disability in adults over the age of 65. Reduced ROM compared to a group of younger normals was noted in the motions of elevation, internal rotation, and external rotation. The older group was further divided into those with disability in ADL and those without. Disability was evaluated using the Katz index of independence, which includes activities such as grooming, bathing, feeding, and dressing. Thirty percent of the group had disability as measured by this index. Those with disability had less ROM in all ranges than the group without disability. Strength was not measured in this study, which is a drawback.

Studies of age-related changes in motion of lower extremity joints presents a mixed picture. Vandervoort et al.[107] found that dorsiflexion ROM decreased as age increased from 55 to 85. Also, passive resistance to stretching increased with age, while maximum voluntary isometric contraction decreased by 30 percent. They hy-

pothesized that the combined factors of decreased strength and increased passive resistance to movement resulted in reduced mobility and suggested that strengthening the dorsiflexors may increase mobility. Whether this could improve function by making gait more efficient and making falling less likely remains to be seen.[107] Blanpied and Smidth[108] also found a probable age-related increase in passive resistance to stretching defined as intrinsic muscle stiffness. They found that strengthening the plantarflexors resulted in reduced passive resistance along with increased plantarflexor torque.

James and Parker[109] measured the ROM of hip, knee, and ankle joints in subjects older than 70 years of age. They found a progressive loss of mobility in all motions, with active and passive motion showing similar patterns of decline. They attributed the decline in motion to a combination of structural changes in periarticular tissues and decreased activity levels. Roach and Miles[110] analyzed goniometric data from the hips and knees of 1,892 subjects. They found that active ROM varies little in age groups younger than 74. They concluded that any substantial loss of joint mobility should be considered abnormal and not be attributed to aging. The differences between their investigation and that of James and Parker were the age and size of the samples. James and Parker used a sample size of 80, divided equally into four age groups from 74–85 and over. Roach and Miles' sample was much larger and ranged in age from 25 to 74, with no less than 400 in each group. It may be that rapid losses in motion occur after the age of 75–80, dependent upon activity levels and other factors.[109,110] Roach and Miles do state that the active ROM values for the oldest group (60–74 years) was less than the youngest (25–39 years), even though the absolute difference was small. Passive ROM was not reported in their study.

Regardless of the degree of lost motion, reduced mobility combined with other factors presents a potential problem in older people. Lost movement capacity, in conjunction with lost strength, tissue degeneration, and generally decreased activity levels, can result in functional loss in ADL involving both upper and lower limbs.

As in other age-related changes such as cardiovascular function, muscle strength, and bone density, mobility in the elderly can be improved with exercise. Exercise programs including low level stretching, relatively low intensity aerobic exercise, and strengthening exercises (kept below the pain threshold[111]) can improve and maintain joint mobility, particularly in the shoulder, hip, and cervical spine areas.[112–115]

POSTURAL CONTROL AND FALLING

One of the greatest limitations to function in the elderly is falling and the fear of falling. Falling has severe potential morbidity, including fracture and head trauma. Fear of falling leads to decreased activity levels with subsequent loss of function of muscle, articular tissues, and information processing. Tinetti and Powell[116] have developed a tool for measuring the fear of falling in the elderly. They identified several factors that contributed to a fear of falling, including slow walking speed, past difficulty in getting up from a fall, medication, depression, and anxiety.

Posture is maintained by a control system that is dependent upon multiple sensory pathways, an intact body scheme, and various feedback and feed-forward loops (see ch.1, Fig. 1-10). Vision is probably the most important contributor of the sensory inputs. Vision identifies objects in the environmental surroundings maintains an awareness of the vertical position of the body in space, and checks for movement errors. Age-related changes in vision include reduced acuity and sensitivity, as well as a reduced visual field.[88,117] Adjusting the environment for reduced visual factors (including higher contrast edges and vertically oriented visual cues) may improve postural performance.[118] Also, placing shelves and other objects that must be visualized for use at eye level or below maintains the head in an optimal vertical position rather than requiring extension of the neck. The extended, head back position reduces postural stability in older women.[118]

Horak et al.[119] described the functional components of postural control. Included are detection of perturbations, perception of the limits of stability, adequate ankle muscle strength, appropriate scaling of response, normal latency of neural tissues, appropriate timing of muscles and postural response, selection of a suitable response, and normal interaction of sensory systems. They consider these elements to be the building blocks of postural control. Briefly, aging results in altered coordination of postural movement patterns,[120] delayed response to postural perturbation,[121] changed motor learning patterns and information processing,[94,120] altered biomechanics as a result of changing tissue and neuromuscular properties,[122] reduced sensory function, and reduced awareness of safe stability limits.[119] The multicomponent nature of falls in the elderly as a result of failing postural control is shown in Fig. 9-3.

There is so much interplay between the motor and sensory components of postural control that it is impossible to separate one from the other. Indeed, it is often difficult to identify a "pure" component. Each sensory element has motor involvement and vice versa. The focus here is to identify the movement changes that underlie postural dyscontrol in the elderly. Most falls occur during a dynamic activity; rarely does a person fall while in a static posture, without some medical cause.

The three basic strategies of postural movement to stabilize the center of gravity are shown in Fig. 9-4. Rogers[123] suggests that the stepping strategy is the primary mechanism of avoiding falls. It is the older individual's inability to appropriately correct posture using a stepping strategy that results in many falls. The reasons for this are several. King et al.[124] found that older people had a smaller functional base of support available to them. They defined functional base of support as the proportion of the anterior-posterior dimension used during leaning activities. This limitation, combined with greater postural sway,[125] reduces the available postural strategies for maintaining balance. Horak et al.[119] suggests that increased postural sway, ankle/calf pathology, and sensory loss reduce the effectiveness of the ankle strategy, while a reduced functional

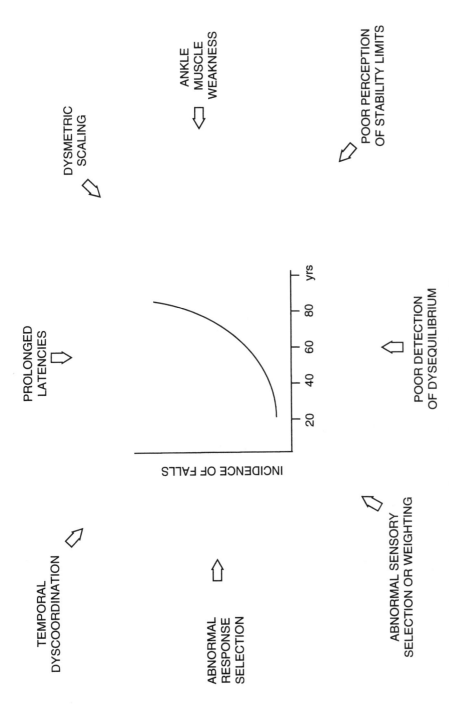

FIGURE 9-3 *Declines in functional postural components that contribute to instability and falls with aging. (From Horak FB,[119] with permission.)*

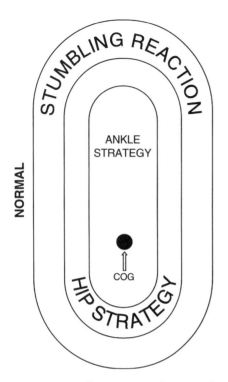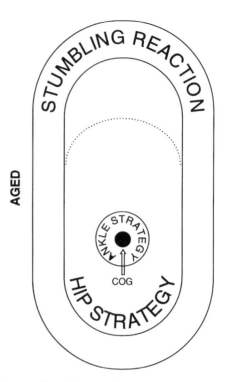

FIGURE 9-4 *Illustration of postural strategy preference based upon the excursion of the center of gravity. Left side shows normal subjects. Right illustration shows limitation of choice in strategy selection with aging. It is possible that the hip strategy is limited as well, making stepping (stumbling reaction) the strategy of choice. (Dotted line to indicate possible limit of hip strategy added.) (From Horak FB,[119] with permission.)*

base of support makes the hip strategy less functional, leaving stepping as the movement strategy of choice, almost by default (Fig. 9-4). Falls can occur when the appropriate movement strategy for a given environment is not available. The available choices may be insufficient to deal with all of the biomechanical and environmetal factors present.

Yet stepping is also affected by age. In some cases, the muscles are unable to generate enough tension to rapidly move the lower limbs. In other instances, somatosensory or visual deficits interfere with a successful stepping strategy, and a fall results. Chen et al.[126] noted that older adults (more than 71 years) had a tendency to adopt a more conservative strategy in stepping over an obstacle; approximately 15 percent of

healthy older adults stepped on an obstacle placed in the way during normal gait. Visual deficits, reduced spatial awareness, and impaired somatosensory information resulting in inappropriate scaling of movement responses[127] can all contribute to a failed stepping strategy before a fall.

Reduced reaction times that accompany aging may interfere with a stepping strategy. Gait is initiated by a stereotypical activation pattern of the leg muscles, particularly gastrocnemius-soleus and anterior tibialis.[128–130] Slower reaction times can upset the coordinated activation of the lower leg muscles and result in an ineffective step. Stelmach et al.[121] and Woolacott and Manchester[120] found that anticipatory postural reactions and reaction times were slower in the older adult, suggesting impaired responses to movement preparation and execution. Morgan et al.[131] also suggest that slower movements exhibited by older (average 69 years) adults is indicative of a decline in motor coordination rather than a simple strategic preference for slower, more cautious movements.

Ineffective postural control strategies, like most functional problems in the elderly result from a variety of causes. Falls can result due to limited or ineffective movement strategies brought on by visual, somatosensory, biomechanical, or CNS processing deficits. Reduced neural function contributing to postural instability is a function of aging and combined pathologies (Fig. 9-5). In general, safe walking in older requires a slower pace, constant scanning of the environment, and close attention to potential ob-

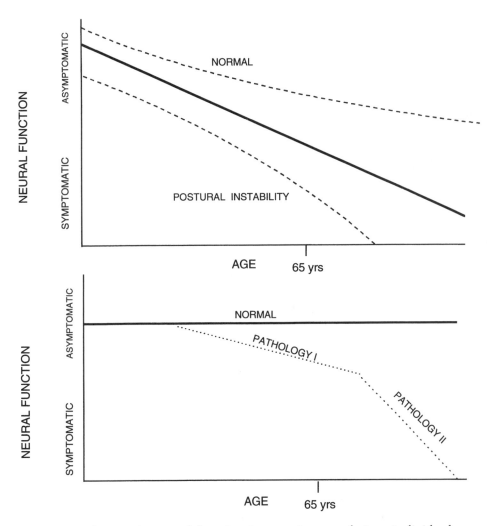

FIGURE 9-5 *Changes in neural function in an aging population. Individuals with postural instability (top graph) or pathology probably have decreased neural function with respect to balance control. Comorbidity (multiple pathology) alters function more than single pathologies. (From Horak FB,[119] with permission.)*

stacles that can require rapid changes in posture or gait.

GAIT

Gait is a basic functional activity that helps to define independence of older adults. Certain characteristics of gait are affected by the aging process, but pathology that is often present in the elderly is more detrimental to gait and function than aging alone. Gait disorders in the elderly can often be attributed to unidentified disease processes.[132] Researchers who study gait in the elderly must carefully screen for pathologic conditions, as many gait disorders attributed to the aging process may be caused by neurologic changes.[132,133]

Healthy older adults show few changes in gait patterns compared to younger subjects. Winter et al.[134] found shorter stride length with longer double-support stance duration, less power generated by the plantar flexors during push-off, and less power absorbed by the quadriceps during late stance and early swing. Hu and Woolacott[133] point out that reduced step length and weaker push-off may be a result of decreased plantar flexion strength, which occurs in the aged.[135] Reduced hip-knee covariance was also noted, a finding that Hu and Woolacott attribute to unidentified balance deficits. Winter et al. refer to the hip-knee covariance as an index of dynamic balance.[134] Other studies of age-related gait changes found a trend to slower gait, higher toe clearance at initial swing, and more conservative gait patterns in general.[126,133]

These strategies may be attempts to reduce the risks associated with walking (Fig. 9-6). Higher toe clearance can reduce the risk of tripping, while slower velocities, shorter stride length, and increased double support phase minimize the risk of slipping and/or falling. These are adaptations designed to maximize the ability of the older adult to compensate for reduced muscle capacity, sensory awareness, and response times. If velocity and stride length are reduced too much, or double support phase is increased excessively, then gait can be adversely affected and become nonfunctional.

Several factors influence gait pattern changes in older adults. A more sedentary lifestyle in general combined with lower cardiovascular and musculoskeletal capacity contributes to reduced walking speeds and endurance. A history of falling causes different gait characteristics, perhaps prompted by cognitive changes or underlying pathology. Slow walking has been implicated as a factor in falling,[116] yet falling results in a slower gait pattern. Pathology feeds into this cycle, resulting in reduced independence in gait. Maki[122] states that it is difficult to establish whether fear of falling is a cognitive problem or whether people with fear of falling have true gait and balance control disturbances. Sensory changes that can affect gait have been discussed earlier.

Other factors that contribute to gait problems in the elderly include severe vestibulopathy and medications. For a review on these topics, the reader is referred to the work of Krebs and Lockert[136] and Chapron,[137] respectively.

UPPER EXTREMITY FUNCTION—PRECISION GRIP

The upper extremity tasks of reaching, grasping, and lifting or manipulating an object are taken for granted by the majority of the population. Little thought is given to the complexity of the sensorimotor coordination that is required for successful completion of these activities. All of the components involved—visual, somatosensory, and muscular function—are affected by aging. Disturbance of gripping and manipulative skills can be as detrimental to overall function and independence as reduced walking capacity. Many ADL tasks performed at home demand use of the upper extremity. These include lifting, dressing, meal preparation, writing, and cleaning.

Manipulation of objects with the hand starts with vision. Accurate reaching and preparation of hand position is a function that is strongly mediated by vision and visual feedback.[138,139] Age-related changes in visual acuity and contrast can affect one's ability to locate and reach for an object. Vision forms the basis of a feed-forward

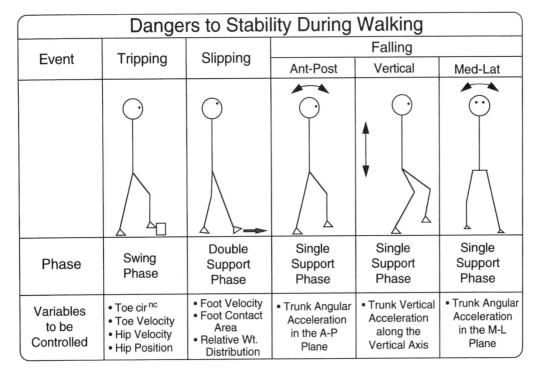

Dangers to Stability During Walking					
Event	Tripping	Slipping	Falling		
			Ant-Post	Vertical	Med-Lat
Phase	Swing Phase	Double Support Phase	Single Support Phase	Single Support Phase	Single Support Phase
Variables to be Controlled	• Toe cir^{nc} • Toe Velocity • Hip Velocity • Hip Position	• Foot Velocity • Foot Contact Area • Relative Wt. Distribution	• Trunk Angular Acceleration in the A-P Plane	• Trunk Vertical Acceleration along the Vertical Axis	• Trunk Angular Acceleration in the M-L Plane

FIGURE 9-6 *Factors that may cause a loss of balance or fall during locomotion along with the variables that need to be controlled by the neuromuscular system to avoid a loss of stability. Successful avoidance may be proactive via identification or prediction of risk followed by avoidance, or a stabilizing response before loss of equilibrium. Reactive control requires adequate detection and stabilization following a perturbation. (From Patla AE,[209] with permission.)*

sensory loop that integrates memory and somatosensory systems during lifting.[140] Accurate identification of an object serves two purposes: to locate the object in order to plan the reaching movement toward it, and to use memory to predict the mechanical parameters of the object to grasp and lift it.

Once an object is touched and grasped, cutaneous receptors indicate the size and shape of the object and begin to modify the muscular force necessary to maintain grip and lift the object. Several mechanisms in the somatosensory system control the force fluctuations of the hand and fingers.[141,142] Variations in aging include greater force fluctuations during grasping and lifting.[143] Decreased muscle function leads to strength loss in both the hand and shoulder muscles. Cognitive skills that relate to motor skills are also impaired, impacting on manual dexterity and function. The time required to manipulate objects by hand in the elderly is significantly increased.[144]

Comorbidity

Comorbidity is the coexistence of several medical conditions simultaneously.[145] Verbrugge et al.[146] studied which chronic conditions and combinations are most prevalent in the elderly. Arthritis is the leading chronic condition of the el-

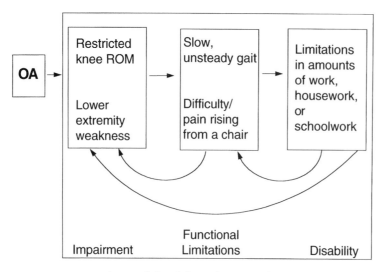

FIGURE 9-7 *Paradigm of disability showing the impairments and limitations that precede disability in osteoarthritis. (From Jette AM,[63] with permission.)*

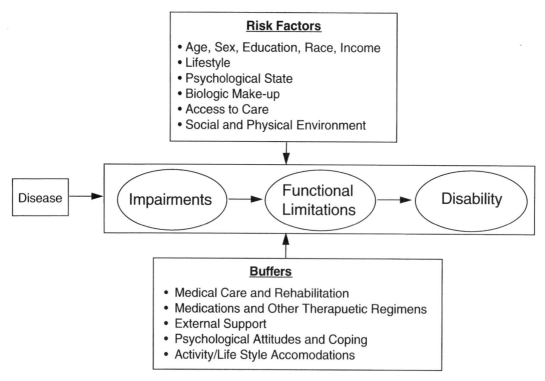

FIGURE 9-8 *Factors that influence the progression of disability in older individuals, Risk factors are those variables that increase disability, while buffers mitigate the disease process. (From Jette AM,[63] with permission.)*

derly in both sexes. Orthopaedic diseases are associated with decreased activity and function, but good health.[145] Arthritis combined with other chronic conditions (heart disease, visual impairment, respiratory disease, etc.) produces the highest level of disability.

The role of multiple impairment of systems should be evaluated by physical therapists. Boissonnault and Bass[147–150] reviewed medical screening for orthopaedic physical therapists. They noted that some of the origins of musculoskeletal pain can originate from various different organ systems as well as from problems at other joints. Although these are not new concepts, the screening process is more important in a population of older adults who may not be aware of medical problems, or whose medical problems can interact with orthopaedic disease processes and, if untreated, may limit their rehabilitation potential.

Dekker et al.[151] described a system of diagnosis and treatment for physical therapists based upon evaluation of existing impairments. Their goal was to develop treatment plans based on identifying all of the existing physical problems and their resulting restrictions of function. Impairments are defined by Jette[63] as abnormalities of specific organs or systems that result from a specific pathology, injury, or accident. Functional limitations are consequences of impairments and are observable losses or changes in performance of a task. Disability is diminished capacity to perform basic ADLs such as feeding, walking, and dressing. An example of this paradigm is given in Figure 9-7. Conduct of other affairs such as shopping, social interaction, financial management, or preparation of meals are part of daily living and would be included in the category of disability. These types of activities are called instrumental ADL. Disability can be modulated by several buffers and exacerbated by various risk factors[63] (Fig. 9-8).

Identifying all of the factors that contribute to physical disability in the elderly can be a thankless task, for not all of the contributors to disability are treatable by physical therapists. Contributions of medical diseases and other aspects of aging to musculoskeletal and movement loss cannot be ignored and should be accounted for within clinical practice.

Evaluation of Function in the Elderly

Several tools have been designed to measure function in the elderly. Many have been used to measure specific aspects of aging, such as gait, falling, and balance. Some of the tests are quick screens for potential problems. An example of this is the Get Up and Go Test, which requires a subject to stand up from a chair, walk 3 m, turn around, and return. The test can be scored subjectively[152] or timed.[153] Tinetti[154] has developed a tool for measuring balance and mobility in the elderly called the Balance and Mobility assessment. Tinetti and Powell[116] also have measured the fear of falling separately from falling itself. Berg[155] reviewed clinical laboratory-based tools used to measure balance, and commented on their reliability and validity. Since balance is a complex motor skill involving several systems, selection of the appropriate balance measurement tool must be based on the population and question being investigated. In a clinical setting, the therapist is encouraged to begin using available tools to evaluate static and dynamic components of balance, at least at the screening level. More advanced (and expensive) devices such as force plates, Neurocom, and Fastex can be used, but clinical validity, reliability, and usage guidelines are still under development. The cost of this equipment may be prohibitive to some clinics.

Functional scoring systems were first developed to measure the results of total joint procedures. The Hospital for Special Surgery knee[162,163] scoring systems and the Harris Hip Score[164] are examples of these. These measurement systems were later adapted to meet the needs of other populations and surgical procedures, particularly in sports medicine and reconstructive procedures (see chs. 4, 6). A second generation of rating scales unrelated to the surgical procedure or diagnosis has evolved to measure function. Examples of these in the elderly population are the Functional Impact Measurement Scale (FIMS),[165,166] Sickness Impact Profile (SIP),[167] and the Arthritis Impact Measurement Scale (AIMS).[168,169] All of these, plus others, measure the physical, mental, ADL, and/or psychosocial level of the patient.

Fractures and Total Joint Arthroplasty

Two of the major orthopaedic problems faced by the elderly are recovery from fractures and joint replacement procedures. Arthritis is the primary cause of disability in the elderly.[63] Fractures of the humerus or hip following a fall can also result in significant impairment, functional limitation, and/or disability.

HIP FRACTURE AND HIP REPLACEMENT

Hip fractures are associated with residual disability that includes physical as well as psychosocial losses. In a meta-analysis of outcomes following displaced hip fracture, Lu-Yao et al.[156] found that operative technique (primary fixation or hip prosthesis) did not have significant impact on outcome, except in pain relief, which was significantly better in the arthroplasty group. Mortality rate, mobility, and reoperation rate tended to be better in the arthroplasty group, but no statistical significance was found.

Reduced ambulatory status is a common result of hip fracture (see section on bone),[19,157] including use of assisstive devices, slower gait, weakness, and contracture of the hip abductors.[88,158] Long et al.[87] noted changes in EMG (electromyographic) parameters of the gluteus medius two years after hip fracture and fixation. With regard to ADL, 15–40 percent of patients returned to their prefracture level of instrumental and regular ADL, respectively, at 1 year after surgery.[159,160] Hip fracture has similar detrimental effects on mental status and psychosocial factors. Patients that are able to maintain social support systems and have a more positive outlook show greater improvement in ambulation following fracture.[157,161]

The Harris Hip Score (Table 9-2) is an integrated scoring system that rated the variables of pain, function (defined by walking, sitting, putting on shoes and socks), ROM, and deformity. The Harris Hip Score had no reliability testing. The author validated the scale by comparing its results to two pre-existing measures of function, the Shepard[170] and Larson[171] scales.

Roush[172] surveyed 43 subjects who underwent elective hip or knee arthroplasty using a questionnaire that asked the subjects' participation in 22 ADLs on a yes/no basis. She found little difference in function following the surgical procedure, and attributed successful surgical results to psychosocial factors. Some drawbacks of her study were the mixed nature of the procedures and diagnoses and the yes/no/better format of the questions. No reliability or validity information was reported with this questionnaire.

Johanson et al.[173] used a self-administered rating questionnaire to assess outcome following total hip replacement (Table 9-3). The reliability was reported to be good to excellent, and validity was established by comparison to established scales (arthritis impact measurement scale and 6-minute walking test). The questionnaire gave equal rating to evaluating arthritis symptoms, walking, pain, and function. The average gain from preoperation to postoperation was approximately 25 points, which was judged to be a significant improvement. The maximum benefit is usually noticed at the 6-month postoperative mark, with little change occurring after that (Fig. 9-9). The greatest functional improvement came in the areas of walking stairs, wearing normal shoes, and housework. Little difference was noted in bathing, mobility, or using public transportation. The largest improvements were in the areas of pain relief and overall impact of arthritis, perhaps indicating that pain is the factor that function most influences in arthritic conditions.

Katz et al.[174] evaluated the validity and reliability of the Total Hip Arthroplasty Outcome Evaluation Questionnaire developed by the American Academy of Orthopaedic Surgeons (AAOS). The system measures pain (degree and

TABLE 9-2 *Harris hip score (synopsis of system)*

Pain (44 possible)	
None or ignores it	44
Slight, occasional, no compromise in activities	40
Mild pain, no effect on average activities, rarely moderate pain with unusual activity, may take aspirin	30
Moderate pain, tolerable but makes concessions to pain. Some limitation of ordinary activity or work. May require occasional pain medication stronger than aspirin	20
Marked pain, serious limitation of activity	10
Totally disabled, crippled, pain in bed, bedridden	0
Function (47 possible)	
Gait (33 possible)	
Limp	
None	11
Slight	8
Moderate	5
Severe	0
Support	
None	11
Cane for long walks	7
Cane for most of the time	5
One crutch	3
Two canes	2
Two crutches	0
Not able to walk (specify reason)	0
Walking Distance	
Unlimited	11
Six blocks	8
Two or three blocks	5
Indoors only	2
Bed and chair	0
Activities (14 possible)	
Stairs	
Normally without using a railing	4
Normally using a railing	2
In any manner	1
Unable to do stairs	0

Shoes and Socks	
With ease	4
With difficulty	2
Unable	0
Sitting	
Comfortably in ordinary chair one hour	5
On high chair for one-half hour	3
Unable to sit comfortably in any chair	0
Enter public transportation	1

Absence of deformity points (4) are given if the patient demonstrates:

Less than 30 degrees fixed flexion contracture
Less than 10 degrees fixed adduction
Less than 10 degrees fixed internal rotation in extension
Limb-length discrepancy less than 3.2 cm

Range of motion (index values are determined by multiplying the degrees of motion possible in each arc by the appropriate index)

Flexion 0–45 degrees $\times$ 1.0
  45–90 degrees $\times$ 0.6
  90–110 degrees $\times$ 0.3
Abduction 0–15 degrees $\times$ 0.8
  15–20 degrees $\times$ 0.3
  over 20 degrees $\times$ 0
External rotation in ext. 0–15 degrees $\times$ 0.4
  over 15 degrees $\times$ 0
Internal rotation in extension any $\times$ 0
Adduction 0–15 degrees $\times$ 0.2

To determine the overall rating for range of motion, multiply the sum of the index values $\times$ 0.05. Record Trendelenburg test as positive, level, or neutral.

(From Harris WH,[164] with permission.)

occurrence), function (work, dressing, stairs, level of activity, sit to stand), walking capacity (time walked with and without support), and satisfaction. Reliability was found to be high (r values from .76–.91 for the different sections). Satisfaction rating showed the greatest fluctuation. Validity was measured by comparing the results to the SIP. Validity was not strong, however, the SIP is a general health measure, while the AAOS form is a specific disease measure. This may have affected the validity of the results.

Laupacis et al.[175] assessed a group of patients for up to 2 years using a battery of scales including the SIP, 6-minute walk test, and sev-

TABLE 9-3 *Self-administered hip-rating questionnaire*

Which hip is affected by arthritis? (Circle one)
Left   Right   Both
Please answer the following questions about the hip(s) you have just indicated.

1. Considering all of the ways that your hip arthritis affects you, mark (X) on the scale for how well you are doing.

0	25	50	75	100
very well	well	fair	poor	very poor

circle one response for each question
(The score here is determined by subtraction of the number marked from 100, with the number being interpolated, if necessary, if the mark is between printed numbers. The result is divided by 4, and the answer is rounded off to the nearest integer. The maximum is 25 points.)

2. During the past month, how would you describe the usual arthritis pain in your hip? (Maximum, 10 points)
   A) Very severe (2 points)
   B) Severe (4 points)
   C) Moderate (6 points)
   D) Mild (8 points)
   E) Never (10 points)

3. During the past month, how often have you had to take medication for your arthritis? (Maximum, 5 points)
   A) Always (1 point)
   B) Very often (2 points)
   C) Fairly often (3 points)
   D) Sometimes (4 points)
   E) Never (5 points)

4. During the past month, how often have you had severe arthritis pain in your hip? (Maximum, 5 points)
   A) Every day (1 point)
   B) Several days per week (2 points)
   C) One day per week (3 points)
   D) One day per month (4 points)
   E) Never (5 points)

5. How often have you had hip arthritis pain at rest, either sitting or lying down? (Maximum, 5 points)
   A) Every day (1 point)
   B) Several days per week (2 points)
   C) One day per week (3 points)
   D) One day per month (4 points)
   E) Never (5 points)

6. How far can you walk without resting because of your hip arthritis pain? (Maximum, 15 points)
   A) Unable to walk (3 points)
   B) Less than one city block (6 points)
   C) 1 to <10 city blocks (9 points)
   D) 10 to 20 city blocks (12 points)
   E) Unlimited (15 points)

7. How much assistance do you need for walking? (Maximum, 10 points)
   A) Unable to walk (1 point)
   B) Walk only with someone's help (2 points)
   C) Two crutches or walker every day (3 points)
   D) Two crutches or walker several days per week (4 points)
   E) Two crutches or walker once per week of less (5 points)
   F) Cane or one crutch every day (6 points)
   G) Cane or one crutch several days per week (7 points)
   H) Cane or one crutch once per week (8 points)
   I) Cane or one crutch once per month (9 points)
   J) No assistance (10 points)

8. How much difficulty do you have going up or down one flight of stairs because of your hip's arthritis? (Maximum 5 points)
   A) Unable (1 point)
   B) Require someone's assistance (2 points)
   C) Require crutch or cane (3 points)
   D) Require banister (4 points)
   E) No difficulty (5 points)

9. How much difficulty do you have putting on your shoes and socks because of your hip arthritis? (Maximum, 5 points)
   A) Unable (1 point)
   B) Require someone's assistance (2 points)
   C) Require long shoehorn and reacher (3 points)
   D) Some difficulty but no devices required (4 points)
   E) No difficulty (5 points)

10. Are you able to use public transportation? (Maximum 3 points)
    A) No, because of my hip arthritis (1 point)
    B) No, for some other reason (2 points)
    C) Yes, able to use public transportation (3 points)

11. When you bathe—either a sponge bath or in a tub or shower—how much help do you need? (Maximum, 3 points)
    A) No help at all (3 points)
    B) Help with bathing one part of your body, like back or leg (2 points)
    C) Help with bathing more than one part of your body (1 point)

12. If you had the necessary transportation, could you go shopping for groceries or clothes? (maximum, 3 points)
    A) Without help (taking care of all shopping needs yourself) (3 points)
    B) With some help (need someone to go with you to help on all shopping trips) (2 points)
    C) Completely unable to do any shopping (1 point)

13. If you had household tools and appliances (vacuum, mops, and so on), could you do your own housework? (Maximum, 3 parts)
    A) Without help (can clean floors, windows, refrigerators, and so on) (3 points)
    B) With some help (can do light housework, but need help with some heavy work) (2 points)
    C) Completely unable to do house work (1 point)

14. How well are you able to move around? (Maximum, 3 points)
    A) Able to get in and out of bed or chairs without the help of another person (3 points)
    B) Need the help of another person to get in and out of bed or chair (2 points)
    C) Not able to get out of bed (1 point)

This is the end of the Hip Rating Questionnaire. Thank you for your cooperation.

(From Johanson NA et al,[175] with permission)

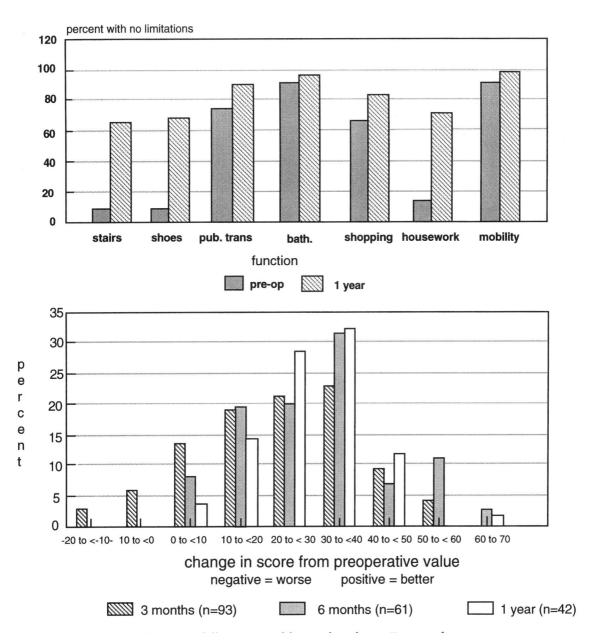

FIGURE 9-9 *Change in function following total hip arthroplasty. Top graph shows changes in ADL. Bottom graph shows changes in functional scores at 3, 6, and 12 months postoperatively. (From Johanson NA,*[173] *with permission.)*

eral scales used in Canada to measure the impact of arthritis. A secondary purpose of the study was to investigate the feasibility of a randomized, clinical trial using two different hip prostheses. The results of that section of the study were not presented, although the authors concluded that such a study is feasible and is underway. There were significant improvements in all measures of function, except for the work section of the SIP, which only showed a trend toward improvement. The distance traveled in the 6-minute walk test had increased 65 percent after a 2-year follow-up. This study showed that the greatest improvement occurred between 3 and 6 months postoperatively and was maintained for up to 2 years following operation.

TOTAL KNEE REPLACEMENT

The Hospital for Special Surgery Knee Score (Table 9-4) was published by Insall et al.[162,163] and subsequently used in several studies to evaluate knee joint function after total knee replacement.[163,177-180] The Knee Society upgraded the HSS system by dividing the rating scale into two separate evaluations, a knee score and a function score[181] (Table 9-5). The knee score measures pain, stability, ROM, and alignment. Deductions are taken for severity of contracture, alignment problems, and extension lag. The function score rates the ability to walk and go up and down stairs. Deductions are taken for the use of a cane or walker. The newer rating system

TABLE 9-4 *Hospital for special surgery knee rating scale*

Pain (30 points)			**Muscle Strength (10 points)**	
No pain at any time	30		Excellent: cannot break the quadriceps power	10
No pain on walking	15		Good: can break the quadriceps power	8
Mild pain on walking	10		Fair: move through the arc of motion	4
Moderate pain on walking	5		Poor: cannot move through the arc of motion	0
Severe pain on walking	0			
No pain at rest	15		**Flexion deformity (10 points)**	
Mild pain at rest	10		No deformity	10
Severe pain at rest	5		Less than 5 degrees	8
Function (22 points)			5-10 degrees	5
Walking and standing unlimited	12		More than 10 degrees	0
Walking distance of 5-10 blocks and standing ability intermittent (<1/2 h)	10		**Instability (10 points)**	
			None	10
Walking 1-5 blocks and standing ability up to 1/2 hour	8		Mild: 0-5 degrees	8
			Moderate: 5-15 degrees	5
Walking less than 1 block	4		Severe: more than 15 degrees	0
Cannot walk	0		**Subtraction**	
Climbing stairs	5		One cane	1
Climbing stairs with support	2		Two canes	2
Transfer activity	5		Two crutches	3
Transfer activity with support	2		Extension lag of 5 degrees	2
Range of Motion (18 points)			Extension lag of 10 degrees	3
1 point for each 8 degrees of arc of motion to a maximum of 18 points	18		Extension lag of 15 degrees	5
			Each 5 degrees of varus	1
			Each 5 degrees of valgus	1

(From Insall JN et al.,[163] with permission.)

TABLE 9-5 *Knee society clinical rating system*

Patient Category
  A. Unilateral or bilateral (opposite knee successfully replaced)
  B. Unilateral, other knee symptomatic
  C. Multiple arthritis or medical infirmity

PAIN	POINTS	FUNCTION	POINTS
None	50	Walking	
Mild or occasional	45	Unlimited	50
Stairs only	40	>10 blocks	40
Walking and Stairs	30	5–10 blocks	30
Moderate		<5 blocks	20
Occasional	20	Housebound	10
Continual	10	Unable	0
Severe	0	Stairs	50
		Normal up and down	
Range of Motion		Normal up; down with rail	40
(5 degrees = 1 point)	25	Up and down with rail	30
		Up with rail; unable down	15
		Unable	0
Stability (maximum movement in any position)			
Anteroposterior		Subtotal	_____
<5 mm	10		
		Deduction (minus)	
5–10 mm	5	Cane	5
10 mm	0	Two canes	10
Mediolateral		Crutches or walker	20
<5 degrees	15		
6–9 degrees	10	Total deductions	_____
10–14 degrees	5		
15 degree	0	Function Score	_____
Subtotal	_____		
Deductions (minus)			
Flexion contracture			
5–10 degrees	2		
10–15 degrees	5		
16–20 degrees	10		
>20 degrees	15		
Extension lag			
<10 degrees	5		
10–20 degrees	10		
>20 degrees	15		
Alignment			
5–10 degrees	0		
0–4 degrees	3 points each degree		
11–15 degrees	3 points each degree		
Other	20		
Total deductions	_____		
Knee score	_____		
(If total is a minus number, score is 0.)			

(From Insall JN et al.,[181] with permission.)

was designed to reflect higher expectations of improvement as a result of surgery. It is also hoped that other medical conditions will have less impact on the evaluation of outcome following total knee arthroplasty. The Knee Society score also categorizes patients according to the number of joints involved (Table 9-5). Neither of the two rating scales has been evaluated for reliability or validity. They are very similar to the HSS hip scale, so one may assume that the two systems would be reliable and valid.

Functional ratings based upon the HSS knee scale show remarkable consistency among studies reporting its use. In general, preoperative scores *average* 45 ± 10 points out of a maximum of 100.[163,177,180,182-185] The range of preoperative scores can be from zero to 65. Postoperatively, scores range average 76 ± 5 points. Postoperative values can be as low as zero or as high as 100.[186] The greatest increase in the functional score is in the area of pain relief.[177]

Functional rating based upon the Knee Society scoring system was reported by Stern and Insall.[184] The average postoperative knee score was 92; however, the average functional score was only 66. Preoperative scores were not given, since this longitudinal study was initiated before development of the Knee Society rating scale. Preoperative HSS scores were 50 (range of 23–74), but HSS scores were not given for the postoperative values. The two rating systems were not compared in this study.

Other measures have been evaluated as a measure of function after total knee arthroplasty and in arthritic knees. Lankhorst et al.[187] found that isokinetic testing was not a good indicator of overall function in individuals with arthritic knees. A functional capacity scale measuring activity, pain, walking, and stair-climbing was a better indicator than isolated strength testing. Berman et al.[176] found that isokinetic measurement at 60 degrees per second of hamstring and quadriceps strength correlated well with gait analysis and HSS knee score. Improvements in strength shadowed improvements in function. No r values were reported. The authors noted that hamstring strength reached its maximum level 7 months after surgery, while quadriceps

torque continued to increase for up to 2 years postoperation. It should be noted that of the original sample of 68, 14 were unable to perform isokinetic testing due to pain or weakness during the first 6 months after surgery.[176]

TOTAL SHOULDER ARTHROPLASTY

There are limited reports on function following shoulder arthroplasty. Lippitt et al.[188] present the results of total shoulder arthroplasty over the course of 12–18 months postoperatively (Fig. 9-10). They noted steady progress of some functions (ROM and ADL) as recovery from surgery progressed. Strength, potential sports activities, and work remain the most difficult to recover after the onset of arthritis resulting in total shoulder arthroplasty. For an explanation of the Simple Shoulder test, please refer to the chapter on upper extremity function in this text. Matsen et al.[189] used both the Simple Shoulder Test and a reliable general health status questionnaire (SF-36[190]). They found that the SST did not correlate strongly with the general health questionnaire, reiterating the issue found in other studies. The general health measurement forms are not sensitive to localized osteoarthritis that may still have a significant impact on function.

The simple shoulder test and the SF-36 questionnaire were used in a second study on the effectiveness of shoulder arthroplasty for patients with primary glenohumeral degenerative joint disease. The major improvements following shoulder replacement were in pain level, general physical function, general health status, and emotional and physical role functions. The latter two variables refer to a person's quality of life perception. Physical function improvement was greatest in overhead activities, strength, and ADL such as washing the opposite shoulder, tucking in a shirt, and sleeping on side. Again, little correlation was found between SF-36 measures of health and specific simple shoulder test indicators of function.[191]

Goldman et al.[185] reported on functional outcome of humeral head replacement after acute three- or four-part proximal humeral fracture. They used the American Shoulder and Elbow

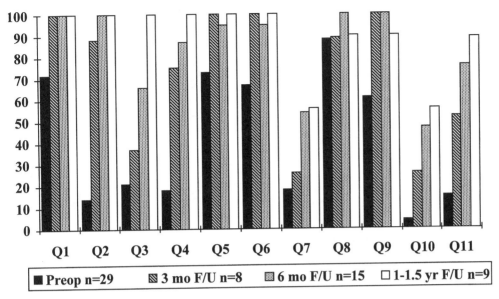

FIGURE 9-10 *Comparison of results of total shoulder arthroplasty at the preoperative, and 3-, 6-, and 12-month postoperative period using the Simple Shoulder Test. (See ch. 4). (From Lippitt SB,[188] with permission.)*

Surgeons evaluation form to rate pain, ROM, strength, and ADL tasks. The average age of the patients was 67 years (48–86 years). No preoperative evaluation was made due to the nature of the injury. Postoperative results were reported as minimal pain, moderate limitation of active motion (average forward elevation to 107 degrees, external rotation to 31 degrees, internal rotation to L2), and 4+/5 strength levels. Almost half of the patients reported difficulty with half of the functional tasks, particularly activities at shoulder level or above, pulling, and sleeping on the surgical shoulder. Most of the limitation was probably due to loss of motion. Younger patients performed better than older patients. No overall functional rating score was reported.

General Health Status Measurements

In addition to the tools that measure function of a joint or extremity following a specific procedure, the physical therapist can also assess the perceived health of the patient. The SIP is a reliable test that has done well in validity trials.[167,192] The SIP measures 12 functional categories including mobility, basic ADL, instrumental ADL, social and effective function, and general health. The SIP measures an individual's perception of how limited they are as a result of sickness or impairment. One of the criticisms of the SIP is that it is too broad a measure. It is probably not sensitive enough to track relatively small changes in patient function, particularly in one functional category, hence the difficulty in using this type of scale for single joint degenerative arthritis.[192]

The FIMS[165,166] is a similar type of profile that is not as broad as the SIP. It measures the level of competency in ADL, mobility, and social function, but not instrumental ADL. This tool has also been tested for reliability and validity (face and content validity).[192]

The AIMS is a multidimensional index that measures the health status of patients with arthritis.[168,169] AIMS is a self-administered test that measures mobility, activity, pain, ADL, dex-

TABLE 9-6 *The Arthritis Impact Scale (AIMS). The questionnaire presented here lists the 9 scale groups included in the AIMS instrument. The AIMS questionnaire contains 7 demographic items and 55 health status items arranged in the scale groups listed below.*

Mobility
4   Are you in bed or chair for most or all of the day?
3   Are you able to use public transportation?
2   When you travel around your community, does someone have to assist you because of your health?
1   Do you have to stay indoors most or all of the day because of your health?

Physical Activity
5   Are unable to walk unless you are assisted by another person or by a cane, crutches, artificial limbs, or braces?
4   Do you have any trouble either walking one block or climbing one flight of stairs because of your health?
3   Do you have any trouble either walking several blocks or climbing a few flights of stairs because of your health?
2   Do you have trouble bending, lifting, or stooping because of your health?
1   Does your health limit the kind of vigorous activities you can do such as running, lifting heavy objects, of participating in strenuous sports?

Dexterity
5   Can you easily write with a pen or pencil?
4   Can you easily turn a key in a lock?
3   Can you easily button articles of clothing?
2   Can you easily tie a pair of shoes?
1   Can you easily open a jar of food?

Social Role
7   If you had to take medicine, could you take all your own medicine?
6   If you had a telephone, would you be able to use it?
5   Do you handle your own money?
4   If you had a kitchen, could you prepare your own meals?
3   If you had laundry facilities (washer, dryer, etc.) could you do your own laundry?
2   If you had the necessary transportation, could you go shopping for groceries or clothes?
1   If you had household tools and appliances (vacuum, mops, etc.), could you do your own housework?

Social Activity
5   About how often were you on the telephone with close friends or relatives during the past month?
4   Has there been a change in the frequency or quality of your sexual relationships during the past month?
3   During the past month, about how often have you had friends or relatives to your home?
2   During the past month, about how often did you get together socially with friends or relatives?
1   During the past month, how often have you visited with friends or relatives at their homes?

Activities of Daily Living
4   How much help do you need to use the toilet?
3   How well are you able to move around?
2   How much help do you need in getting dressed?
1   When you bathe, either a sponge bath, tub, or shower, how much help do you need?

Pain
4   During the past month, how often have you had severe pain from your arthritis?
3   During the past month, how would you describe the arthritis pain you usually have?
2   During the past month, how long has your morning stiffness usually lasted from the time you wake up?
1   During the past month, how often have you had pain in two or more joints at the same time?

Depression
6   During the past month, how often did you feel that others would be better off if you were dead?
5   How often during the past month have you felt so down in the dumps that nothing could cheer you up?
4   How much of the time during the past month have you felt downhearted and blue?
3   How often during the past month did you feel that nothing turned out for you the way that you wanted it to?
2   During the past month, how much of the time have you been in low or very low spirits?
1   During the past month, how much of the time have you enjoyed the things you do?

Anxiety
6   During the past month, how much of the time have you felt tense or "high strung"?
5   How much have you been bothered by nervousness or your "nerves" during the past month?
4   How much of the time during the past month did you find yourself having difficulty trying to calm down?
3   How much of the time during the past month were you able to relax without difficulty?
2   How much of the time during the past month have you felt calm and peaceful?
1   How much of the time during the past month did you feel relaxed and free of tension?

(From Meenan RF et al.,[169] with permission.)

terity, and four psychosocial categories (Table 9-6) AIMS was developed primarily for use in patients with rheumatoid arthritis (RA), rather than osteoarthritis. It has been shown to be reliable and may be sensitive enough to track long-term outcomes of treatment of RA.[169] The AIMS2 was developed to be consistent with the World Health Organization standards.[192]

The general status scales are rarely reported in the rehabilitation literature. It remains to be seen if these tools will be useful in determining the efficacy of physical therapy interventions in the elderly population.

Athletics in Older Adults

Older people are participating in sports activities in larger numbers than ever before at all levels of competition.[193] This phenomenon is to be en-couraged as exercise appears to be the best treatment for aging, both from a physical and psycho-social point of view. One must consider the changes that affect the older athlete in light of the demands of the sports chosen for participation. Also, realistic expectations of performance and recovery from injury, if it occurs, must be emphasized in the older athlete.

Changes in reaction time,[194] proprioception, strength, and vision all place the older athlete at risk of injury in sports that require movement such as tennis and skiing. General loss of range of motion, changes in the intervertebral disk, and fatigue of the spinal muscles place limits on endurance activities such as running.[104,195,196] Degenerative changes in articular cartilage,[2,16,197] tendon,[44,198] bone,[15,199] and muscle reduce the force-generating and absorbing capacity of the musculoskeletal system and make the older athlete prone to overuse injuries.

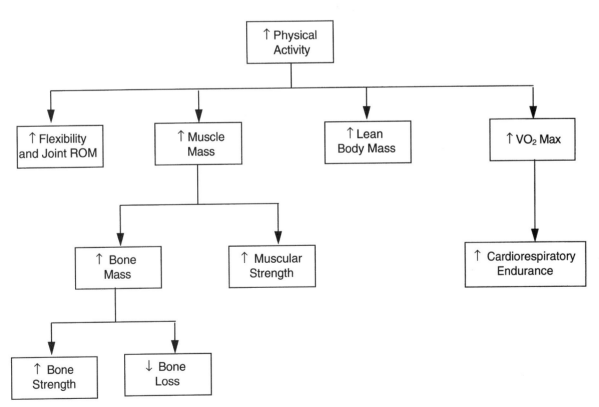

FIGURE 9-11 *Influence of physical activity on older individuals. (From Seto JL and Brewster CE,[200] with permission.)*

In general, participation in sports (golf, tennis, swimming, cycling, dance, etc.) that promote an active lifestyle is to be encouraged as long as it is not contraindicated. Attention to intensity, proper conditioning, and adequate warm-up are essential to minimize the risk of injury or aggravate underlying medical conditions.[200,201]

Treatment

Some of the sequelae of the aging process can be treated only with medical or surgical intervention. Yet many of the functional problems caused by the aging process can be ameliorated by exercise. Muscle strength, cardiac function, sensory loss, postural control, and cognition can all be improved by exercise and practice. Indeed, many of the symptoms related to aging can also be attributed to disuse. The primary age-related change is a general decrease in physical activity levels. The ability of the systems related to movement to respond to exercise may be limited, but in healthy older adults a training response is possible.

Figure 9-11 summarizes the impact of physical activity on the older individual.[200] Exercise prescription must take into account the lower ultimate strength and regenerative capacity of the musculoskeletal tissues and the capacity of the cardiovascular system. Figures 9-12 to 9-14 show the intensity, duration, and frequency effects of exercise in the elderly.[201] Orthopaedic complications to exercise can be minimized by proper warm-up and stretching[200] and avoiding

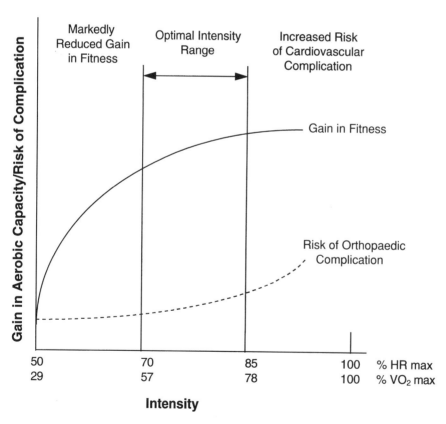

FIGURE 9-12 *Influence of intensity of exercise on gain in fitness. (From Kay GL,[201] with permission.)*

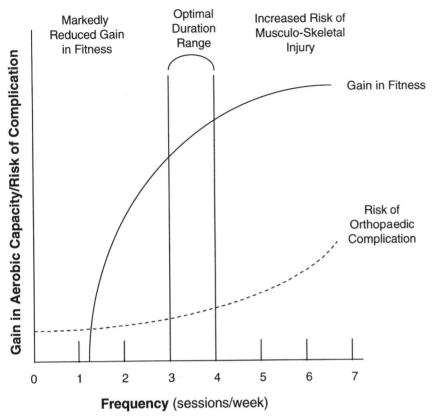

FIGURE 9-13 *Influence of frequency of exercise on gain in fitness. (From Kay GL,[201] with permission.)*

overtraining. These restrictions to exercise in the healthy, but sedentary, older adult are the same that apply to patients and athletes of all ages.

Improving posture control and reducing the incidence of falling requires more specific exercise direction. Hu and Woolacott[202,203] investigated the effect of multisensory training on standing balance in older adults. They trained their subjects using a variety of support surfaces and sensory paradigms (eyes open or closed, head position neutral or extended). Their results included improved postural stability and fewer falls in the trained group. The improvement was attributed to a training effect on redundant systems via manipulation of sensory and somatosensory inputs. The authors found that training only the sensory (visual and vestibular) systems produced postural improvements without simul-

taneous training of the somatosensory system. Wolfson et al.[53] have undertaken a study to evaluate the effects of strength training, balance platform training, or both on postural control and falling. Their program will also include a 6-month follow-up program of tai chi to continue the strength, balance, and movement improvements that may occur as a result of training. Jarnlo[204] found that women over the age of 70 were able to improve their balance following a program of exercise, including dance, balance, and coordination training. No mention was made of the impact of this program on the incidence of falls.

Other interventions that incorporate multisensory training include the Neurocom and the Fastex devices. The Neurocom can be used to alter the support platform under a subject's feet

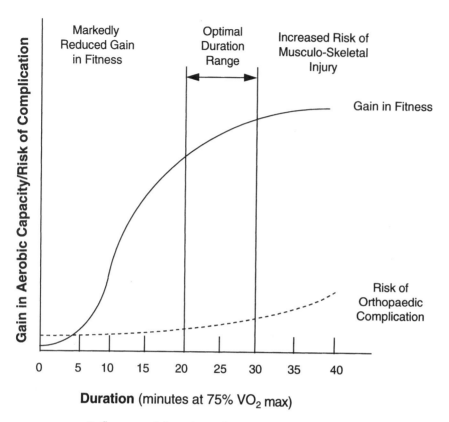

FIGURE 9-14 *Influence of duration of exercise on gain in fitness. (From Kay GL,[201] with permission.)*

in order to challenge the somatosensory systems. Visual and vestibular inputs can be altered during the use of this device. The Fastex can challenge the patient by requiring various different movement skills including balance, reaction time, obstacle avoidance, and visual response. Less sophisticated training can be accomplished using different foam surfaces for balance training.

Physical fitness may also have an effect on cognitive function. Individuals with cardiovascular disease do not perform as well on cognitive and perceptual-motor tasks.[205,206] Older people who are athletically active perform better on choice reaction tests and tests that are more complex or demand rapid processing. Some evidence exists that cognitive performance can improve along with improvements in aerobic ca-

pacity following an exercise program, but these results are not definitive.[206] Proposed mechanisms for improved cognitive performance with higher levels of physical fitness include enhanced cerebral circulation[207] and changes in neural responses.[208]

References

1. Pendergast DR, Fisher NM, Calkins E: Cardiovascular, neuromuscular, and metabolic alterations with age leading to frailty. J Gerontol 48: 61–67, 1993
2. Buckwalter JA, Woo SL-Y, Goldberg VM et al: Current concepts review. Soft tissue aging and musculoskeletal function. J Bone Joint Surg 75A: 1533–1548, 1993

3. Jette AM, Branch LG: The Framingham disability study: II. Physical disability among the elderly. Am J Pub Health 71:1211–1216, 1981

4. National Center for Health Statistics: Health statistics on older persons, 1987. In Ory MG et al: Frailty and injuries in later life: the FICSIT trials. J Am Geriatr Soc 41:283–296, 1993

5. Hinton RY, Lennox DW, Ebert FR et al: Relative rates of fracture of the hip in the United States. J Bone Joint Surg 77A:695–702, 1995

6. Burke RE, Hodgson JL: Age and power aerobic: the rate of change in men and women. Fed Proc 46:1824–1829, 1987

7. Hagberg JM: Effect of training on the decline of VO$_2$ max with aging. Fed Proc 46:1830–1833, 1987

8. Badenhop DT, Clearly PA, Schaal SF et al: Physiological adjustments to higher or lower intensity exercise in elders. Med Sci Sports Exer 15:496–502, 1983

9. Seals DR, Hagberg JM, Hurley BF et al: Endurance training in older men and women. I. Cardiovascular responses to exercise. J Appl Physiol 57:1024–1029, 1984

10. Belman MJ, Gaesser GA: Exercise training below and above the lactate threshold in the elderly. Med Sci Sports Exer 23:562–569, 1991

11. Pescatello LS, Judge JO: The impact of physical activity and physical fitness on functional capacity in older adults. p. 325. In Spivack BS (ed): Evaluation and Management of Gait Disorders. Marcel Dekker, New York, 1995

12. Shepard RJ: Can we identify those for whom exercise is hazardous? Sports Med 1:75–84, 1984

13. Pescatello LS, DiPetro L, Fargo AE et al: The impact of physical activity and physical fitness on health outcomes in older adults. J Aging Phys Activ

14. Guccione AA. Geriatric Physical Therapy. CV Mosby, St. Louis, 1993

15. McCalden RW, McGeough JA, Barker MB et al: Age-related changes in the tensile properties of cortical bone. J Bone Joint Surg 75A:1193–1205, 1993

16. Buckwalter JA, Kuettner KE, Thonar EJ-M: Age-related changes in articular cartilage proteoglycans: electronmicroscopic studies. J Orthop Res 3:251–257, 1985

17. Klitgaard H, Mantoni M, Schfiaffino S et al: Function, morphology and protein expression of aging skeletal muscle, a cross section of elderly men with different training backgrounds. Acta Physiol Scand 140:41–54, 1990

18. Whipple R, Wolfson L, Derby C et al: Altered sensory function and balance in older persons. J Gerontol 48:71–76, 1993

19. Koval KJ, Zuckerman JD: Current concepts review. Functional recovery after fracture of the hip. J Bone Joint Surg 76A:751–758, 1994

20. Evans JG, Prudham D, Wandless I: A prospective study of fractured proximal femur: incidence and outcome. Public Health 93:235, 1979

21. Grabiner MD, Enoka RM: Changed in movement capabilities with aging. Exer Sport Sci Rev 23:65–104, 1994

22. Frykman SF, Nelson RF: Fractures and traumatic conditions of the wrist. p. 267. In Hunter JM et al (eds): Rehabilitation of the Hand, 3rd ed. CV Mosby, St. Louis, 1990

23. Poss R: Natural factors that affect the shape and strength of the aging human femur. Clin Orthop Rel Res 274:194–201, 1992

24. Riggs BL, Melton LJ: Involutional osteoporosis. N Engl J Med 314:1676–1689, 1988

25. Smith CB, Smith DA: Relationship between age, mineral density, and mechanical properties of human femoral compacta. Acta Orthop Scand 47:496–502, 1976

26. Cummings SR, Nevitt MC: A hypothesis: the causes of hip fractures. J Gerontol 44:M107–111, 1989

27. Mosekilde LI, Mosekilde ME, Danielsen CC: Biomechanical competence of vertebral trabecular bone in relation to ash density and age in normal individuals. Bone 8:79–87, 1987

28. Weinstein RS, Hutson MS: Decreased trabecular width and increased trabecular spacing contribute to bone loss with aging. Bone 8:137–143, 1987

29. Nash MS, Spielholz NI: The effect of aging and exercise on bone and skeletal muscle. Orthop Phys Ther Clin North Am 2:225–240, 1993

30. Nilsson BE, Weslin NE: Bone density in athletes. Clin Orthop 77:179–186, 1971

31. Lane NE, Block D, Jones H et al: Long distance running, osteoporosis and osteoarthritis. JAMA 255:1147–1150, 1986

32. Talmage RV, Stinnet SS, Landwehr JT et al: Age-related loss of bone mineral density in non-athletic women. Bone Min 1:115–121, 1986

33. Dalsky G, Stocke KS, Eshani AA: Weight bearing exercise training and lumber bone mineral content in postmenopausal women. Ann Intern Med 108:224, 1988

34. Ayalon J, Simkin A, Leichter I et al: Dynamic

bone loading exercises for postmenopausal women. Arch Phys Med Rehab 68:280–283, 1987

35. Krolner B, Toft B, Neilson SP et al: Physical exercise as a prophylaxis against involutional bone loss: a controlled trial. Clin Sci 64:541–546, 1983

36. Cavanaugh DJ, Cann CE: Brisk walking does not stop bone loss in postmenopausal women. Bone 9:201–204, 1988

37. Rubin CT, Lanyon LE: Regulation of bone mass by mechanical strain magnitude. Calcif Tissue Int 37:411–418, 1985

38. Laurencin CT, Gelberman RH: Overview of disease and treatment related to aging of tendons and ligaments. p. 259. In Buckwalter JA, Goldberg VM, Woo SL-Y (eds): Musculoskeletal Soft Tissue Aging: Impact on Mobility. AAOS, Rosemont III, 1993

39. Butler DL: Mechanical properties of the ACL (in situ) and in vivo forces as a function of age. p. 289. In Buckwalter JA, Goldberg VM, Woo SL-Y (eds): Musculoskeletal Soft Tissue Aging: Impact on Mobility. AAOS, Rosemont III, 1993

40. Noyes FR, Grood ES: The strength of the anterior cruciate ligament in human and rhesus monkeys: age-related and species-related changes. J Bone Joint Surg 58A:1074–1082, 1976

41. Woo SL-Y, Hollis JM, Adams DJ et al: Tensile properties of the human femur-anterior cruciate ligament-tibia complex: the effect of specimen age and orientation. Am J Sports Med 19:217–225, 1991

42. Woo SL-Y, Orlando CA, Gomez MA et al: Tensile properties of the medial collateral ligament as a function of age. J Orthop Res 4:133–141, 1986

43. Wang CW, Weiss JA, Albright J et al: Lifelong exercise and aging effects on the canine medial collateral ligament. Orthop Trans 14:488–489, 1990

44. Kannus P, Józsa L: Histopathological changes preceding spontaneous rupture of a tendon. J Bone Joint Surg 73A:1507–1525, 1991

45. Vogel KG: Biochemical changes associated with aging in tendon and ligament. p. 277. In Buckwalter JA, Goldberg VM, Woo SL-Y (eds): Musculoskeletal Soft Tissue Aging: Impact on Mobility. AAOS, Rosemont III, 1993

46. Ralphs JR, Benjamin M: The joint capsule: structure, composition, ageing, and disease. J Anat 503–509, 1994

47. Skinner HB, Barrack RL, Cook SD: Age-related decline in proprioception. Clin Orthop Rel Res 184:208–211, 1984

48. Barrett DS, Cobb AG, Bentley G: Joint proprioception in normal, osteoarthritic, and replaced knees. J Bone Joint Surg 73B:53–56, 1991

49. O'Connor BL, Palmoski MJ, Brandt KD: Neurogenic acceleration of degenerative joint lesions. J Bone Joint Surg 67A:562–572, 1985

50. Finsterbush A, Friedman B. The effect of sensory denervation on rabbits' knee joints. J Bone Joint Surg 57A:949–952, 1975

51. Buchner DM, Cress ME, Wagner EH et al: The Seattle FICSIT/Move It study: the effect of exercise on gait and balance in older adults. J Am Geriatr Soc 41:321–325, 1993

52. Wolf SL, Kutner NG, Green RC et al: The Atlanta FICSIT study: two exercise interventions to reduce frailty in elders. J Am Geriatr Soc 41:329–332, 1993

53. Wolfson L, Whipple R, Judge J et al: Training balance and strength in the elderly to improve function. J Am Geriatr Soc 41:341–343, 1993

54. Lohmander S: Osteoarthritis: a major cause of disability in the elderly. p. 99. In Buckwalter JA, Goldberg VM, Woo SL-Y (eds): Musculoskeletal Soft Tissue Aging: Impact on Mobility. AAOS, Rosemont III, 1993

55. Praemer A, Furner S, Rice DP: Musculoskeletal Conditions in the United States. AAOS, Park Ridge, IL, 1992

56. Dahlberg L, Ryd L, Heinegard D et al: Proteoglycan fragments in joint fluid: influence of arthrosis and joint inflammation. Acta Orthop Scand 63:417–423, 1992

57. Elliott RJ, Gardner DL: Changes with age in the glycosamonoglycans of human articular cartilage. Ann Rheum Dis 38:371–377, 1979

58. Sweet MBE, Thonar EJ-MA, Marsh J: Age-related changes in proteoglycan structure. Arch Biochem Biophys 198:439–448, 1979

59. Venn MF: Variation of chemical composition with age in human femoral head cartilage. Ann Rheum Dis 37:168–174, 1977

60. Brandt KD, Fife RS: Ageing in relation to the pathogenesis of osteoarthritis. Clin Rheum Dis 12:117–130, 1986

61. Radin EL, Paul IL, Tolkoff MJ: Subchondral bone changes in patients with early degenerative joint disease. Arthritis Rheum 13:400–405, 1970

62. Guccione AA: Arthritis and the process of disablement. Phys Ther 74:408–414, 1994

63. Jette AM: Musculoskeletal impairments and associated physical disability in the elderly: insights from epidemiologic research. p. 7. In

Buckwalter JA, Goldberg VM, Woo SL-Y (eds). Musculoskeletal Soft Tissue Aging: Impact on Mobility. AAOS, Rosemont, III, 1993

64. Yelin E, Lubeck D, Holman H et al: The impact of rheumatoid arthritis and osteoarthritis: the activities of patients with rheumatoid arthritis and osteoarthritis compared to controls. J Rheumatol 14:710–717, 1987

65. Verbrugge LM, Lepkowski JM, Konkol LL: Levels of disability among U.S. adults with arthritis. J Gerontol 46:S71–83, 1991

66. Davis MA, Ettinger WH, Neuhaus JM et al: Knee osteoarthritis and physical functioning evidence from the NHANES I epidemiologic follow-up study. J Rheumatol 18:591–598, 1991

67. Yelin E: Arthritis: the cumulative impact of a common chronic condition. Arthritis Rheum 35: 489–497, 1992

68. Coventry MB, Ghormley RK, Kernohan JW: The intervertebral disk: its microscopic anatomy and pathology; changes in the intervertebral disk concomitant with age. J Bone Joint Surg 27: 233–247, 1945

69. Vernon-Roberts B, Pirie CJ: Degenerative changes in the intervertebral disk of the lumbar spine and their sequelae. Rheumatol Rehab 16: 13–21, 1977

70. Holm S: Pathophysiology of disc degeneration. Acta Orthop Scand 64(suppl 251):13–15, 1993

71. Kellgren JH, Lawrence JS: Rheumatism in miners: an x-ray study. Br J Int Med 9:197–207, 1952

72. Caplan PS, Freedman LM, Connely TP: Degenerative joint disease of the lumbar spine in coal miners: a clinical and x-ray study. Arthritis Rheum 9:693–702, 1967

73. Wiltse LL: The effect of common anomalies of the lumbar spine upon disc degeneration and low back pain. Orthop Clin North Am 2:569–582, 1971

74. Gower WE, Pedrini V: Age-related variations in protein polysaccharides from human nucleus pulposus, annulus fibrosis, and costal cartilage. J Bone Joint Surg 51A:1154–1162, 1969

75. Hassler O: The human intervertebral disk. A micro-angiographical study on its vascular supply at various ages. Acta Orthop Scand 40: 765–772, 1969

76. Farfan HF, Cossette JW, Robertson GH et al: The effects of torsion on the lumbar intervertebral joints: the role of torsion in the production of disk degeneration. J Bone Joint Surg 52A: 468–497, 1970

77. Lexell J, Taylor CC, Sjöström M: What is the cause of aging atrophy? Total number, size and proportion of different fiber types studied in whole vastus lateralis muscle from 15- to 83-year old men. J Neurol Sci 84:275–294, 1988

78. Grimby G, Danneskiold-Samsoe B, Hvid K et al: Morphology and enzymatic capacity in arm and leg muscles in 78–81 year old men and women. Acta Physiol Scand 15:125–134, 1982

79. Tomonga M: Histochemical and ultrastructural changes in senile human muscle. J Am Geriatr Soc 25:125–131, 1977

80. Larsson L: Morphological and functional characteristics of the aging skeletal muscle in man. A cross sectional study. Acta Physiol Scand 457(suppl):1–36, 1978

81. Larsson L: Physical training effect on muscle morphology in sedentary males at different ages. Med Sci Sports Exerc 14:203–206, 1982

82. Agre JC, Pierce LE, Raab D et al: Light resistance and stretching exercise in elderly women: effect upon strength. Arch Phys Med Rehab 69: 273–276, 1988

83. Frontera WR, Hughes VA, Lutz KJ et al: A cross sectional study of muscle strength and mass in 45 to 78 year old men and women. J Appl Physiol 71:644–650, 1991

84. Vandervoort AA: Effects of ageing on human neuromuscular function: implications for exercise. Can J Sports Sci 17:178–184, 1992

85. Brown M: Physical and orthopaedic limitations to exercise in the elderly. p. 209. In Buckwalter JA, Goldberg VM, Woo SL-Y (eds): Musculoskeletal Soft Tissue Aging: Impact on Mobility. AAOS, Rosemont III, 1993

86. Skinner HB, Barrack RL, Cook SD et al: Joint position sense in total knee arthroplasty. J Orthop Res 1:276–283, 1984

87. Long WT, Dorr LD, Healy B et al: Functional recovery of noncemented total hip arthroplasty. Clin Orthop Rel Res 288:73–77, 1993

88. Sekuler R, Hutman LP, Owsley CJ: Human aging and spatial vision. Science 209:1255–1256, 1980

89. Bergstöm B: Morphology of the vestibular nerve III. Analysis of the calibers of the myelinated vestibular nerve fibers in men of various ages. Acta Otolaryngol 76:331–338, 1973

90. Rosenhall U, Rubin W: Degenerative changes in the human vestibular sensory epithelia. Acta Otolaryngol 79:67–81, 1975

91. Woolacott MA, Shumway-Cook A, Nashner LM: Aging and posture control: changes in sensory

organization and muscular coordination. Int J Neurosci 23:97–114, 1986

92. Brandt T, Daroff RB: The multisensory physiological and pathological vertigo syndromes. Ann Neurol 7:195–197, 1979

93. Shumway-Cook A, Woolacott MA: Aging and postural control. p. 169. In Shumway-Cook A, Woolacott MA, (eds): Motor Control: Theory and Practical Applications. Williams and Wilkins, Baltimore, 1995

94. Light KE: Information processing for motor performance in aging adults. Phys Ther 70:820–826, 1990

95. Hines T, Poon LW, Cerella J et al: Age related changes in the time course of encoding. Exp Aging Res 8:175–178, 1982

96. Botwinick J: Sensory-perceptual factors in reaction time in relation to age. J Genet Psychol 121:173–174, 1972

97. Stelmach GE, Worringham C: Sensorimotor deficits related to postural stability: implications for falling in the elderly. Clin Geriatr Med 1:679–694, 1985

98. Rabbitt PMA: Set and age in a choice-response task. J Gerontol 19:301–306, 1964

99. Rabbitt PMA, Vyas SM: Selective anticipation for events in old age. J Gerontol 35:913–919, 1980

100. Salthouse TA, Somberg BL: Isolating the age deficit in speeded performance. J Gerontol 37:59–63, 1982

101. Goggin NL, Meeuwsen HJ: Age-related differences in the control of spatial aiming movements. Res Q Exerc Sport 63:366–372, 1992

102. Light KE, Spirduso WW: Effects of adult aging on the movement complexity factor of response programming. J Gerontol 45:107–109, 1990

103. Baylor AM, Spirduso WW: Systematic aerobic exercise and components of reaction time in older women. J Gerontol 43:121–126, 1988

104. Netzer O, Payne VG: Effects of age and gender on functional rotation and lateral movements of the neck and back. Gerontology 39:320–326, 1993

105. Einkauf DK, Gohdes ML, Jensen GM et al: Changes in spinal mobility with increasing age in women. Phys Ther 67:370–375, 1987

106. Chakravarty K, Webley M: Shoulder joint movement and its relationship to disability in the elderly. J Rheumatol 20:1359–1361, 1993

107. Vandervoort AA, Chesworth BM, Cunningham DA et al: Age and sex effects on mobility of the human ankle. J Gerontol 47:M17–M21, 1992

108. Blanpied P, Smidt G: The difference in stiffness of the active plantarflexors between young and elderly human females. J Gerontol 48:M59–M63, 1993

109. James B, Parker AW: Active and passive mobility of the lower limb joints in elderly men and women. Am J Phys Med 68:162–167, 1989

110. Roach KE, Miles TP: Normal hip and knee active range of motion: the relationship to age. Phys Ther 71:656–665, 1991

111. Amundsen LR: The effect of aging and exercise on joint mobility. Orthop Phys Ther Clin North Am 2:241–249, 1993

112. Raab DM, Agre JC, McAdam M et al: Light resistance and stretching exercise in elderly women: effect on flexibility. Arch Phy Med Rehab 69:268–272, 1988

113. Hopkins DR, Murrah B, Hoeger WW et al: Effect of low impact aerobic dance on the functional fitness of elderly women. Gerontologist 30:189–192, 1990

114. Morey MC, Cowper PA, Feussner JR et al: Two-year trends in physical performance following supervised exercise among community-dwelling older veterans. J Am Geriatr Soc 39:549–554, 1991

115. Misner JE, Massey BH, Bemben M et al: Long term effects of exercise on the range of motion of aging women. J Orthop Sports Phys Ther 16:37–42, 1992

116. Tinetti ME, Powell L: Fear of falling and low self-efficacy: a cause of dependence in elderly persons. J Gerontol 48:35–38, 1993

117. Simoneau GG, Cavanagh PR, Ulbrecht JS et al: The influence of visual factors on fall-related kinematic variables during stair descent by older women. J Gerontol 46:M188–195, 1991

118. Simoneau GG, Leibowitz HW, Ulbrecht JS et al: The effects of visual factors and head orientation on postural steadiness in women aged 55 to 70. J Gerontol 47:M151–M158, 1992

119. Horak FB, Shupert CL, Mirka A: Components of postural dyscontrol in the elderly: a review. Neurobiol Aging 10:727–738, 1989

120. Woolacott MH, Manchester D: Anticipatory postural adjustments in older adults: are changes in response characteristics due to changes in strategy? J Gerontol 48:M64–M70, 1993

121. Stelmach GE, Populin L, Müller F: Postural onset and voluntary movement in the elderly. Neurosci Letters 117:188–193, 1990

122. Maki BE: Biomechanical approach to quantify-

ing anticipatory postural adjustments in the elderly. Med Biol Eng Comput 31:355–362, 1993

123. Rogers M: Interaction of posture and locomotion during the initiation of protective stepping: implications for falls in older adults. Presented at Multisegmental Motor Control: Interfaces of Biomechanical, Neural, and Behavioral Approaches, New Hampshire, 1995

124. King MB, Judge JO, Wolfson L: Functional base of support decreases with age. J Gerontol 49:M258–M263, 1994

125. Teasdale N, Bard C, LaRue J et al: On the cognitive penetrability of posture control. Exp Aging Res 19:1–13, 1993

126. Chen H-S, Ashton-Miller JA, Alexander NB et al: Stepping over obstacles: gait patterns of healthy young and old adults. J Gerontol 46:M196–203, 1991

127. Inglis JT, Horak FB, Shupert CL et al: The importance of somatosensory information in triggering and scaling automatic postural responses in humans. Exp Brain Res 101:159–164, 1994

128. Cook T, Cozzens B: Human solutions for locomotion. III. The initiation of gait. p. 65. In Herman RM, Grillner S, Stein PSG, et al (eds): Neural Control of Locomotion. Plenum Press, New York, 1976

129. Crenna P, Frigo C: A motor programme for the initiation of forward oriented movements in man. J Physiol 437:635–653, 1991

130. Elble RJ, Moody C, Leffler K, et al: The initiation of normal walking. Movement Dis 9:139–146, 1994

131. Morgan M, Philips JG, Bradshaw JL et al: Age-related motor slowness: simply strategic? J Gerontol 49:M133–M139, 1994

132. Sudarsky L, Ronthal M: Gait disorders among elderly patients: a survey study of 50 patients. Arch Neurol 40:740–743, 1983

133. Hu M-H, Wollacott M: Characteristic patterns of gait in older persons. p. 67. In Spivack BS (ed): Evaluation and Management of Gait Disorders Marcel Dekker, New York, 1995

134. Winter DA, Patla AE, Frank JS et al: Biomechanical walking pattern changes in the fit and healthy elderly. Phys Ther 70:340–347, 1990

135. Vandervoort AA, McComas AJ. Contractile changes in opposing muscles of the human ankle joint with aging. J Appl Physiol 61:361–367, 1986

136. Krebs DE, Lockert J: Vestibulopathy and gait. p. 93. In Spivak BS (ed): Evaluation and Management of Gait Disorders. Marcel Dekker, New York, 1995

137. Chapron DJ: Adverse effects of medications on gait and mobility in the elderly. p. 223. In Spivak BS (ed): Evaluation and Management of Gait Disorders. Marcel Dekker, New York, 1995

138. Jeannerod M: The interaction of visual and proprioceptive cues in controlling reaching movements. p. 277. In Humphrey DR, Freund H-J, (eds): Motor Control: Concepts and Issues. John Wiley & Sons, New York, 1991

139. Jeannerod M: A neurophysiological model for the directional coding of reaching movements. p. 49. In Paillard J, (ed.) Brain and Space. Oxford University Press, Oxford, 1991

140. Johansson RS, Cole KJ. Sensory-motor coordination during grasping and manipulative actions. Curr Op Neurobiology 2:815–823, 1992

141. Johansson RS, Riso R, Bäckström L: Somatosensory control of precision grip during unpredictable pulling loads. I. Changes in load force amplitude. Exp Brain Res 89:181–191, 1992

142. Johansson RS, Häger C, Riso R: Somatosensory control of precision grip during unpredictable pulling loads. II. Changes in load force rate. Exp Brain Res 89:192–203, 1992

143. Cole KJ, Beck CI: The stability of precision grip force in older adults. J Motor Beha 26:171–177, 1994

144. Jebsen RH, Taylor N, Treischmann RB et al: An objective and standardized test of hand function. Arch Phys Med Rehab 50:311–319, 1969

145. Cagle PE: Effect of comorbidities on the rehabilitation of patients with musculoskeletal disorders. Orthop Phys Ther Clin North Am 2:289–300, 1993

146. Verbrugge LM, Lepkowski JM, Imakaka Y: Comorbidity and its impact on disability. Milbank Q 67:450–484, 1989

147. Boissonnault WG, Bass C: Pathological origins of trunk and neck pain: part I—pelvic and abdominal visceral disorders. J Orthop Sport Phys Ther 12:192–207, 1990

148. Boissonnault WG, Bass C: Pathological origins of trunk and neck pain: part II—disorders of the cardiovascular and pulmonary systems. J Orthop Sport Phys Ther 12:208–215, 1990

149. Boissonnault WG, Bass C: Pathological origins of trunk and neck pain: part III—diseases of the musculoskeletal system. J Orthop Sport Phys Ther 12:216–221, 1990

150. Boissonnault WG, Bass C: Medical screening ex-

amination: not optional for physical therapists. J Orthop Sport Phys Ther 14:241–242, 1992

151. Dekker J, van Baer ME, Curfs EC et al: Diagnosis and treatment in physical therapy: an investigation of their relationship. Phys Ther 73:568–580, 1993

152. Mathias S, Nayak U, Isaacs B: Balance in elderly patients: the "get up and go" test. Arch Phys Med Rehab 67:387–389, 1986

153. Podsialdo D, Richardson S: The timed "get up & go": a test of basic functional mobility for frail elderly persons. J Am Geriatr Soc 39:142–148, 1991

154. Tinetti M: Performance-oriented assessment of mobility problems in elderly patients. J Am Geriatr Soc 34:119–126, 1986

155. Berg K: Balance and its measure in the elderly: a review. Physiother Canada 41:240–246, 1989

156. Lu-Yao GL, Keller RB, Littenberg B et al: Outcomes after displaced fractures of the femoral neck. A meta-analysis of one hundred and six published reports. J Bone Joint Surg 76A:15–25, 1994

157. Craik RL: Disability following hip fracture. Phys Ther 74:388–398, 1994

158. Barnes B, Dunovan K: Functional outcomes after hip fracture. Phys Ther 67:1675–1679, 1987

159. Jette AM, Harris BA, Cleary PD et al: Functional recovery after hip fracture. Arch Phys Med Rehab 68:735–740, 1987

160. Magaziner J, Simonsick EM, Kashner TM et al: Predictors of functional recovery one year following hospital discharge for hip fracture: a prospective study. J Gerontol 45:101–107, 1990

161. Borgquist L, Nordell E, Lindelow G et al: Outcome after hip fracture in different health care districts: rehabilitation of 837 consecutive patients in primary care 1986–88. Scand J Prim Health Care 9:244–251, 1991

162. Ranawat CS, Shine JJ: Duo-condylar total knee arthroplasty. Clin Orthop Rel Res 94:185–195, 1973

163. Insall JN, Ranawat CS, Aglietti P et al: A comparison of four models of total-knee replacement prostheses. J Bone Joint Surg 58A:754–765, 1976

164. Harris WH: Traumatic arthritis of the hip after dislocation and acetabular fractures: treatment by mold arthroplasty. J Bone Joint Surg 51A: 737–755, 1969

165. Linacre JM, Heinemann AW, Wright BD et al: The structure and stability of the functional independence measure. Arch Phys Med Rehab 75: 127–132, 1994

166. Long WB, Sacco WJ, Coombes SS et al: Deter-

mining normative standards for functional independence measure transitions in rehabilitation. Arch Phys Med Rehab 75:144–148, 1994

167. Bergner M, Bobbitt RA, Carter WB et al: The sickness impact profile: development and final revision of a health status measure. Medical Care 19:787–805, 1981

168. Meenan RF, Gertman PM, Mason JH: Measuring health status in arthritis. The arthritis impact measurement scales. Arth Rheum 23:146–152, 1980

169. Meenan RF, Gertman PM, Mason JH et al: The arthritis impact measurement scales. Further investigations of a health status measure. Arth Rheum 25:1048–1053, 1982

170. Shepard MM: Further review of the results of operations on the hip joint. J Bone Joint Surg 42B:177–204, 1960

171. Larson CB: Rating scale for hip disabilities. Clin Orthop Rel Res 31:85–93, 1963

172. Roush SE: Patient-perceived functional outcomes associated with elective hip and knee arthroplasties. Phys Ther 65:1496–1500, 1985

173. Johanson NA, Charlson ME, Szatrowski TP et al: A self-administered hip-rating questionnaire for the assessment of outcome after total hip replacement. J Bone Joint Surg 74A:587–597, 1992

174. Katz JN, Phillips CB, Poss R et al: The validity and reliability of a total hip arthroplasty outcome evaluation questionnaire. J Bone Joint Surg 77A:1528–1534, 1995

175. Laupacis A, Bourne R, Rorabeck C et al: The effect of elective total hip replacement on health related quality of life. J Bone Joint Surg 75A: 1619–1626, 1993

176. Berman AT, Bosacco SJ, Israelite C: Evaluation of total knee arthroplasty using isokinetic testing. Clin Orthop Rel Res 271:106–113, 1991

177. Ranawat CS, Insall JN, Shine J: Duo-condylar knee arthroplasty. Clin Orthop Rel Res 120: 76–82, 1976

178. Faris PM, Herbst SA, Ritter MA et al: The effect of preoperative knee deformity on the initial results of cruciate-retaining total knee arthroplasty. J Arthroplasty 7:527–530, 1992

179. Hsu RW, Pan GF, Ho WP: A follow-up study of porous-coated anatomic knee arthroplasty. J Arthroplasty 10:29–36, 1995

180. Ranawat CS, Flynn WF, Deshmukh RG: Impact of modern technique on long-term results of total condylar knee arthroplasty. Clin Orthop Rel Res 309:131–135, 1994

181. Insall JN, Dorr LD, Scott RD et al: Rationale of the knee society clinical rating system. Clin Orthop Rel Res 248:13–14, 1989

182. Malkani AL, Rand JA, Bryan RS et al: Total knee arthroplasty with the kinematic condylar prosthesis. J Bone Joint Surg 77A:423–431, 1995

183. Haas SB, Insall JN, Montgomery W et al: Revision total knee arthroplasty with use of modular components with stems inserted without cement. J Bone Joint Surg 77A:1700–1707, 1995

184. Stern SH, Insall JN: Posterior stabilized prosthesis. Results after follow-up of nine to twelve years. J Bone Joint Surg 74A:980–986, 1992

185. Goldman RT, Koval KJ, Cuomo F et al: Functional outcome after humeral head replacement for acute three- and four-part proximal humeral fractures. J Shoulder Elbow Surg 4:81–86, 1995

186. Colizza WA, Insall JN, Scuderi GR: The posterior stabilized knee prosthesis. Assessment of polyethylene damage and osteolysis after a ten-year-minimum follow-up. J Bone Joint Surg 77A:1713–1720, 1995

187. Lankhorst GJ, Van de Stadt RJ, Van der Korst JK: The relationships of functional capacity, pain, and isometric and isokinetic torque in osteoathrosis of the knee. Scand J Rehab Med 17:167–172, 1985

188. Lippitt SB, Harryman DT, Matsen FA: A practical tool for evaluating function: the simple shoulder test. p. 501. In Matsen FA, Fu FH, Hawkins RJ (eds): The Shoulder: A Balance of Mobility and Stability. AAOS, Rosemont, 1993

189. Matsen FA, Ziegler DW, DeBartolo SE: Patient self-assessment of health status and function in glenohumeral degenerative joint disease. J Shoulder Elbow Surg 4:345–351, 1995

190. McHorney CA, Ware JE, Lu R et al: The MOS 36-item short-form health survey (SF 36): III. Tests of data quality, scaling assumption, and reliability across diverse patient groups. Med Care 32:40–66, 1994

191. Matsen FA: Early effectiveness of shoulder arthroplasty for patients who have primary glenohumeral degenerative joint disease. J Bone Joint Surg 78A:260–264, 1996

192. Sullivan MG, Guccione AA: Measuring outcomes in geriatric orthopaedics. Orthop Phys Ther Clin North Am 2:301–311, 1993

193. Wilmore JH: The aging of bone and muscle. Clin Sports Med 10:231–244, 1991

194. Lewis RD, Brown RMM: Influence of muscle activation dynamics on reaction time in the elderly. Eur J Appl Physiol 69:344–349, 1994

195. Gogia PP, Sabbahi MA: Electromyographic analysis of neck muscle fatigue in patients with osteoarthritis of the cervical spine. Spine 19:502–506, 1993

196. Ahrens SF: The effect of age on intervertebral disc compression while running. J Orthop Sports Phys Ther 20:17–21, 1994

197. Murata H, Ikuta Y, Murkami T: An anatomic investigation of the elbow joint, with special reference to aging of the articular cartilage. J Shoulder Elbow Surg 2:175–181, 1993

198. Hattrup SJ: Rotator cuff repair: relevance of patient age. J Shoulder Elbow Surg 4:95–100, 1995

199. Burstein AH, Reilly DT, Martens M: Aging of bone tissue: mechanical properties. J Bone Joint Surg 58-A:82–86, 1976

200. Seto JL, Brewster CE: Musculoskeletal conditioning of the older athlete. Clin Sports Med 10:401–429, 1991

201. Kay GL: Athletic participation after myocardial revascularization. Possibilities and benefits. Clin Sports Med 10:371–389, 1991

202. Hu M-H, Woolacott MH: Multi-sensory training of standing balance in older adults: I. Postural stability and one-leg balance. J Gerontol 49:M52–M61, 1994

203. Hu M-H, Woolacott MH: Multi-sensory training of balance in older adults: II. Kinematic and electromyographic postural responses. J Gerontol 49:M62–M71, 1994

204. Jarnlo G-B: Hip fracture patients. Background factors and function. Scand J Rehab Med suppl 24:1–31, 1991

205. Reitan RN: Intellectual and affective changes in essential hypertension. Am J Psychiatry 110:817–824, 1954

206. Chodzko-Zajko WJ, Moore KA: Physical fitness and cognitive functioning in aging. Exer Sport Sci Rev 22:195–220, 1994

207. Rogers RL, Meyers JS, Mortel KF: After reaching retirement age physical activity sustains cerebral perfusion and cognition. J Am Geriatr Soc 38:123–128, 1990

208. Dustman RE, Emmerson RY, Ruhling RO et al: Age and fitness effects on EEG, ERPs, visual sensitivity, and cognition. Neurobiol Aging 11:193–200, 1990

209. Patla AE: A framework for understanding mobility problems in the elderly. In Craik RL, Oatig CA (eds). Mosby Year Book, St. Louis, 1995

Appendix

Functional Outcomes in Orthopaedic and Sports Physical Therapy

Outcomes research has taken on almost mythic stature in the past few years. The rush to demonstrate efficacy of treatment is driven by changes in reimbursement, competition between large providers (corporations and networks of practitioners) for contracts, changes in clinical treatment and management, and research interest.

The financial pressure is obvious. Risk management in health care demands that treatments have definable limits and results. The specificity of these limits is open to interpretation and varies widely. Insurance companies can control costs by limiting both access and reimbursement. Unfortunately, neither variable has been linked directly to better outcomes.

Marketing has taken on a greater emphasis as networks of private and associated clinics compete for managed care contracts. Presumably, the groups that can demonstrate consistent, more or less predictable results at a stable cost have a competitive advantage. Knowledge of expected treatment intensity (with respect to manpower and other requirements) and duration helps the provider predict costs and negotiate profitable contracts. Insurance companies have an abundance of data on the cost of physi-

cal therapy treatments, but they must rely on the therapist and therapy groups to provide outcome data.

Clinical treatment, management, and research are all driven by the same data—what treatments are effective in restoring maximum function? The purpose of measuring results in each case is different. Although all are used to identify optimal treatments and the circumstances that may demand a different approach, the goals of each may differ. Innovation in treatment requires some method of comparing old versus new and determining the efficacy of techniques under varying clinical conditions. It is the place of clinical managers to encourage innovation and enable therapists to develop new clinical skills. These and other management issues are discussed earlier in the text.

Interpretation of outcomes data is subject to several limitations. A functional evaluation provides a snapshot of the patient's evolving status. It is difficult to design a questionnaire or series of tests that are appropriate for all patients. In orthopaedic and sports medicine, the functional, work, and athletic demands vary widely among groups of patients. Subjective responses to in-

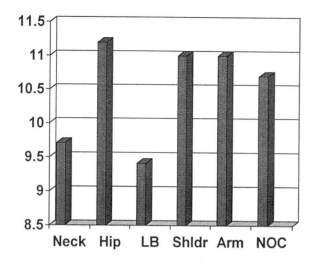

FIGURE A-1 *Visits Per Category.*

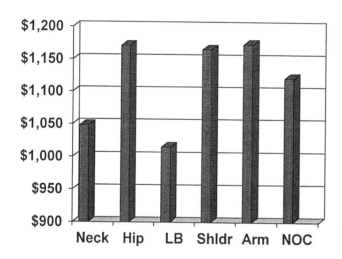

FIGURE A-2 *Net Revenue Per Category.*

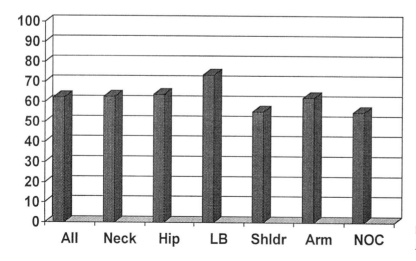

FIGURE A-3 *Outcome Index Per Category.*

TABLE A-1 *Impairment category*

	PATIENT ADMISSIONS	PERCENTAGE
Cervical	4,596	16
Hip, Lower Extremity	6,032	21
Lumbar Spine	9,766	34
Shoulder	3,159	11
Arm and hand	1,723	6
Not Otherwise Classified (refers to diagnoses not limited to a single joint and other classifications)	3,447	12
Total admissions	28,723	

TABLE A-3 *Statistical outcomes for all categories*

	LOW	MEAN	HIGH
Average Visits	1	10.3	89
Average Net Revenue	$46	$1095	$8995
Days	1	31.8	290
Intensity		2.27	

15,735 (55%) patients discharged; impairment mix same as admission. Percent discharged noncompliant: 6.04%. Percent discharged goals met: 61.9%.

Other data
Male	43%
Female	57%
Average Age	44 years
Percent ≥ 45 years	55%
Percent <45 years	43%

jury are not consistent. These are significant factors in designing or selecting a valid functional evaluation tool (see Chs. 4, 5, 6, 7, and 9). Tools that measure ADL for sedentary individuals are not valid for competitive athletes or professional performers and vice versa. Co-morbidities and other non-medical factors may muddle the overall picture when addressing the geriatric or pediatric populations. Tools that evaluate global function may not be sensitive enough to detect outcome changes caused by recovery from an orthopaedic injury, while tools that focus on the orthopaedic aspects alone cannot distinguish or evaluate the effects of other physiologic, emotional, or social influences (see Ch. 9).

Can we make clinical decisions based upon functional scores? Certainly, some decisions are

TABLE A-2 *Admission severity*

	SLIGHT (%)	MODERATE (%)	SEVERE (%)	VERY SEVERE (%)
Overall	21	14	16	49
Cervical	28	15	17	40
Hip	24	14	18	44
Lumbar	11	9	13	67
Shoulder	29	17	15	39
Arm and Hand	23	16	21	40
Not Classified	26	15	17	42

Severity is a risk-adjusted indicator based upon SF–36 score at intake, age, and gender.

possible. On the most obvious level, the therapist can note general improvement. A patient has either improved or not, assuming the measuring tool is a valid one. Functional scores may be able to differentiate treatment programs. A patient with lower functional ratings may require a less aggressive initial program or may require greater attention to symptoms other than weakness, such as inflammation. Physicians may be able to predict which patients will require surgery based upon initial testing and a trial of rehabilitation, although that type of analysis has not been done using functional scores.

Regardless of these issues, this appendix contains data from two separate sources regarding general outcomes in physical therapy. Each source uses a different method of measuring functional outcomes. It is not possible to compare the data sets directly. The data is broken down by body region, age, and sex. Some data regarding outcomes of specific surgical procedures is presented.

Interpretation of functional data must be done carefully. Functional scores are highly dependant upon the tools used to generate data, the subjective response to injury, relative severity of injury—both anatomic and behavioral, the treatment used and the patient's response to treatment. Grouping of patients is compromised by

TABLE A-4 *Outcomes for foot/ankle diagnoses*

	AGE RANGE	NUMBER	MEAN VISITS	ADMIT FUNCTION	D/C FUNCTION	% CHANGE
Nonsurgical	<20	1855	6.8	57.7	74.9	29.8
	20–29	625	6.8	62.3	76.9	23.5
	30–39	761	7.5	55.1	74.3	34.8
	40–49	718	8.5	56.9	73.2	28.6
	50–59	453	7.9	54.2	72.3	33.4
	60–69	192	8.7	52.8	72.2	36.7
	70–79	116	8.1	50.4	63.5	26.1
	80–89	68	8.0	52.0	69.0	32.7
	Total	4788	7.4	57.0	74.1	30.0
Surgical	<20	145	11.1	51.5	72.3	40.5
	20–29	67	10.3	59.3	76.8	29.5
	30–39	112	12.1	51.1	64.8	26.8
	40–49	101	14.5	57.0	64.6	13.3
	50–59	67	11.3	41.4	70.2	69.6
	60–69	29	10.9	56.7	70.0	23.5
	70–79	15	10.1			
	80–89	11	8.1			
	Total	547	11.8	50.0	66.1	32.2

TABLE A-5 *Outcomes for knee/hip diagnoses*

	AGE RANGE	NUMBER	MEAN VISITS	ADMIT FUNCTION	D/C FUNCTION	% CHANGE
Non surgical	<20	3,609	9.0	57.4	72.2	25.8
	20–29	1,379	9.6	59.7	75.7	26.9
	30–39	1,727	9.9	58.0	70.8	22.0
	40–49	1,617	9.5	54.5	68.6	25.9
	50–59	946	9.2	52.0	66.7	28.3
	60–69	630	9.3	51.9	65.5	26.2
	70–79	468	8.4	48.2	58.3	20.9
	80–89	207	8.2	57.1	66.3	16.2
	Total	10,583	9.3	56.1	70.3	25.2
Surgical	<20	3,001	13.0	43.5	67.8	55.9
	20–29	1,363	14.6	44.8	70.9	58.2
	30–39	1,932	14.7	43.0	67.8	57.7
	40–49	1,830	13.1	41.1	65.7	59.8
	50–59	1,240	11.9	41.9	63.7	52.1
	60–69	835	12.2	41.1	61.9	50.6
	70–79	519	12.0	42.5	59.6	40.1
	80–89	168	9.2	45.6	66.3	45.6
	Total	10,888	13.2	42.8	66.5	55.4

TABLE A-6 *Outcomes for shoulder diagnoses*

	AGE RANGE	NUMBER	MEAN VISITS	ADMIT FUNCTION	D/C FUNCTION	% CHANGE
Non surgical	<20	2,230	9.2	53.9	67.6	25.3
	20–29	577	9.2	55.8	70.0	25.6
	30–39	1,035	9.3	53.6	67.0	25.0
	40–49	1,625	11.4	53.9	67.0	24.4
	50–59	1,602	12.1	51.9	67.3	29.6
	60–69	1,090	11.8	50.9	66.6	30.8
	70–79	794	11.7	50.3	65.2	29.6
	80–89	280	9.4	45.9	60.2	31.4
	Total	9,233	10.6	52.7	67.0	27.0
Surgical	<20	701	15.4	41.3	65.1	57.6
	20–29	240	15.1	45.8	67.5	47.4
	30–39	398	16.5	36.9	65.4	77.2
	40–49	544	18.1	39.7	62.0	56.3
	50–59	587	20.1	37.6	62.4	66.2
	60–69	489	19.5	38.6	64.2	66.5
	70–79	318	19.3	40.9	62.6	53.2
	80–89	56	15.5	33.8	50.0	47.8
	Total	3,333	17.8	39.6	63.7	60.9

TABLE A-7 *Outcomes for spine diagnoses, including cervical, thoracic, lumbar, and sacro iliac*

	AGE RANGE	NUMBER	MEAN VISITS	ADMIT FUNCTION	D/C FUNCTION	% CHANGE
Non surgical	<20	3,999	8.7	60.2	75.8	25.9
	20–29	1,307	9.1	61.2	76.7	25.5
	30–39	2,913	9.6	60.5	76.6	26.6
	40–49	3,244	9.5	60.0	75.3	25.4
	50–59	2,127	9.8	60.9	74.8	22.7
	60–69	1,432	9.1	62.5	73.7	17.9
	70–79	1,109	9.4	57.6	70.9	23.1
	80–89	484	8.3	58.8	71.5	21.6
	Total	16,615	9.2	60.4	75.1	24.5
Surgical	<20	747	12.0	51.9	66.5	28.1
	20–29	158	12.3	61.1	74.6	22.1
	30–39	674	13.5	56.5	71.3	26.1
	40–49	853	12.6	54.5	68.6	25.7
	50–59	507	12.6	53.1	64.4	21.4
	60–69	298	12.6	57.2	69.0	20.7
	70–79	224	11.1	51.9	65.0	25.1
	80–89	72	10.9	64.1	71.1	10.9
	Total	3,533	12.5	54.7	68.2	24.7

TABLE A-8 *Outcomes for all diagnoses by age*

	AGE RANGE	NUMBER	MEAN VISITS	ADMIT FUNCTION	D/C FUNCTION	% CHANGE
Non surgical	<20	11,693	8.6	57.8	73.0	26.4
	20–29	3,888	8.9	60.0	75.4	25.7
	30–39	6,436	9.4	58.1	73.2	26.1
	40–49	7,204	9.8	57.1	71.7	25.6
	50–59	5,128	10.2	55.9	70.7	26.6
	60–69	3,344	10.0	56.2	69.7	24.2
	70–79	2,487	9.9	53.2	66.4	24.8
	80–89	1,039	8.6	54.5	67.2	23.4
	Total	41,219	9.3	57.2	71.9	25.8
Surgical	<20	4,594	13.1	44.8	67.3	50.3
	20–29	1,828	14.3	46.9	71.0	51.4
	30–39	3,116	14.6	45.4	68.1	50.0
	40–49	3,328	13.8	44.8	65.8	46.9
	50–59	2,401	14.0	43.2	63.7	47.6
	60–69	1,651	14.4	13.5	64.0	47.1
	70–79	1,076	13.9	43.4	60.8	40.0
	80–89	307	10.7	46.1	62.1	34.6
	Total	18,301	13.9	44.7	66.3	48.3

TABLE A-9 *Outcomes for ACL reconstruction*

AGE RANGE	NUMBER	MEAN VISITS	ADMIT FUNCTION	D/C FUNCTION	% CHANGE
<20	180	18.4	41.0	69.8	70.1
20–29	139	20.7	38.3	75.6	97.6
30–39	146	24.1	47.0	67.3	43.1
40–49	65	21.0	38.7	70.2	81.2
50–59	9	21.9	39.7	67.3	69.6
60–69	2	10.5	43.5	49.5	13.8
80–89	2	10.5			
Total	543	20.8	41.5	70.3	69.4

TABLE A-10 *Outcomes for total hip replacement*

AGE RANGE	NUMBER	MEAN VISITS	ADMIT FUNCTION	D/C FUNCTION	% CHANGE
<20	312	10.4	51.5	63.9	24.1
20–29	26	10.3	55.6	75.2	35.3
30–39	70	11.4	53.6	69.5	29.7
40–49	138	14.4	49.9	63.3	26.8
50–59	119	11.1	47.3	61.8	30.7
60–69	164	8.6	51.4	63.4	23.4
70–79	138	8.6	49.1	58.1	18.4
80–89	59	8.0	40.3	53.1	32.0
Total	1,026	10.4	50.1	62.8	25.4

TABLE A-11 *Outcomes for total knee replacement*

AGE RANGE	NUMBER	MEAN VISITS	ADMIT FUNCTION	D/C FUNCTION	% CHANGE
<20	111	15.9	42.7	56.7	32.6
20–29	4	17.5	57.5	76.5	33.0
30–39	10	17.1	38.3	73.7	92.2
40–49	13	24.2	32.0	49.7	55.2
50–59	46	18.8	30.1	47.6	57.8
60–69	101	17.8	37.0	55.8	51.1
70–79	90	16.6	39.1	57.2	46.3
80–89	23	12.6	36.0	42.3	17.6
Total	398	17.0	38.3	55.1	43.9

TABLE A-12 *Outcomes for total shoulder replacement*

AGE RANGE	NUMBER	MEAN VISITS	ADMIT FUNCTION	D/C FUNCTION	% CHANGE
<20	12	12.4	48.4	59.6	23.1%
20–29	3	33.0			
30–39	1	7.0	54.0	85.0	57.4%
40–49	8	12.8	58.5	65.5	12.0%
50–59	6	21.8	44.0	72.0	63.6%
60–69	5	22.8			
70–79	10	12.9	60.0	65.0	8.3%
80–89	3	9.0	54.0	59.0	9.3%
Total	48	15.8	44.4	53.8	21.3%

TABLE A-13 *Outcomes for ankle sprain (all grades) with ICD-9 code 845.0*

	AGE RANGE	NUMBER	MEAN VISITS	ADMIT FUNCTION	D/C FUNCTION	% CHANGE
Non surgical	<20	611	6.2	57.9	76.7	32.7
	20–29	240	6.5	61.3	77.6	26.7
	30–39	281	7.5	51.3	73.3	42.8
	40–49	242	7.9	55.2	75.4	36.7
	50–59	127	7.0	56.8	77.0	35.6
	60–69	39	9.2	50.5	81.0	60.4
	70–79	17	7.4	47.0	76.0	61.7
	80–89	13	7.9			
	Total	1,570	6.9	55.9	75.5	35.1
Surgical	<20	25	12.7	56.6	72.8	28.6
	20–29	18	7.4	61.5	79.5	29.3
	30–39	22	12.5	47.3	54.7	15.5
	40–49	16	8.4	68.5	78.0	13.9
	50–59	9	13.7	49.0	65.0	32.7
	60–69	5	11.6	65.0	81.0	24.6
	70–79	4	10.8			
	80–89	0				
	Total	99	11.0	54.8	67.6	23.3

TABLE A-14 *Outcomes for medial meniscus tear with ICD-9 code 836.0*

	AGE RANGE	NUMBER	MEAN VISITS	ADMIT FUNCTION	D/C FUNCTION	% CHANGE
Non surgical	<20	308	9.7	53.1	68.0	28.0
	20–29	78	8.7	56.1	71.0	26.6
	30–39	161	9.8	54.3	66.4	22.3
	40–49	201	9.4	52.0	67.4	29.7
	50–59	137	9.1	48.6	63.6	30.9
	60–69	98	9.8	46.7	66.7	42.8
	70–79	52	8.4	42.9	59.6	39.0
	80–89	18	7.4	62.5	74.5	19.2
	Total	1,053	9.4	51.8	66.9	29.2
Surgical	<20	789	10.5	41.8	68.4	63.7
	20–29	214	10.6	45.8	71.7	56.6
	30–39	469	10.9	45.3	68.7	51.6
	40–49	577	10.3	40.1	67.0	67.3
	50–59	499	10.4	41.2	64.3	56.0
	60–69	304	10.6	41.1	64.4	56.7
	70–79	135	10.7	45.4	63.0	38.7
	80–89	43	9.1	43.8	64.8	48.0
	Total	3,030	10.5	42.3	67.0	58.5

TABLE A-15 *Outcomes for rotator cuff sprain with ICD-9 code 840.4*

	AGE RANGE	NUMBER	MEAN VISITS	ADMIT FUNCTION	D/C FUNCTION	% CHANGE
Non surgical	<20	396	9.2	53.3	67.3	26.2
	20–29	67	9.8	55.8	65.8	17.8
	30–39	151	10.4	53.3	68.7	28.8
	40–49	180	12.2	54.3	67.4	24.0
	50–59	180	12.2	46.3	64.1	38.4
	60–69	155	12.5	46.4	64.8	39.4
	70–79	142	13.0	50.0	63.5	27.1
	80–89	57	8.5	45.7	57.0	24.8
	Total	1,328	10.9	51.1	65.8	28.7
Surgical	<20	237	18.3	38.5	66.6	73.1
	20–29	30	16.1	48.0	73.4	52.9
	30–39	92	20.1	33.5	63.7	89.9
	40–49	178	20.5	35.0	63.4	80.8
	50–59	246	22.0	34.4	63.0	83.3
	60–69	238	20.7	36.9	66.7	80.8
	70–79	158	20.9	40.3	68.7	70.6
	80–89	26	17.4	36.5	70.0	91.8
	Total	1,205	20.2	36.9	65.7	78.2

TABLE A-16 *Outcomes for lumbar disc injury with ICD-9 code 722.10*

	AGE RANGE	NUMBER	MEAN VISITS	ADMIT FUNCTION	D/C FUNCTION	% CHANGE
Non surgical	<20	413	9.6	58.4	72.3	23.9
	20–29	183	9.3	53.5	76.4	42.9
	30–39	489	10.1	54.2	72.2	33.2
	40–49	475	9.5	52.9	73.8	39.4
	50–59	249	10.2	56.5	76.9	36.1
	60–69	128	9.0	56.2	65.9	17.2
	70–79	66	9.6	45.8	73.6	60.7
	80–89	63	7.8	56.5	78.3	38.5
	Total	2,066	9.6	54.9	73.4	33.7
Surgical	<20	256	12.1	49.1	66.8	36.2
	20–29	70	10.9	61.1	78.5	28.4
	30–39	276	14.3	55.6	70.7	27.0
	40–49	317	12.9	51.7	62.8	21.5
	50–59	146	12.9	47.6	61.1	28.4
	60–69	66	12.7	52.1	67.5	29.6
	70–79	30	10.6	40.5	61.3	51.2
	80–89	16	9.2	70.3	81.3	15.7
	Total	1,177	12.8	52.1	66.7	28.1

TABLE A-17 *Outcomes for patellofemoral chondrosis with ICD-9 Code 717.7*

	AGE RANGE	NUMBER	MEAN VISITS	ADMIT FUNCTION	D/C FUNCTION	% CHANGE
Non surgical	<20	918	7.4	62.9	74.3	18.1
	20–29	360	8.1	65.3	75.0	14.9
	30–39	437	7.9	65.2	73.0	12.0
	40–49	390	8.1	58.6	70.2	19.9
	50–59	202	7.6	54.7	64.7	18.4
	60–69	86	9.3	58.4	70.9	21.5
	70–79	34	7.7	53.7	64.4	20.0
	80–89	34	5.4	73.0	68.0	(6.8)
	Total	2,461	7.8	62.2	72.4	16.5
Surgical	<20	304	6.7	56.8	76.4	34.6
	20–29	142	11.1	52.0	68.8	32.3
	30–39	241	12.8	50.6	68.6	35.6
	40–49	240	13.5	45.7	65.3	43.0
	50–59	115	12.3	45.1	61.3	35.9
	60–69	55	12.3	37.9	67.4	77.8
	70–79	13	9.0	34.7	52.7	51.9
	80–89	4	9.5	55.0	80.0	45.5
	Total	1,114	10.9	50.0	69.1	38.1

TABLE A-18 *Outcomes for tendinitis/bursitis of the shoulder with ICD-9 code 726.10*

	AGE RANGE	NUMBER	MEAN VISITS	ADMIT FUNCTION	D/C FUNCTION	% CHANGE
Non surgical	<20	622	8.9	56.6	69.1	22.1
	20–29	183	8.8	57.3	71.3	24.4
	30–39	307	8.8	56.1	69.4	23.7
	40–49	481	10.7	57.0	69.0	21.1
	50–59	478	11.2	56.5	68.5	21.2
	60–69	285	11.1	54.7	68.0	24.2
	70–79	206	10.3	55.7	65.5	17.7
	80–89	52	8.9	57.2	68.3	19.5
	Total	2,614	10.0	56.4	68.7	21.9
Surgical	<20	122	14.0	44.7	61.7	37.9
	20–29	33	14.1	44.3	75.3	69.9
	30–39	69	16.8	36.9	72.5	96.5
	40–49	102	15.7	45.1	63.9	41.6
	50–59	105	20.3	40.1	61.6	53.6
	60–69	76	22.2	38.6	61.7	59.8
	70–79	47	15.6	45.3	60.8	34.3
	80–89	5	27.2			
	Total	559	17.2	41.7	63.6	52.3

TABLE A-19 *Outcomes for adhesive capsulitis with ICD-9 Code 726.0*

	AGE RANGE	NUMBER	MEAN VISITS	ADMIT FUNCTION	D/C FUNCTION	% CHANGE
Non surgical	<20	495	10.2	52.3	66.5	27.1
	20–29	57	9.4	58.4	71.9	23.0
	30–39	147	9.5	50.0	60.7	21.4
	40–49	437	12.9	53.8	66.0	22.7
	50–59	543	13.7	49.9	66.7	33.6
	60–69	315	11.9	50.5	67.8	34.4
	70–79	167	11.4	48.9	68.9	41.0
	80–89	57	10.7	46.5	63.0	35.5
	Total	2,218	11.9	51.3	66.5	29.5
Surgical	<20	86	14.8	45.9	66.6	45.1
	20–29	14	16.7	46.0	72.0	56.5
	30–39	32	12.4	23.7	46.0	94.3
	40–49	83	17.2	42.0	67.7	61.3
	50–59	87	19.4	46.2	63.4	37.2
	60–69	49	17.3	41.8	61.5	47.0
	70–79	22	17.8	52.3	64.3	22.9
	80–89	7	8.6	47.0	31.0	(34.0)
	Total	380	16.6	43.1	63.1	46.4

the factors noted earlier in the appendix. An important variable in the rating tool itself are the weighting of factors (pain, strength, ROM, performance, etc.). For a greater discussion of this area, please refer to the functional testing sections of the lower extremity and upper extremity chapters.

The first six tables are data from FOTO (Focus On Therapeutic Outcomes, Knoxville, TN 1–800–482–3686). FOTO is a national entity which compiles outcomes scores from its member organizations and clinics. The remaining tables are compiled from HealthSouth Corporation (Birmingham, Alabama) (used with permission). The data in tables 7–11 include the top 50 diagnoses (by ICD–9 code) for each body part. HealthSouth uses a proprietary rating system for each region of the body.

Index

Note: Page numbers followed by f indicate figures, and those folowed by t indicate tables.